Special Procedures in Foot and Ankle Surgery

Amol Saxena

Editor

Special Procedures
in Foot and Ankle Surgery

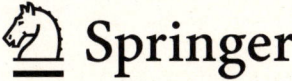 Springer

Editor
Dr. Amol Saxena, D.P.M.
Department of Sports Medicine
Palo Alto Foundation Medical Group-Palo
Alto Division
Palo Alto, CA
USA

ISBN 978-1-4471-4102-0   ISBN 978-1-4471-4103-7   (eBook)
DOI 10.1007/978-1-4471-4103-7
Springer London Heidelberg New York Dordrecht

Library of Congress Control Number: 2012943941

Springer is part of Springer Science+Business Media (www.springer.com)

Foreword

As a colleague and friend of Amol Saxena, I feel honoured to write the foreword to *International Advances in Foot and Ankle Surgery*.

During my 20 years of experience, I found the specialty of foot and ankle surgery growing unexpectedly. This was due to international collaboration between podiatric, orthopaedic, and trauma surgeons from around the globe.

As a German trauma surgeon I had little to no exposure to reconstructive foot andankle surgery at the time I was trained; the first hallux valgus repair I performed was with Dr. Brian Holcomb, a podiatric surgeon in Georgia. Years later this led to the formation of the German-based foundation, the Association for Foot Surgery. Among others, this foundation created a global platform for all disciplines to train together and shares ideas and experiences concerning foot pathologies. Amol Saxena was one of the invited speakers to the scientific conference in Munich, where he shared all his experience with the surgeons.

As a speaker at many international conferences he took it upon himself to gather international contributing authors for this book. All the authors have extraordinary personal experience with the procedures they describe.

While this book does not exclude scientific background, it emphasizes a practical, hands-on approach. To meet the demand of all foot and ankle surgeons, the book encompasses forefoot and rearfoot deformities as well as trauma and reconstructive surgery of the diabetic foot.

With that in mind I strongly recommend this book for all foot and ankle surgeons of any subspecialty from any nation as this book will shortly be recognized as the state of the art.

Bad Schwartau, Germany   Kai Olms

Preface

It is with great pleasure and gratitude that I am able to edit *International Advances of Foot and Ankle Surgery*. The idea for this book came about through my contact and subsequent friendships with two well-known and innovative foot and ankle surgeons – Nicola Maffulli, M.D., Ph.D., and Kai Olms, M.D. – as we discussed the need to share international thought leaders' concepts. As the world progressed into a global economy and the Internet helped connect people of similar interests in the early twenty-first century, I began communicating, writing, and lecturing with these two individuals across the globe. Through these two individuals with their zeal for traveling, teaching, and learning (but not necessarily in that order!), professional friendships and further contacts developed, ideas were shared, and many of the authors of this book became connected.

The globalization of foot and ankle surgery may not be readily apparent; however in this book there are many examples. Recently I personally experienced this as I performed a "Stainsby" procedure on a patient whose second toe was severely dislocated despite metatarsal osteotomy, hammertoe, and soft tissue lengthening. In the past I may have performed an isolated partial metatarsal head resection. However, I was able to relocate the toe, preventing a possible transfer lesion with the Stainsby, which I learned from German authors of chapters in this text, which they in turn "imported" from the British surgeon it is named after. The Italian surgeon Valente Valenti performed a resectional arthroplasty for hallux rigidus in the mid-1970s. His procedure was "imported" to the United States in the mid-1980s and subsequently "exported" back to Germany early in the twenty-first century.

Many older procedures have been re-popularized with regional modifications such as the Hohmann osteotomy first described in Germany in the early 1900s. In the United States, the procedure was performed on the first and fifth metatarsal with no fixation as a minimally invasive technique during the 1970s. Subsequently with the increased utilization of AO fixation from Europe, the desire to have more stability, and predictable healing time, the Hohmann procedure was adapted with inclusion of screw fixation. As the Europeans (particularly the Latin-based speaking countries of Italy, France, and Spain) increased their desire to have smaller incisions, this osteotomy has been increasingly utilized using percutaneous fixation.

Other examples are Ilizarov fixation from Russia, arthroscopy from Japan, and the Weil osteotomy from the United States being adopted by other parts of the world. This often came about by motivated surgeons visiting other surgeons with similar interests and the desire to better serve their patients.

I believe all the authors in this text share this commonality as our patients drive us to learn and excel, and I am grateful for the opportunity to pull this select group together. I am cognizant that many authors created chapters on topics that could be entire texts in their own right. Furthermore, the need to publish in a foreign language provides additional stress, along with combining different writing styles in chapters where similar topics were "blended" together. This adds to this text's uniqueness.

Everyone's life journey, including their career, is a story formed by happenstance and instances of luck, misfortune, and guidance. As a young and often injured runner I found myself in the offices of two early forefathers of sports medicine, Fred Behling, M.D., and Gordon Campbell, M.D., in my hometown of Palo Alto, California. It was through their encouragement and possibly lack of interest in foot surgery, that I pursued podiatry as a profession, as they desired a partner proficient in treating the sports medicine aspects of the foot and ankle. They professed and practiced subspecialization as a way of achieving excellence in patient care. I subsequently joined their practice in 1993 just as they were retiring from the Palo Alto Medical Clinic's Sports Medicine Department, where I currently have three orthopedic sports medicine and one pediatric sports medicine colleagues. All four are among the most productive in their respective fields in the United States, covering professional and high school sports teams, writing chapters, and having high-volume practices. With the support of our department, combined with my other podiatric colleagues within our clinic, I have been able to offer a fellowship for post-residency training in sports medicine and foot and ankle surgery. These fellows have been able to further share in exchanges with some of the international authors of this book and I have hosted colleagues from other countries as well.

As I stated, luck has a part in one's journey and subsequently their training. I am extremely fortunate to have had the training from not only one of the most versatile foot and ankle surgeons but great teacher and human being in John Grady, D.P.M. There are other highly respected authors I've met through contacts that are mentors writing here as well. I was also fortunate to be able to connect and shadow with another legend and thought leader in the foot and ankle world, Sigvard T. Hansen, M.D., early on, whose philosophy on foot and ankle surgeons paralleled mine in life, in that everyone is equal until proved otherwise. It is also exciting to have many of the current and future bright minds of the orthopedic, podiatric, and trauma worlds of foot and ankle surgery all contributing in the name of advancing foot and ankle surgery.

Finally, I am indebted to my family, teachers, and friends for being supportive of not only this project but how my career developed. I am richer for all their positive encouragement, able to be fulfilled professionally, but also personally. I am sure I could not have completed this and other accomplishments without them.

CA, USA   Amol Saxena

Contents

Contributors

Eliza Addis-Thomas, D.P.M. Connecticut Orthopaedic Specialists PC, Hamden, CT, USA

David G. Armstrong, D.P.M., M.D., Ph.D. Southern Arizona Limb Salvage Alliance (SALSA), Department of Surgery, University of Arizona, Tucson, AZ, USA

Nicholas J. Bevilacqua, D.P.M. Associate, Foot and Ankle Surgery, North Jersey, Orthopaedic Specialists, Teaneck, NJ, USA

Adam William Brynizcka, D.P.M. Northwest Podiatry Center, Ltd., Wheaton, IL, USA

David S. Caminear, D.P.M. Connecticut Orthopaedic Specialists, PC, Hamden, CT, USA

Vincenzo Denaro, M.D. Department of Trauma and Orthopaedic Surgery, University Campus Bio-Medico of Rome, Rome, Italy

Lawrence A. DiDomenico, D.P.M., F.A.C.F.A.S. Department of Surgery, Northside Medical Center, Youngstown, OH, USA

Andreas Dietze, M.D., Ph.D. Department of Orthopaedic Surgery, Sykehuset i Vestfold — Tønsberg, Tønsberg, Norway

Nicholas Antonio Ferran, M.B.B.S., M.R.C.S.Ed. Department of Trauma and Orthopaedics, Lincoln County Hospital, Lincoln, Lincolnshire, UK

Ludger Gerdesmeyer, M.D. Department of Orthopaedic and Trauma Surgery, Mare Klinikum Kiel, Kiel-Kronshagen, Germany

Hans Gollwitzer, M.D., C.C.R.P. Klinik für Orthopädie und Sportorthopädie, Klinikum rechts der Isar, Technische Universität München, Munich, Germany

Reiner Gradinger, M.D. Clinic for Orthopaedics and Traumatology, Klinikum rechts der Isar, Technische Universität München, Munich, Germany

Allison N. Granot, P.T., M.P.T., O.C.S., C.S.C.S. Department of Physical Therapy, Palo Alto Medical Foundation, Palo Alto, CA, USA

Thomas W. Groner, D.P.M., A.A.C.F.A.S. Department of Surgery, Ankle and Foot Care Center, Alliance, OH, USA

Sig T. Hansen Jr., B.A., M.D. Department of Orthopaedics (and Sports Medicine), Harborview Medical Center, STH Foot and Ankle Institute, Seattle, WA, USA

Andrew Haskell, M.D. Department of Orthopedics, Palo Alto Medical Foundation, Palo Alto, CA, USA

Department of Orthopaedic Surgery, University of California, San Francisco, CA, USA

Umile Giuseppe Longo, M.D. Department of Trauma and Orthopaedic Surgery, University Campus Bio-Medico of Rome, Rome, Italy

Nicola Maffulli, M.D., M.S., Ph.D., F.R.C.S (Orth). Queen Mary University of London, Barts and The London School of Medicine and Dentistry, Centre for Sports and Exercise Medicine, Mile End Hospital, London, UK

Francesco Oliva, M.D., Ph.D. Department of Trauma and Orthopaedic Surgery, University of Rome "Tor Vergata", Rome, Italy

Joseph S. Park, M.D. Department of Orthopaedic Surgery, Union Memorial Hospital, Baltimore, MD, USA

Hans Rechl, M.D., D.V.M. Klinik für Orthopädie und Unfallchirurgie, Technische, Universität München, Munich, Germany

Lee C. Rogers, D.P.M. Amputation Prevention Center, Valley Presbyterian Hospital, Van Nuys, CA, USA

Amol Saxena, D.P.M. PAFMG-Palo Alto Division, Department of Sports Medicine, Palo Alto, CA, USA

Lew C. Schon, M.D. Department of Orthopaedics, Union Memorial Hospital, Baltimore, MD, USA

Ralph Springfeld, M.D. Head of Orthopedic Clinic, Klinik Dr. Guth, Hamburg, Germany

Jeffrey A. Szczepanski, D.P.M. PLLC Munson Medical Center, Traverse City, MI, USA

Andreas K. Toepfer, M.D. Klinik für Orthopädie und Unfallchirurgie, Technische Universität München, Munich, Germany

Chapter 1
The Lapidus Procedure

Eliza Addis-Thomas, David S. Caminear, and Amol Saxena

In 1934, Dr. Paul Lapidus described a procedure for correcting hallux valgus. It was first described as a fusion of the base of the first and second metatarsal and the medial cuneiform combined with distal soft tissue alignment.[1] As with surgical procedures, it has been modified over the years, particularly with the advent of internal fixation. There are numerous benefits to performing the Lapidus procedure. The Lapidus procedure addresses hallux valgus at the apex of the deformity, increases the efficacy of the peroneal longus tendon, and stabilizes the medial longitudinal arch.[2,3]

1.1 Indications

The original indication for the procedure as described by Lapidus was for the correction of metatarsus primus adductus with severe hallux abductovalgus (HAV). However, the major indication for this procedure is moderate to severe hallux valgus deformity; this is defined as a hallux valgus angle of at least 30° and an intermetatarsal angle of at least 16°[4] (Figs. 1.1 and 1.2). Today, the indications have been expanded to include hypermobility of the first ray, medial angulation of the metatarsocuneiform joint of 30° or greater, medial column instability, subluxation and degeneration of the metatarsocuneiform joint, and failed HAV surgery.[5]

E. Addis-Thomas, D.P.M. (✉)
Connecticut Orthopaedic Specialists, PC,
2408 Whitney Avenue, Hamden, CT 06518, USA
e-mail: eaddisthomas@gmail.com

D.S. Caminear, D.P.M.
Connecticut Orthopaedic Specialists PC, Hamden, CT, USA

A. Saxena, D.P.M.
Department of Sports Medicine, PAFMG-Palo Alto Division,
Palo Alto, CA, USA

A. Saxena (ed.), *Special Procedures in Foot and Ankle Surgery*,
DOI 10.1007/978-1-4471-4103-7_1, © Springer-Verlag London 2013

Fig. 1.1 This is a clinical photograph of a patient with severe hallux abductus valgus. Note the large medial bony prominence at the first metatarsal phalangeal joint

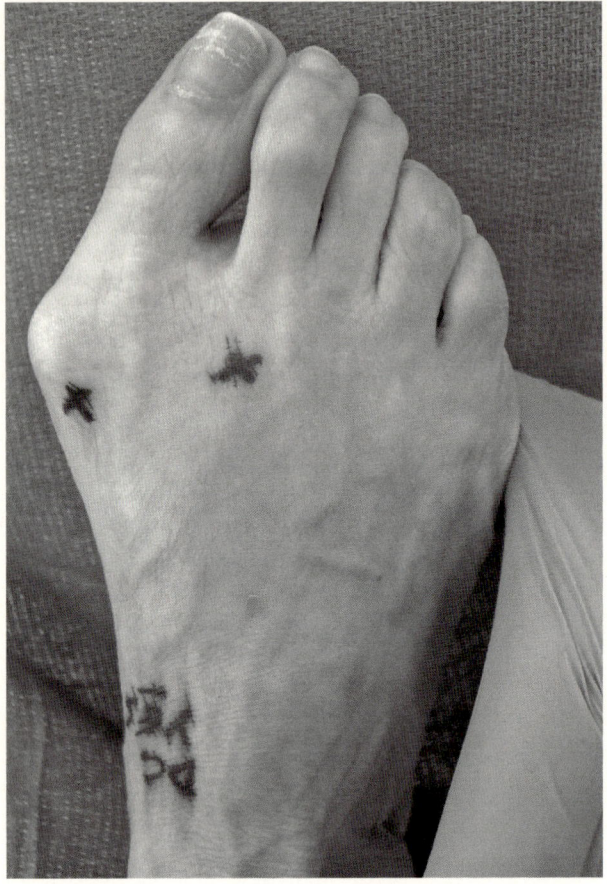

The concept of hypermobility of the first ray is very difficult to describe objectively. Sangeorzan and Hansen quantified hypermobility as relatively increased first ray dorsiflexion with a soft end point on exam along with second metatarsal overload.[6] This is also described as excessive dorsal/plantar excursion of the first metatarsal above the level of the lesser metatarsal.[7] First ray hypermobility is often seen with a medially orientated cuneiform metatarsal articulation and hypertrophy of the second metatarsal.[6] Hypermobility can also be demonstrated by radiographic evaluation by a first metatarsal cuneiform fault with plantar gapping or a navicular-cuneiform fault.[7] Often a sub-second metatarsal hyperkeratotic lesion is seen.

Hypermobility is also called hyperlaxity, hyperextensibility, and hyperflexibilty.[8] Root et al. attempted to explain hypermobility by writing that during gait, if the foot is in a pronated position during late midstance, the peroneus longus is unable to stabilize the first ray against ground reactive forces.[8] Hypermobility is often associated with ligamental laxity and the development of HAV; this has not been definitively correlated in the literature. In one study, a statistically significant relationship was

Fig. 1.2 In this X-ray, it is clear that this patient has a large intermetatarsal angle of greater than 16° and a very large hallux abductus angle. The medial cuneiform appears to be mildly atavistic. The sesamoids are significantly displaced laterally into the first interspace

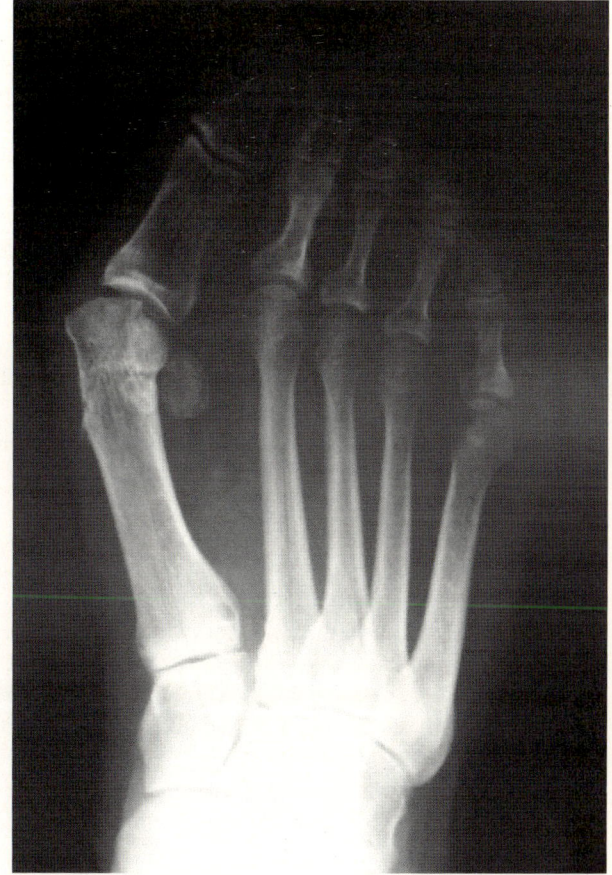

found between women with symptomatic HAV and mild hypermobility when compared to a similar control group.[9] In another study assessing first metatarsal cuneiform motion, the only significant correlation to first ray hypermobility was found to be hyperflexibility of the thumb; sex, age, intermetatarsal angle, skin elasticity, and patient size were found to have no relationship with first ray hypermobility.[10]

1.2   Contraindications

The presence of a short first metatarsal, juvenile hallux valgus with open epiphysis, and mild or moderate hallux valgus deformity without the presence of hypermobility are all contraindications to performing the Lapidus procedure.[4,11] Additionally, degenerative joint disease at the first metatarsal phalangeal joint is also a relative contraindication; a distal osteotomy can be performed to increase motion at the first metatarsal phalangeal joint.[5]

1.3   Surgical Technique

The Lapidus procedure can be performed under general anesthesia or local block with monitored anesthesia care. The patient is positioned supine and a bump can be placed under the ipsilateral hip for better exposure. A thigh or ankle tourniquet can be used depending on whether general or local anesthesia is utilized, respectively.

There have been multiple incisional approaches described for the Lapidus procedure. A three-incision approach utilizes incisions over the first tarsometatarsal joint, the medial first metatarsophalangeal joint, and over the first interspace.[12] The two-incisional approach uses the first tarsometatarsal joint incision as well as an incision over the medial first metatarsophalangeal joint. Finally, the single incision approach extends approximately 10 cm in length from the middle of the hallux proximal phalanx to the midportion of the medial cuneiform in a linear orientation medial and parallel to the extensor hallucis longus tendon. This is the approach preferred by the authors. The incision is carried through the skin and subcutaneous tissue using sharp and blunt dissection, respectively. Care is taken to avoid neurovascular structures. Often the medial dorsal cutaneous nerve is seen in the incision crossing from lateral to medial and should be retracted. Biasing the incision medio-plantarward proximally can aid in placement of the hardware as preferred by the authors (i.e., use of a plantar to dorsal screw).

Although not performed by all surgeons, the authors perform a lateral release through anatomic dissection. This includes transection of the deep transverse intermetatarsal ligament, elevation and excision of the adductor hallucis tendon from its insertion and the fibular sesamoid, and complete release of the fibular sesamoid. At the surgeon's discretion, a lateral capsulotomy is completed based on the extent of the soft tissue contracture. Dissection of the first metatarsal phalangeal joint is carried out using an inverted L capsulotomy. The joint is inspected but resection of the medial eminence is reserved until fixation of the fusion procedure is complete. This is done to avoid overexuberant resection of the bunion prominence and prevent hallux varus. (Portions of this resected bone can be used as autograft in the fusion site if needed.) It is important to ensure that the structures surrounding the first metatarsal phalangeal joint are adequately released.

Attention is then directed to the first metatarsal cuneiform joint. A periosteal-capsular incision is made dorsally across the base of the first metatarsal to the midportion of the medial cuneiform exposing the first metatarsal cuneiform joint. The periosteum and its associated blood supply are preserved on the shaft of the first metatarsal. Lamina spreaders are used to expose the joint surface and initial preparation for the fusion involves curettage (Figs. 1.3 and 1.4). The first intermetatarsal angle is reduced and provisionally stabilized with a Kirschner wire applied transversely between the first and second metatarsal heads (Fig. 1.5). Biasing the placement of this wire in a medial-proximal to a distal-lateral direction in the transverse plane allows for the subsequent compression screw to work more appropriately. The fusion interface is then reciprocally planed to achieve maximum bone apposition

Fig. 1.3 Joint preparation is key to this procedure. The authors suggest using a lamina spreader to obtain best visualization and access to the first metatarsal cuneiform joint. Initially, curettage of the joint surfaces is done to remove cartilage

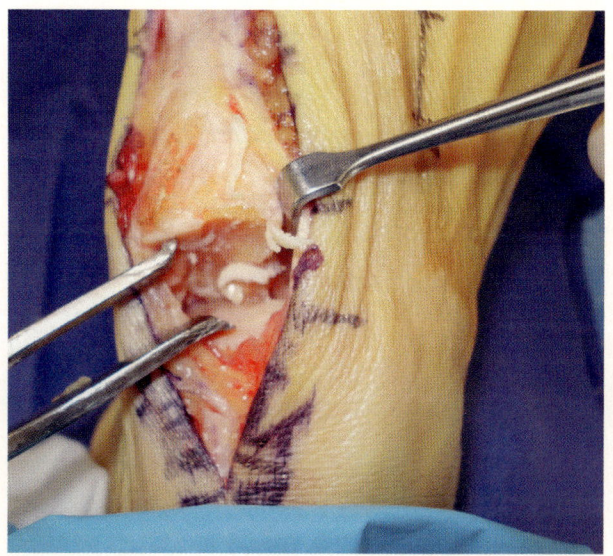

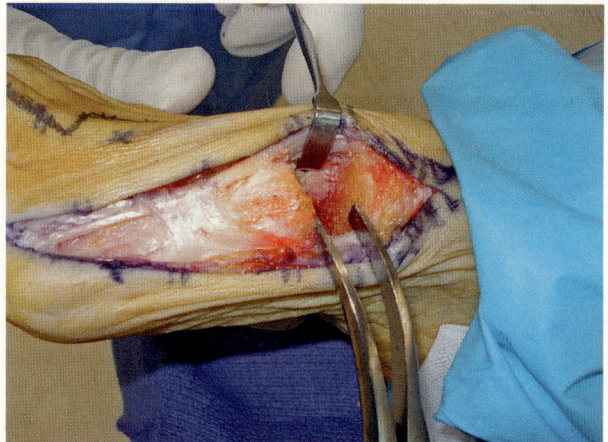

Fig. 1.4 In this lateral photograph, the depth of the first metatarsal cuneiform is visualized. This is essential to ensure adequate joint preparation at the most plantar aspect of the joint. Failure to remove the cartilage at the plantar aspect of the first metatarsal cuneiform joint can result in malunion or nonunion. Also, apparent is the subchondral fenestration to promote good joint fusion. There is periosteum present at the shaft of the first metatarsal to help preserve blood flow to the metatarsal. Again, note the use of the lamina spreader

between the first metatarsal and the medial cuneiform. Often times, if the medial cuneiform is medially and obliquely oriented, a bone wedge from the cuneiform may need to be removed to facilitate reduction of the intermetatarsal angle. Joint fusion preparation is complete after exposure of the subchondral plate is noted and

Fig. 1.5 (**a**) Once reduction of the intermetatarsal angle has been achieved, provisional fixation is utilized. A K-wire can be used to fixate the joint, taking care to keep it out of the way of the permanent fixation devices. Note "Springfeld maneuver" of keeping the intermetatarsal angle reduced with the fifth finger (Photo courtesy of Ralph Springfeld, MD). (**b**) A K-wire is placed from the head of the first metatarsal to the second metatarsal to maintain correction (seen here with a white pin cap in place). Finally, the orientation of the so-called "tension-band screw" can be seen in this photograph. It is oriented from the plantar-distal-medial surface of the first metatarsal to the dorsal-proximal-lateral aspect of the medial cuneiform

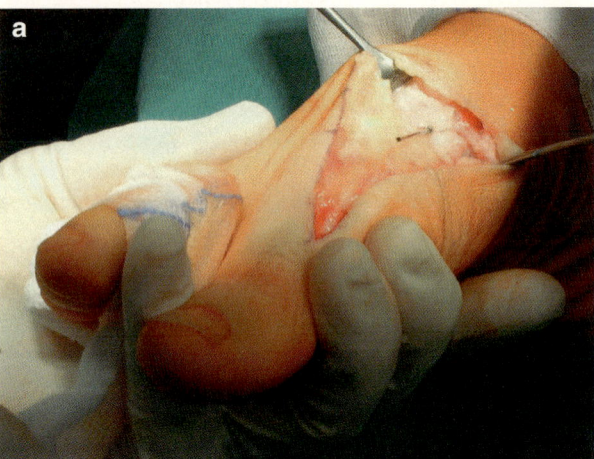

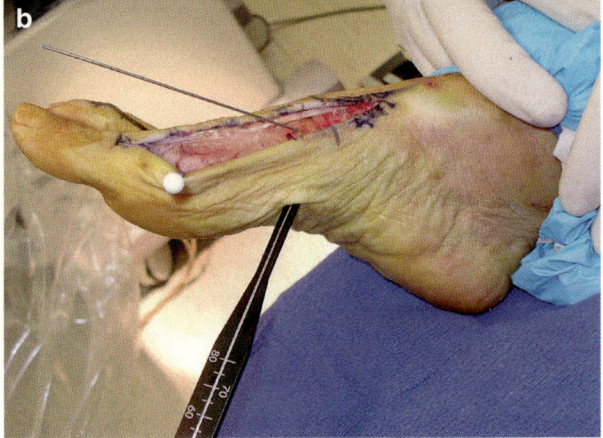

may be enhanced by fenestration if necessary. The reduction and temporary stabilization of the first metatarsal-cuneiform joint is then performed with a K-wire (Fig. 1.5).

1.4   Fixation

Multiple forms of fixation have been described for the Lapidus procedure. Numerous variations of screw and plate fixation have been reported. Improved fixation strength is thought to improve rates of fixation. Lapidus initially reported using temporary fixation to increase stability across the fusion site.[1] Kirschner wires and Steinmann pins have been utilized because they are relatively quick and easy to use. Two wires are preferred and less dissection is required than with screws.

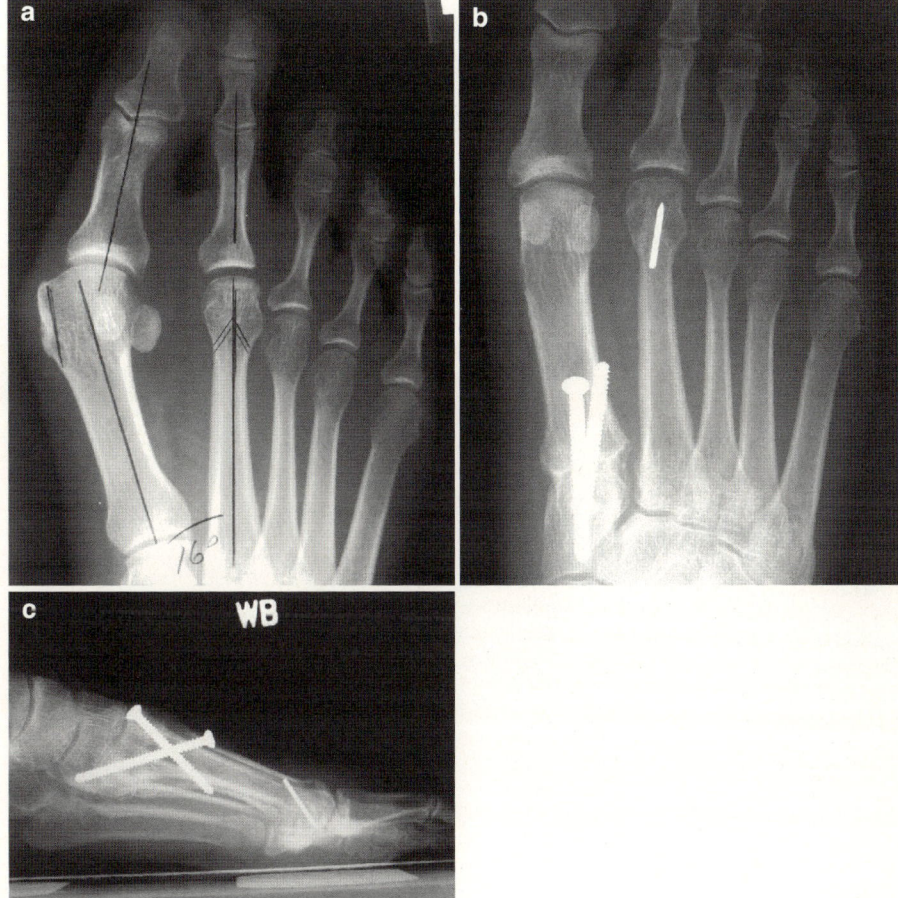

Fig. 1.6 (**a**) Preoperative AP; (**b, c**) Postoperative screw fixation (Photos courtesy of Richard Bouché, DPM)

Since Sangeorzan and Hansen reported using two screws for fixation, there have been significant advances in fixation. Compression screws provide excellent stability. Typically, 3.5- or 4.0-fully or partially threaded cortical or cancellous screws are used in a lag fashion. Cannulated screws can also be used. Myerson, in his textbook, describes the screw orientation he uses; the first screw is orientated from the dorsal proximal medial cuneiform to distal and plantar aspect of the first metatarsal. The second screw is directed from the dorsal aspect of the first metatarsal to proximal, plantar, and lateral to the first screw (Fig. 1.6).[13] Another technique orients the first screw from the dorsal aspect of the base of the first metatarsal in a plantar direction into the medial cuneiform.[14] The other screw starts at the medial aspect of the first metatarsal and ends at the lateral proximal aspect of the medial

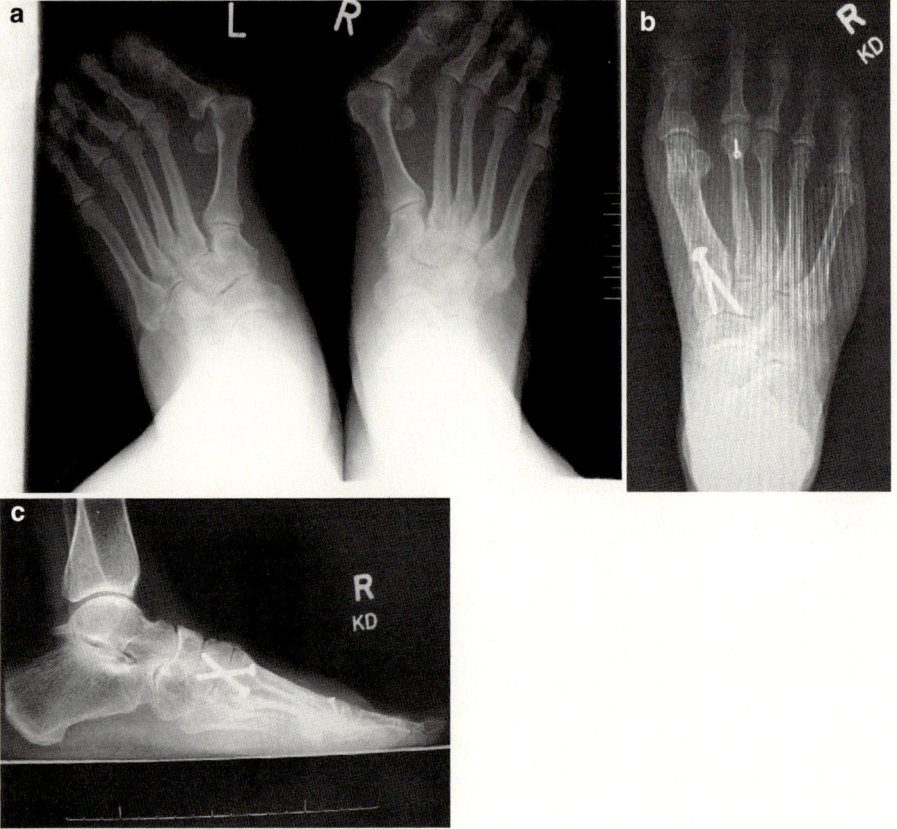

Fig. 1.7 (**a**) Preoperative AP; (**b**, **c**) Postoperative screw fixation with a plantar lag screw and "home run screw"

cuneiform (Fig. 1.7). Finally, if there is either sagittal or transverse plane instability present, a third lag screw can be inserted from the base of the first metatarsal to the intermediate cuneiform or from the medial cuneiform into the intermediate cuneiform.[14]

Plates have been developed and used for the Lapidus procedure as well. Plates are indicated when more stability is wanted, especially if a bone graft is being used. With the addition of a plantar interfragmentary screw, even more stability is obtained. When compared to two-screw fixation, Cohen et al. found that plate fixation had a lower resistance to failure.[15] In another cadaveric study, a Lapidus-specific plate was compared with a interfragmentary screw versus the crossed-screw technique in which they found the load to failure was higher with the Lapidus plate.[15] Finally, in a study by Saxena et al. crossed screws were compared with a locking plate with a plantar lag screw.[16] They found no difference in complications between the two fixation methods but did find that the patients with the plate with plantar lag screw were able to bear weight earlier (4 weeks versus 6 weeks).

Fig. 1.8 Next, a distal-medial locking plate is applied. At minimum, a four-hole plate should be used. The provisional fixation from the head of the first metatarsal to the second metatarsal remains in place

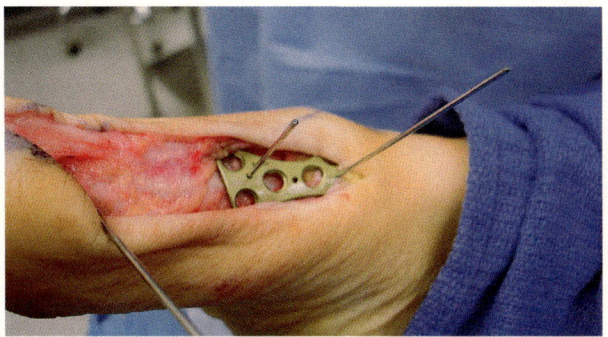

External fixation has also been reported for fixating the Lapidus procedure. In a cadaveric study, internal and external fixation of the Lapidus procedure was comparatively studied.[17] External fixation was found to be clinically as strong a construct as two crossed screws. However, in clinical studies, data has not been as supportive. In one study, 8/11 patients developed complications when a mini-external fixator was used for fixation.[18] The complications included pin loosening, pin-tract infections and cellulitis, need for recontouring of the fixator, and sub-second metatarsal callus. It also reported an 18% nonunion rate; however the small size of the study must be taken into account.

The authors' preferred method of fixation involves application of a plantar compression screw and a dorsal-medial locking plate. The authors' refer to the plantar compression screw as a "tension-band screw" because it in effect compresses the tension side (plantar) of the fusion interface, thus, acting in accordance with the tension band principle. A 3.5 or 4.0 mm cannulated screw is orientated from the plantar-distal-medial surface of the first metatarsal to the dorsal-proximal-lateral aspect of the medial cuneiform. Next, a minimum four hole, 2.7 mm or greater screw size, dorsal-medial locking plate is contoured and applied (Figs. 1.8 and 1.9). Intraoperative fluoroscopy is used for guidance. Finally, any prominent medial eminence is resected and a layered closure is performed (Fig. 1.10). Final radiographs demonstrate a reduced intermetatarsal angle and realignment of the first metatarsal phalangeal joint (Figs. 1.11 and 1.12).

1.5 Postoperative Course

Postoperatively, patients are placed in a modified Jones compression posterior splint for approximately 2 weeks. Then patients are placed in a non-weight-bearing, short leg cast for 4 weeks and then transitioned to a removable walking boot and full weight-bearing in another 2–4 weeks. Radiographs are evaluated serially for consolidation at the fusion site. At 8–10 weeks, patients are allowed to return to normal shoe gear with gradual return to regular activity. A physical therapy regimen for the Lapidus procedure is presented in Chap. 15.

Fig. 1.9 In this photograph, fixation has been achieved and the provisional K-wire has been removed distally. In this case, a mixture of locking and non-locking screws were placed in the plate

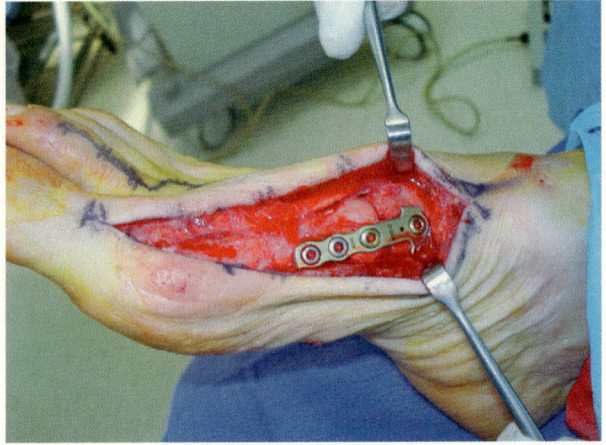

Fig. 1.10 To avoid overcorrection and hallux varus, resection of the medial eminence of the first metatarsal head is left until the end of the procedure. Often, such dramatic correction of the hallux abductovalgus deformity has been achieved that no resection is required

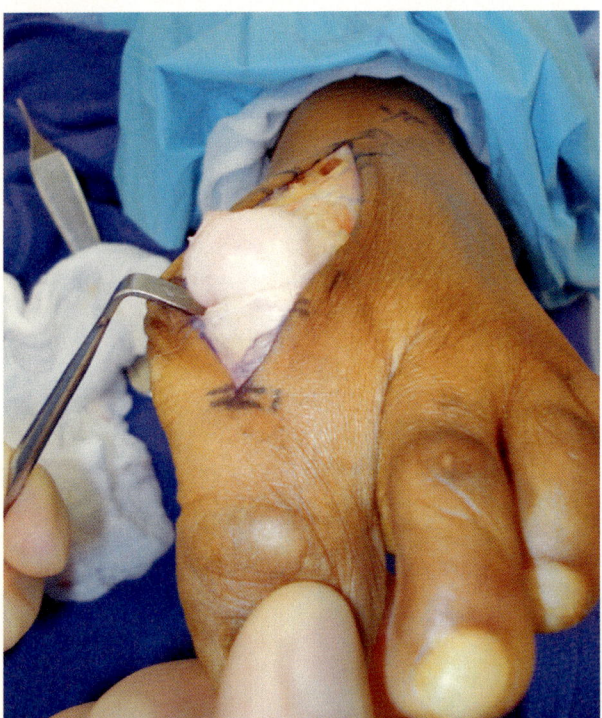

Fig. 1.11 Radiographically, the bunion deformity has been corrected. The intermetatarsal angle has been reduced to approximately 2°. Realignment at the first metatarsal phalangel joint has occurred with return of the sesamoids to underneath the first metatarsal head. There is no gapping or malposition at the first metatarsal cuneiform joint and the fixation is in adequate position

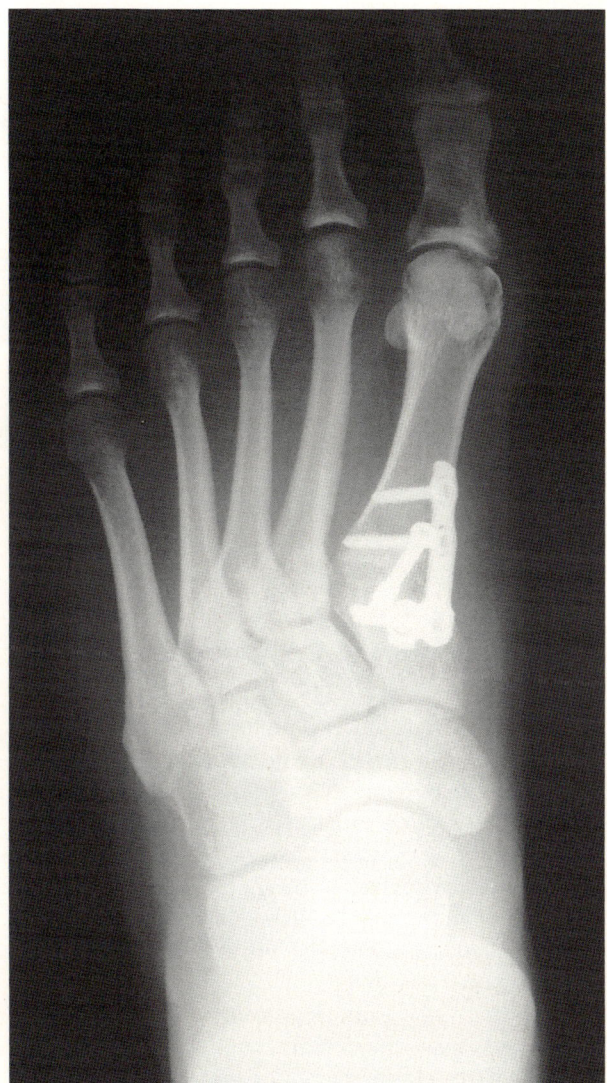

Fig. 1.12 Again, the plantar lag screw and plate are in acceptable positions. There is no dorsiflexion noted

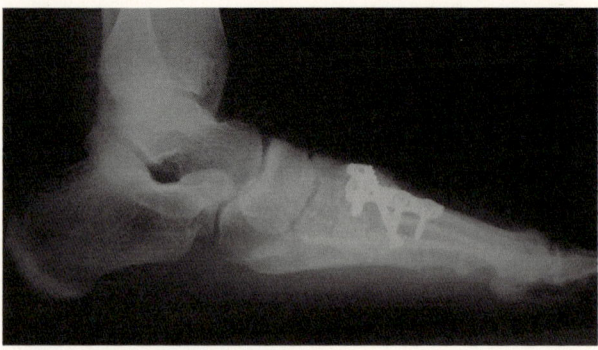

In a recent study, patients were allowed to fully weight-bear using a wedge shoe immediately after surgery using crutches only for balance.[19] Successful union was reported in all 27 patients in 6–24 weeks. However, the small size of the study must be considered.

1.6   Outcomes and Complications

In a study by Myerson et al. intermetatarsal angles improved from an average of 14.3° to 5.8°.[20] Another study demonstrated improvement of preoperative intermetatarsal angles by an average 11.7°.[8] Of the 67 patients in the study by Myerson et al., 77% reported to have achieved total resolution of symptoms.[20] In another study, American Organization of Foot and Ankle Surgeons (AOFAS) Hallux Metatarsophalangeal Interphalangeal Scale scores improved from 52 preoperative to 87 postoperative points.[21] Rink-Brüe reported that 70.5% of patients in her study were satisfied with the procedure and 80.2% would have the same procedure performed again.[22]

Historically, the Lapidus procedure has been considered technically difficult and has been associated with high complication rates. In a large study by Lagaay et al. the rate of revision surgery for the Lapidus procedure was found to be 8.19% (28/342).[7] Of the 342 patients who underwent the Lapidus procedure, 10 had recurrence, 1 had a hallux varus, 7 had retained, painful hardware, 7 patients had a nonunion, and 3 had symptomatic first metatarsal phalangeal joint. Sangeorzan and Hansen found a 13% revision rate for nonunion, hallux varus, and malunion combined.[6]

Hallux varus has also been reported as a late complication. In their studies, Kopp et al. and Mauldin et al. report incidences of hallux varus of 10% and 16%, respectively.[23,24] Hallux varus can be the result of overaggressive resection of the medial eminence of the first metatarsal head (staking the metatarsal head) or by creating a negative intermetatarsal angle.

Nonunions have been described as common complications. Nonunion rates have been reported between 2% and 12% for unilateral procedures and 33% for bilateral procedures.[25,26] It is not recommended to attempt simultaneous bilateral procedures. In 2000, Myerson and Badekas performed a large, multicenter study that reported a nonunion rate of 5.3% using curettage as the method of joint preparation.[26] Patel et al. reported a similar nonunion rate of 5.3% in 227 ft that underwent the Lapidus procedure.[27] Coetzee and Wickum write that the high nonunion rate is thought to be due to the orientation of the joint perpendicular to the weight-bearing axis of the foot that results in shearing forces across the joint.[21] This procedure also requires patients to comply with prolonged non-weight-bearing; nonunions are often found in patients who begin weight-bearing too early in their postoperative courses.

Transfer metatarsalgia has been described as the result of malunion. As the Lapidus procedure results in shortening of the first metatarsal, pressure can be redistributed to the lesser metatarsals causing symptoms. In a retrospective analysis, an average of 3.9 mm of shortening of the first metatarsal was reported after the Lapidus procedure.[22] In the study, 20 of these patients with long metatarsals were intentionally shortened. Additionally, elevation of the first metatarsal was found in seven patients; among these patients, only three of these patients experienced lesser metatarsal symptoms and all of these were successfully treated with orthotics. Dorsiflexion of the first metatarsal is often the result of poor joint preparation; the first metatarsal cuneiform joint is 30 mm deep and if proper joint exposure is not obtained, the plantar cartilage is left intact.[21] Table 1.1 summarizes complications (such as nonunion) found in pertinent studies.

Two considerations are critical but underreported when assessing the "success" and "failure" of the Lapidus procedure: activity level and postoperative time frame. Athletically active patients may not be ideal candidates for the procedure as the fusion site may be prone to breakdown.[16,28] Though performed in active patients who do sports, elite athletes without arthrosis of the first metatarsal cuneiform articulation may not be ideal candidates for the Lapidus procedure. This may not be noted until 2 or more years postoperative. Therefore, studies that report union rates in shorter time frames (such as reported by Patel et al.[27]) may not reveal the true nonunion rate from the Lapidus procedure.[16,27] Other studies with longer follow-up listed in Table 1.1 reveal an approximately 10% nonunion rate which may be unavoidable with the Lapidus procedure.[6,8,13,21,22]

1.7   Conclusion

The Lapidus procedure is indicated in patients with HAV with an intermetatarsal angle greater than 16° with associated hypermobility of the first ray. The Lapidus procedure has the advantage of being able to correct the deformity in all three planes. It has been found to adequately decrease intermetatarsal angles in HAV

Table 1.1 A review of the literature comparing lapidus fixation methods and the incidence of nonunion

Authors (year)	Number of feet (patients)	Preoperative intermetatarsal angle	Postoperative intermetatarsal angle	Fixation technique	Incidence of nonunion (%)
McInnes and Bouche (2001)	31 (26)	16.7°	8.2°	2 crossed screws	15.6
Catanzariti et al. (1999)	47 (39)	13.8°	2.1°	2 stacked screws	6.4
Coetzee and Wickum (2004)	105 (91)	18°	8.2°	2 crossed screws	6.7
Kopp et al. (2005)	35 (29)	16°	6°	2 crossed screws	0
Patel et al. (2004)	227 (211)	NE	NE	2 crossed screws	5.3
Rink-Brüne (2004)	106 (106)	22.55°	10.1°	Screw and threaded K-wire	1.8
Sangeorzan and Hansen (1989)	40 (32)	14°	6°	2 crossed screws	10
Saxena et al. (2009)	19 (19)	15.6°	5.9°	2 crossed screws	5.26
	21 (21)	15°	4.24°	Plate with plantar lag screw	0
Thompson et al. (2005)	201 (182)	NE	NE	2 crossed screws	4

NE not examined

deformities with hypermobility as well as have high rates of patient satisfaction. Potential complications include nonunion, malunion, and hallux varus.

References

1. Blitz NM. The versatility of the Lapidus arthrodesis. Clin Podiatr Med Surg. 2009;26:427-41.
2. Bierman RA, Christensen JC, Johnson CH. Biomechanics of the first ray. Part III. Consequences of Lapidus arthrodesis on peroneus longus function: a three-dimensional kinematic analysis in a cadaver review. J Foot Ankle Surg. 2001;37:125-31.
3. Avino A, Patel S, Hamilton GA, Ford LA. The effect of the Lapidus arthrodesis on the medial longitudinal arch: a radiographic review. J Foot Ankle Surg. 2008;47:510-4.
4. Mann RA, Coughlin MJ. Hallux valgus. In: Coughlin MJ, Mann RA, Saltzman CL, editors Surgery of the foot and ankle. 8th ed. Philadelphia: Mosby Elsevier; 2007. p.298-300.
5. Frankel JP, Larsen DC. The misuse of the Lapidus procedure: re-evaluation of the preoperative criteria. J Foot Ankle Surg. 1996;35:355-61.
6. Sangeorzan BJ, Hansen ST. Modified Lapidus procedure for hallux valgus. Foot Ankle. 1989;9:262-6.
7. Lagaay PM, Hamilton GA, Ford LA, Williams ME, Rush SM, Schuberth JM. Rates of revision surgery using chevron-Austin osteotomy, Lapidus arthrodesis, and closing base wedge osteotomy for correction of hallux valgus deformity. J Foot Ankle Surg. 2008;47:267-72.
8. Catanzariti AR, Mendicino RW, Lee MS, Gallina MR. The modified Lapidus arthrodesis: a retrospective analysis. J Foot Ankle Surg. 1999;38:322-32.
9. Carl A, Ross S, Evanski P, Waugh T. Hypermobility in hallux valgus. Foot Ankle. 1988;8:264-70.
10. Fritz GR, Prieskorn D. First metatarsocuneiform motion: a radiographic and statistical analysis. Foot Ankle Int. 1995;16:153-7.
11. Bacardi B, Boysen T. Considerations for the Lapidus operation. J Foot Surg. 1986;25:133-8.
12. Mote GA, Yarmel D, Treaster A. First metatarsal-cuneiform arthrodesis for the treatment of first ray pathology: a technical guide. J Foot Ankle Surg. 2009;48:593-601.
13. Myerson MS. The modified lapidus procedure. In: Myerson MS, editors Reconstructive foot and ankle surgery. 1st ed. Philadelphia: Elsevier Saunders; 2005. p. 21-30.
14. Haas Z, Hamilton G, Sundstrom D, Ford L. Maintenance of correction of first metatarsal closing base wedge osteotomies versus modified Lapidus arthrodesis for moderate to severe hallux valgus deformity. J Foot Ankle Surg. 2007;46:358-65.
15. Scranton PE, Coetzee JC, Carreira D. Arthrodesis of the first metatarsocuneiform joint: a comparative study of fixation methods. Foot Ankle Int. 2009;30:341-5.
16. Saxena A, Nguyen A, Nelsen E. Lapidus bunionectomy: early evaluation of crossed lag screws versus locking plate with plantar lag screw. J Foot Ankle Surg. 2009;48:170-9.
17. Webb B, Nute M, Wilson S, Thomas J, Van Gompel J, Thompson K. Arthrodesis of the first metatarsocuneiform joint: a comparative cadaveric study of external and internal fixation. J Foot Ankle Surg. 2009;48:15-21.
18. Treadwell J. Rail external fixation for stabilization of closing base wedge osteotomies and Lapidus procedures: a retrospective analysis of sixteen cases. J Foot Ankle Surg. 2005;44:429-36.
19. Kazzaz S, Singh D. Postoperative cast necessity after a Lapidus arthrodesis. Foot Ankle Int. 2009;30:746-51.
20. Myerson M, Allon S, McGarvey W. Metatarsocuneiform arthrodesis for management of hallux valgus and metatarsus primus varus. Foot Ankle. 1992;13:107-15.
21. Coetzee JC, Wickum D. The Lapidus procedure: a prospective cohort outcome study. Foot Ankle Int. 2004;25:526-31.
22. Rick-Brüne O. Lapidus arthrodesis for management of hallux valgus – a retrospective review of 106 cases. J Foot Ankle Surg. 2004;43:290-5.

23. Kopp FJ, Patel MM, Levine DS, Deland JT. The modified Lapidus procedure for hallux valgus; a clinical and radiographic analysis. Foot Ankle Int. 2005;26:913-7.

24. Mauldin DM, Sanders M, Whitmer WW. Correction of hallux valgus with metatarsocuneiform stabilization. Foot Ankle. 1990;13:59-66.

25. Hamilton GA, Mullins S, Schuberth JM, Rush SM, Ford L. Revision Lapidus arthrodesis: rate of union in 17 cases. J Foot Ankle Surg. 2007;46:447-50.

26. Myerson NS, Badekas A. Hypermobility of the first ray. Foot Ankle Clin. 2000;5:469-84.

27. Patel S, Ford FA, Etcheverry J, Rush SM, Hamilton GA. Modified Lapidus arthrodesis: rate of nonunion in 227 cases. J Foot Ankle Surg. 2004;43:37-42.

28. McInnes B, Bouché R. Critical evaluation of the modified Lapidus procedure. J Foot Ankle Surg. 2001;40(2):71-90.

Chapter 2
Revision Hallux Valgus Surgery

David S. Caminear, Eliza Addis-Thomas, Adam William Brynizcka, and Amol Saxena

Foot and ankle surgeons routinely perform surgery of the first ray, such as correction of hallux valgus deformity. The complication rate in hallux valgus surgery ranges between 10% and 55%.[1] Although hallux valgus surgery is common, several common complications can occur that necessitate revision.

There are several causes of hallux valgus surgery failure; often, potential complications can be avoided by performing a thorough and careful preoperative evaluation of the patient. The presence of preexisting, but unexpected, osteoarthritis of the first metatarsal phalangeal joint (MTP) can lead to postoperative stiffness or arthrofibrosis. Recurrence of a previously corrected condition, hallux varus, avascular necrosis, and bone union problems are all some of the causes of revisional hallux valgus surgery. Excluded in this chapter is the discussion of the following conditions that also lead to complications of hallux valgus surgery: infection, hematoma, nerve injury, thrombophlebitis, complex regional pain syndrome, trauma, and disruption of the soft tissue envelope about the first ray.

D.S. Caminear, D.P.M. (✉)
Connecticut Orthopaedic Specialists, PC,
2408 Whitney Ave, Hamden, CT 06518, USA
e-mail: dcaminear@gmail.com

E. Addis-Thomas, D.P.M.
Connecticut Orthopaedic Specialists, PC, Hamden, CT, USA

A.W. Brynizcka, D.P.M.
Northwest Podiatry Center, Ltd., Wheaton, IL, USA

A. Saxena, D.P.M.
Department of Sports Medicine, PAFMG-Palo Alto Division,
Palo Alto, CA, USA

A. Saxena (ed.), *Special Procedures in Foot and Ankle Surgery*,
DOI 10.1007/978-1-4471-4103-7_2, © Springer-Verlag London 2013

2.1 Preoperative Evaluation

Revision surgery can be challenging to the most experienced foot and ankle surgeon. These challenges can often be avoided with an accurate preoperative evaluation. The importance of the initial evaluation is tantamount to the surgical technique in an effort to achieve a successful outcome. If the initial evaluation process is not accurate and detailed, a steep downward slope can ensue for the remainder of the treatment course and may ultimately lead to a need for revision surgery.

The preoperative evaluation begins with a detailed and accurate history and physical examination. There are numerous documented surgical procedures for hallux valgus correction dating back to the nineteenth century.[2] The procedure selected needs to coincide with the patient's age, functional limitations, and lifestyle demands. For example, it would be unwise to choose a complex realignment osteotomy for a sedentary, geriatric patient with limited functional requirements. On the other hand, a minimally invasive procedure may not provide adequate enough correction for a young, active patient.

Patients' goals and expectations should be elucidated. In revision surgery of the first ray, bony and clinical alignment may appear to be "normal" to the surgeon, yet the patient may feel the index procedure was a failure. Going beyond the potential anatomical correction to find out what the patient actually wants is very important in revision surgery. For the first ray, is the patient concerned about the Hallux position: is it too straight, too angled, too stiff or fused in an uncomfortable position? Surgeons need to ask "What is it you hope to achieve from another surgery?," not only to themselves but the patient and possibly even their family members.

Many surgeons are adept at performing an excellent history and physical examination; however, they are uncomfortable performing the necessary procedure to achieve the desired correction. Often times, as a result of lack of training and inexperience, surgeons become habitually familiar with too few available surgical options. This could lead to performing the improper procedure for a given deformity. In short, the surgical procedure should fit the deformity, rather than forcing the deformity to fit the procedure (Fig. 2.1).

The radiographic examination is equally as important as the history and physical examination. Key evaluation parameters include: the first intermetatarsal angle, metatarsal parabola, the presence or absence of metatarsus adductus, and the integrity of the joints of the first ray (hallux interphalangeal, first metatarsal phalangeal, and first metatarsal cuneiform joints).[2] The first intermetatarsal angle is arguably the most important structural parameter that determines osteotomy selection. Undercorrection can lead to recurrence of deformity, while overcorrection can lead to hallux varus.

The metatarsal parabola is frequently underappreciated. Over lengthening the first metatarsal by osteotomy can cause a soft tissue imbalance and retrograde buckling resulting in recurrence, whereas, lesser metatarsalgia is a frequent problem following excessive shortening of the first metatarsal.

Fig. 2.1 An opening base wedge procedure was performed on this patient along with an aggressive medial capsuloraphy. Clearly, the deformity is not adequately reduced. The metatarsal was overly lengthened causing retrograde forces to act at the first metatarsal phalangeal joint; these forces caused the soft tissues to cause the deformity to recur

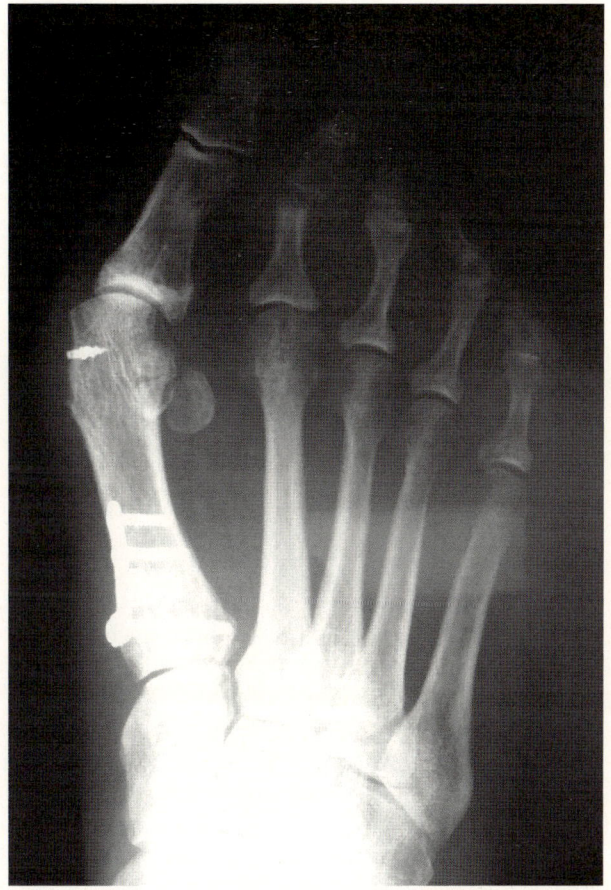

The metatarsus adductus angle should not be overlooked because the true inter-metatarsal angle equals the measured intermetatarsal angle plus the influence of any increase over accepted normal of the metatarsus adductus angle. A large metatarsus adductus angle can give the illusion of a relatively small first intermetatarsal angle, and if not addressed properly, the resultant procedure selection will inadequately correct the deformity.

2.2 Arthrofibrosis

A common postoperative complication of hallux valgus surgery is joint stiffness or arthrofibrosis. The cause can be commonly attributed to unrecognized preoperative osteoarthritis that is identified intraoperatively (Fig. 2.2). Frequently, the sesamoids are degenerated as well. Metabolic disorders, such as diabetes mellitus, advanced

Fig. 2.2 In this clinical picture, degeneration of the first metatarsal head is seen. This is often an unexpected intraoperative finding. Early range of motion is helpful in preventing arthrofibrosis

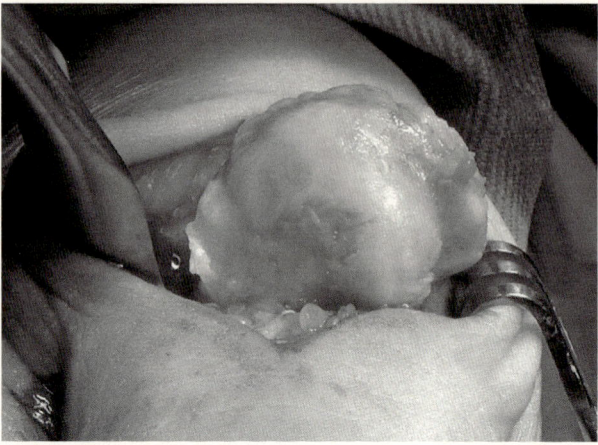

age, postoperative infection, noncompliance, and the patient's intrinsic propensity to form scar can also lead to arthrofibrosis.

Preventative treatment for arthrofibrosis is difficult to achieve. Early active range of motion and institution of an aggressive postsurgical physical therapy program are the mainstays of prevention. A novel approach to the treatment of debilitating post-surgical arthrofibrosis is manipulation of the first metatarsal phalangeal joint under anesthesia. The authors follow the guidelines established by Solan et al., whereby, following sedation of the patient and aseptic preparation of the foot, the great toe joint is infiltrated with a combination of 40 mg of Depomedrol and 2 mL of 1% Xylocaine plain.[3] Joint distention is observed under fluoroscopy and the great toe is manually manipulated to achieve a normal range of motion. This is often character-ized by a palpable and audible breakup of the scar tissue. The sesamoid apparatus should be freely mobile during range of motion as visualized under fluoroscopy.

2.3 Recurrence

Recurrence of hallux valgus deformity after surgical correction is multifactorial. The incidence has been reported as high as 16%.[4] One of the more common expla-nations for hallux valgus recurrence is due to incomplete initial correction (Fig. 2.3). Furthermore, anatomical and biomechanical factors can predispose a patient to recurrent deformity. Unfortunately, despite careful analysis, the cause of recurrent deformity may be idiopathic.

Incomplete initial correction is a direct result of failure to properly analyze all pertinent preoperative parameters. Clinical considerations include evaluating the patient's age, Body Mass Index (BMI), functional demands, and unique physiologic and anatomic configurations. For example, a failure to identify a patient with liga-mentous laxity may lead to an underappreciation of potential deforming forces

Fig. 2.3 A common cause of recurrence is incomplete initial correction. This picture reveals an uncorrected intermetatarsal angle with recurrent deformity

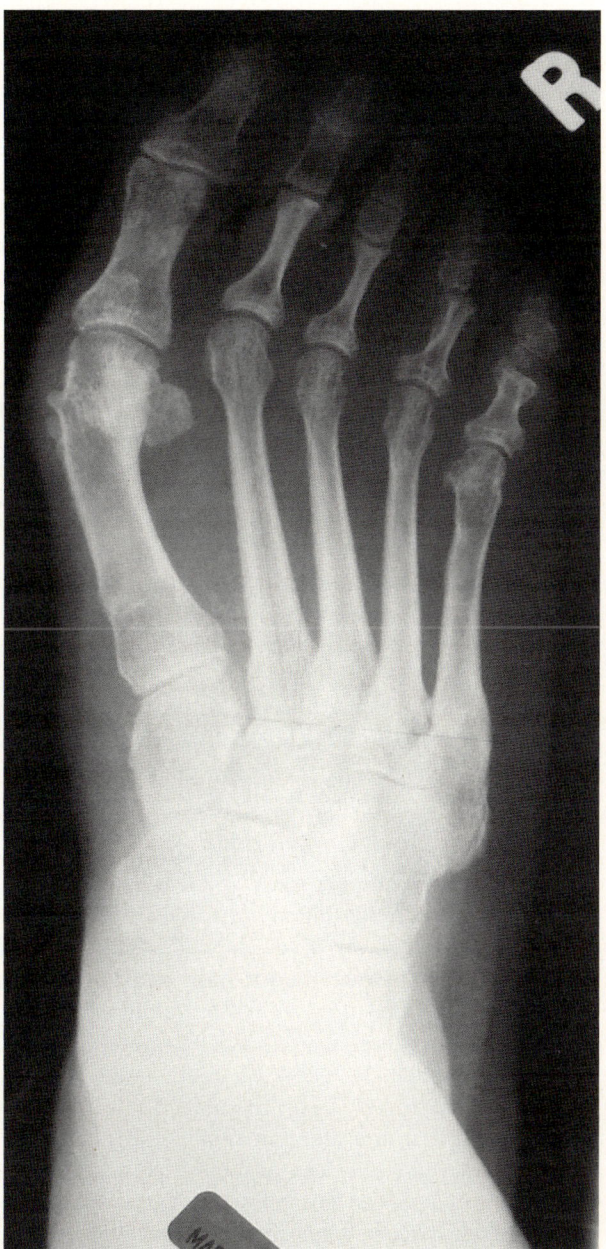

resulting in an inability to maintain correction. Also, the surgeon must pay careful attention to radiographic structural details such as first intermetatarsal angle, proximal articular set angle, congruence of the first metatarsal phalangeal and hallux interphalangeal joints, the length of the first metatarsal, and sesamoid position.[2]

Following a thorough clinical and radiographic evaluation, the surgeon then must determine what he/she wishes to accomplish with a given procedure or osteotomy. Osteotomies are powerful procedures and are able to correct many parameters of a hallux valgus deformity. The purpose of an osteotomy is to normalize the alignment of the first ray to restore its function in weight-bearing and ambulation.[5] For example, an osteotomy can accomplish transposition of the metatarsal either plantarly, dorsally, medially, or laterally. Furthermore, specific osteotomies can provide angular correction to reduce the intermetatarsal angle and/or proximal articular set angle. Finally, osteotomies can de-rotate the first metatarsal and may also have a linear effect by either lengthening or shortening the metatarsal as necessary.

Adhering to the following general osteotomy principles can mitigate recurrent hallux valgus caused by incomplete initial surgical correction:

• Understand that every osteotomy has a maximal corrective effect.
• Variations in technique or application of an osteotomy generally diminish the primary corrective effect of the osteotomy.
• Determine the desired correction and then select the osteotomy that will allow you to obtain the correction.
• Avoid the temptation of becoming procedure bound.
• The procedure should fit the deformity, rather than the deformity fit the procedure (Jacobs A., 2005, personal correspondence) (Fig. 2.4).

Anatomic factors such as metatarsus adductus or medial column adductus can lead to recurrent hallux valgus deformity. Choosing an osteotomy yet failing to recognize inherent metatarsus adductus or medial column adductus will likely to lead to either an undercorrected deformity or recurrence. The presence of metatarsus adductus gives the radiographic illusion that the hallux valgus deformity is less severe than it is in reality. The effective first intermetatarsal angle equals the measured true intermetatarsal angle plus any degree of metatarsus adductus greater than 15°.[6] For example, a patient with a 10° first intermetatarsal angle and also 26° of metatarsus adductus has an effective first intermetatarsal angle of 21°; the selection of the procedure should be based on this effective first intermetatarsal angle (Fig. 2.5).

Biomechanical influences can predispose a patient to recurrent hallux valgus. Excessive pronation can destabilize the first ray and cause medial migration of the first metatarsal with concomitant lateralization of the great toe.[7] Therefore, control of pathologic pronatory deforming forces will minimize the chance for recurrence. Ankle equinus contracture is known to lead to hyperpronation. Therefore, ankle equinus is important to recognize and treat in conjunction with the hallux valgus procedure.[8] Surgical management of ankle equinus is based upon the Silverskold maneuver and can include either tendo-Achilles lengthening or gastrocnemius recession. Finally, patients with excessive pronation who demonstrate heel valgus, longitudinal arch collapse, and

Fig. 2.4 (**a**) The Z-type osteotomy has been strictly translated. The surgeon was not satisfied with correction. (**b**) The osteotomy has been subsequently translated with rotation of the capital fragment. The rotation of the capital fragment allows for a more complete correction of the deformity but compromises the amount of translation that can be achieved

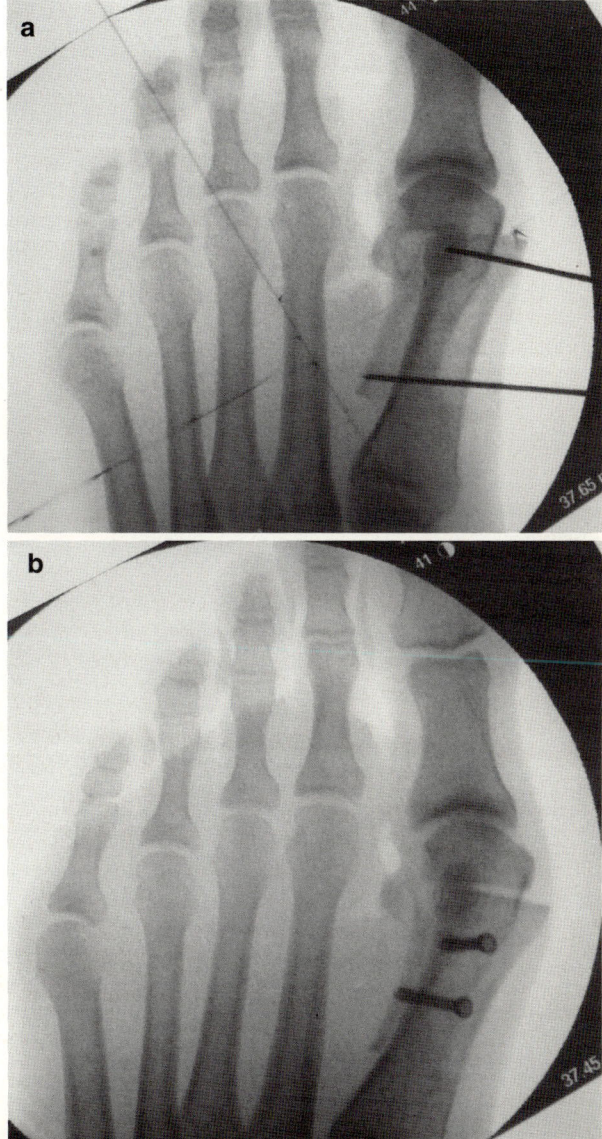

Fig. 2.5 It is imperative to take metatarsus adductus into account when assessing the hallux valgus deformity. The metatarsus adductus can mask the severity of the bunion deformity

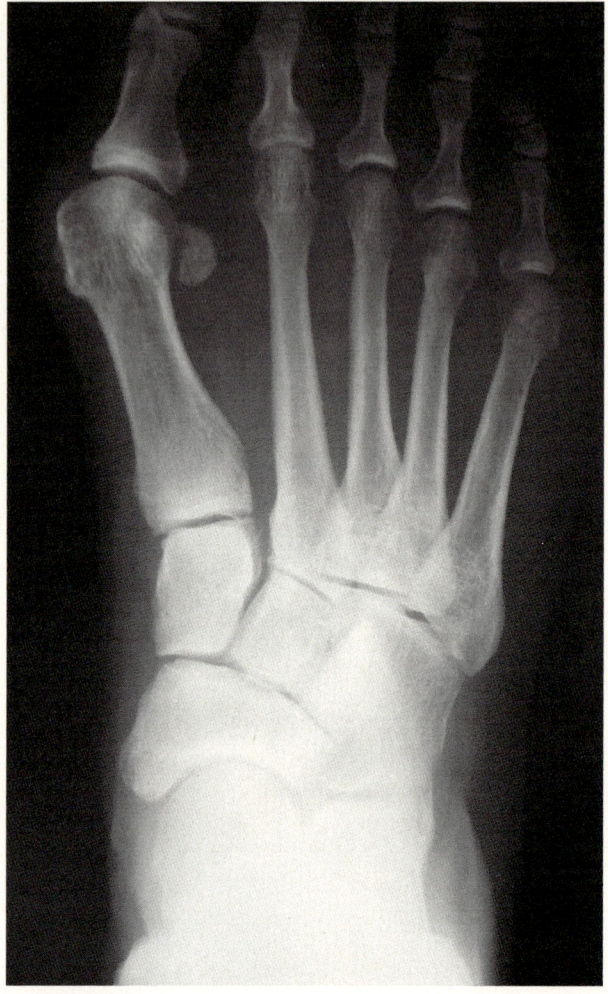

midfoot abductus may also benefit from custom foot controlling orthoses postoperatively as a measure of protection to guard against hallux valgus recurrence.

2.4 Hallux Varus

Hallux varus most commonly occurs after a proximal metatarsal osteotomy (Fig. 2.6). The incidence rate of hallux varus has been reported to be as high as 10–12%.[4] Paradoxically, many patients with hallux varus are asymptomatic and do not require treatment, particularly if the hallux varus measures less than 10°.[9] However, when symptoms occur, they usually result from an associated hallux

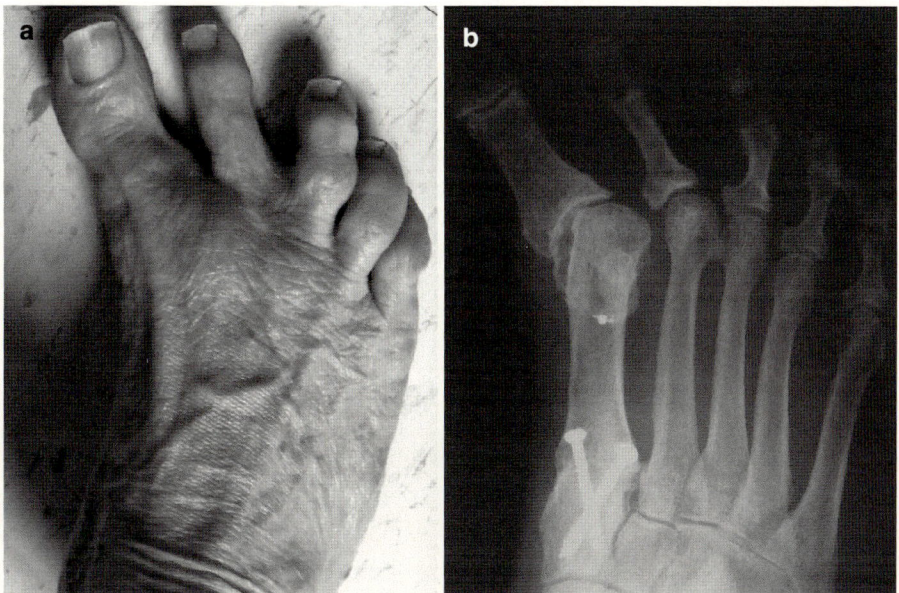

Fig. 2.6 (a) In this photograph, the hallux varus deformity is clear. This deformity can make wearing shoe gear quite uncomfortable for the patient. (b) A Lapidus procedure was performed with an overaggressive resection of the medial eminence. The staking of the first metatarsal head resulted in hallux varus

malleus, a rigid deformity that limits footwear, and arthrosis of the first metatarsal phalangeal joint.

The causes of hallux varus have been attributed to scar contracture, fibular sesamoidectomy with excessive plication of the medial capsule, aggressive resection of the medial eminence (staked first metatarsal head), and the overcorrection of the first intermetatarsal angle.[10] Avoiding these surgical pitfalls can prevent the development of hallux varus.

Nonsurgical management of hallux varus includes early recognition, physical therapy, and soft tissue mobilization. For example, passive abduction exercises of the great toe performed in conjunction with dynamic buddy splinting may arrest a developing deformity.

When surgical correction is indicated for a flexible hallux varus, a methodical stepwise approach is followed. A thorough sequential release of the deformity is performed from superficial to deep anatomic structures. Beginning with the skin, a Z-plasty or other similar plastic-type skin incision should be considered. Next, extensor and/or abductor hallucis tendon lengthening is performed followed by first metatarsal phalageal joint capsule release. This may be all that is required for a mild deformity.

An intraoperative decision is then made to follow either a soft tissue or osseous pathway.

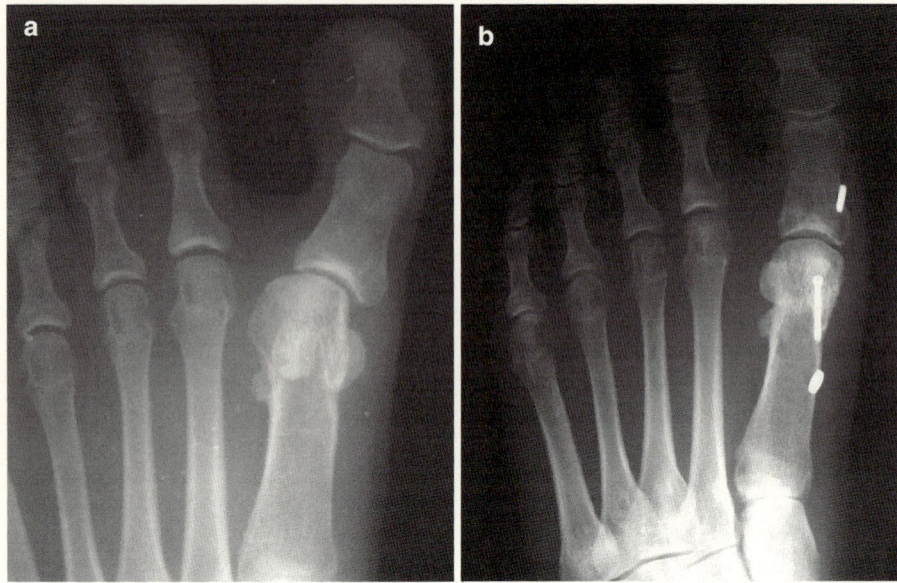

Fig. 2.7 (**a**) Note the hallux varus deformity with peaking of the tibial sesamoid. (**b**) In this surgical correction of the hallux varus deformity, an Arthrex Mini-Tightrope was used. The joint has been realigned and the sesamoid apparatus has been relocated

The authors' preferred soft tissue approach is to follow the technique described by Juliano, Meyerson, and Cunningham whereby the extensor hallucis brevis (EHB) tendon is divided proximally and routed deep to the transverse metatarsal ligament and through a drill hole in the first metatarsal.[11] The procedure may be modified by using a Mini-Tightrope (Arthrex) in place of the EHB for tendon augmentation (Fig. 2.7).

The osseous pathway makes use of a distal first metatarsal osteotomy. A reverse chevron with internal fixation is often sufficient to realign the first metatarsal phalangeal joint (Fig. 2.8).

In cases where the hallux varus is long-standing, rigid, and/or demonstrates arthrosis of the first metatarsal phalangeal joint, a first metatarsal phalangeal joint arthrodesis is the procedure of choice. However, a Keller arthroplasty can also be considered for geriatric patients.

2.5 Avascular Necrosis

Although uncommon, avascular necrosis (AVN) of the first metatarsal head following hallux valgus surgery can lead to loss of function of the first metatarsophalangeal joint. AVN most commonly follows distal first metatarsal osteotomies and is caused by a disruption of the blood supply to the metatarsal head.[12] The resultant cascade of avascularization with subsequent revascularization of the head can lead to articular collapse and degeneration of the joint.

The blood supply to the first metatarsal includes the nutrient artery, metaphyseal vessels, and periosteal network. The vessels are branches of the first dorsal metatarsal artery that originate from the dorsalis pedis artery, the first plantar metatarsal artery, and the medial plantar artery.[13] The dorsal vessels supply the superior two thirds of the first metatarsal head and the plantar vessels supply the inferior one third of the head. The lateral and dorsal aspects of the first metatarsal head have a better blood supply compared to the remainder of the head.[14] The nutrient artery divides into a proximal and distal branch with the later anastomosing with the capital vessels.[12]

Much has been written about soft tissue lateral release as a cause of AVN. Meier and Kenzora reported a 20% AVN rate with osteotomy alone and 40% when combined with lateral release.[15] More recently, several studies indicate that a lateral release may be performed without compromising blood supply.[16]

All metatarsal osteotomies have the potential to cause AVN secondary to a disruption of blood flow to the metatarsal head. Distal osteotomies can compromise the flow from the nutrient artery. In these circumstances, the remaining blood flow to the head stems from the capsular vessels. If the capsular network is breached, the overall blood supply to the head is altered and AVN can occur. Furthermore, lateral transposition of the capital fragment of an osteotomy can stretch the vasculature and potentially compromise perfusion to the head. Finally, thermal necrosis from the modern saw blade can not only result in osseous damage but also jeopardize the metatarsal blood supply.

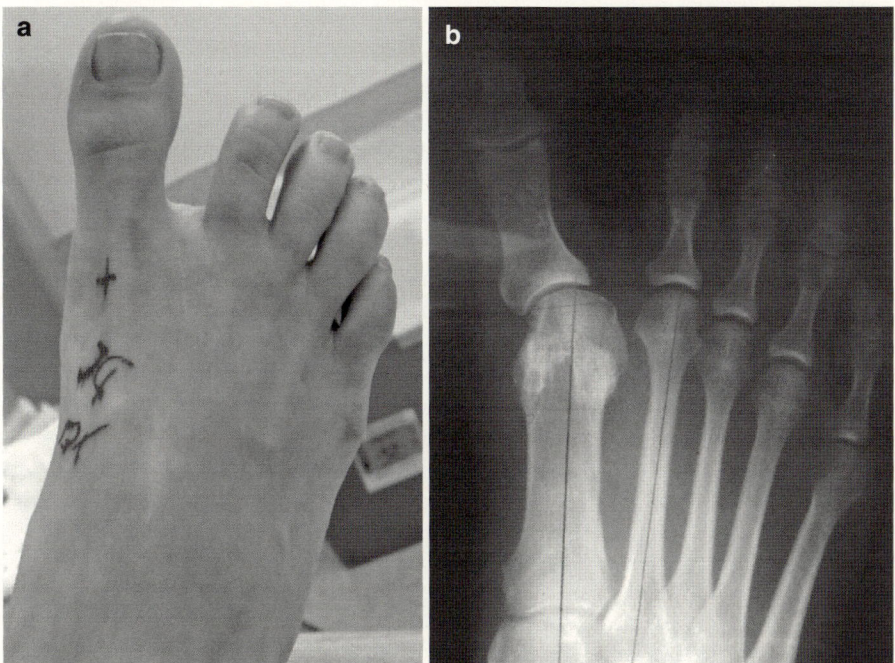

Fig. 2.8 Preoperative clinical photograph (**a**) and radiograph (**b**) following a hallux valgus surgery. Again, staking of the first metatarsal head has occurred. (**c, d**) Postoperatively, the iatrogenic hallux varus has been corrected. As this was a more moderate deformity, an osseous procedure was selected. A reverse chevron was performed and fixated with two screws

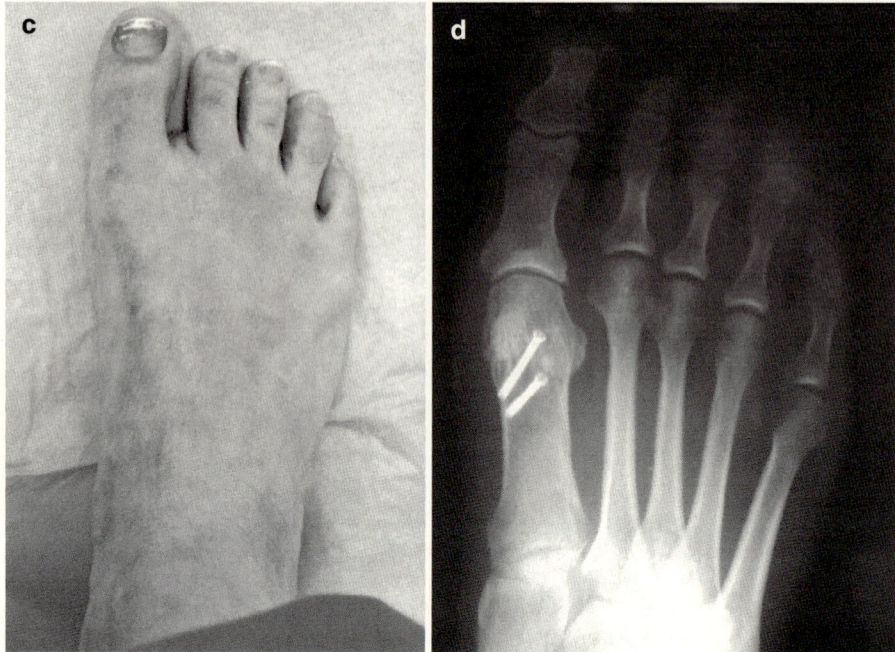

Fig. 2.8 (continued)

Preservation of the capsular network is critical for the prevention of AVN. Meticulous soft tissue technique and maintenance of the dorsal synovial fold that contains the capsular vessels is advocated. It is recommended to avoid multiple saw blade passes and use of worn saw blades when performing an osteotomy.[17]

The predominant early clinical findings of AVN are pain and joint swelling but can occur at variable times after surgery. For example, one should expect AVN if such findings are noted at follow-up at a time when the osteotomy is expected to be healed. Later, there may be stiffness and transfer metatarsalgia.

Radiographs at the time of clinical presentation, more often than not, demonstrate articular collapse with varying degrees of arthrosis. It is difficult to recognize the pre-collapse stages; these stages are more easily recognizable in retrospect.

Because many AVN cases are asymptomatic, nonoperative treatment may be employed. Mildly symptomatic patients may improve with joint debridement and synovectomy.[17] When surgical intervention is required, a Keller arthroplasty or a first metatarsophalangeal joint arthrodesis with or without bone graft may be performed.[17]

2.6 Nonunion

Osteotomies are commonly utilized to correct hallux valgus. Reports of nonunion following first metatarsal osteotomy are rare, and vary depending on the procedure. As most procedures are performed through the metaphyseal region of the bone, healing is predictable.[4] Modern improvements in fixation have also reduced nonunion rates.

Fig. 2.9 Hypertrophic nonunions
are characterized by exuberant bone
callous. This callous is evident
in the radiograft

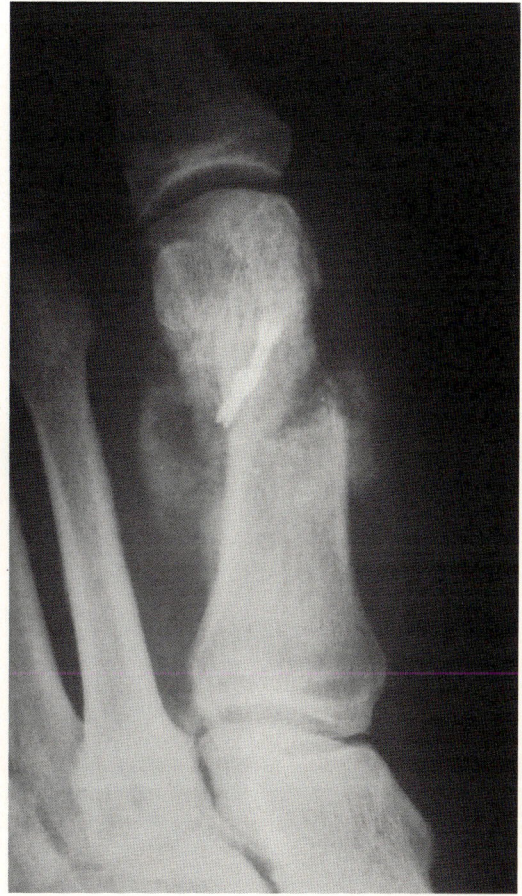

There are two basic causes of nonunions: biomechanical and biological. Because of the orientation of the first metatarsal, osteotomies are subjected to loads perpendicular to the long axis of the metatarsal; this results in unique forces acting across the osteotomy sites.[18] Proximal osteotomies are more likely to lead to nonunion than distal osteotomies as there is an increased moment arm through which loads are applied. Any osteotomy is intrinsically unstable if it has a single plane that is directed from dorsal proximal to plantar distal (i.e., Ludloff); also, any osteotomy that is made perpendicular to the shaft of the first metatarsal is unstable (i.e., closing abductory base wedge).[18]

Appropriate fixation should also be utilized to reduce the potential for nonunion; the more inherently unstable the osteotomy, the more essential fixation is. In the event that stability is compromised and motion occurs at the osteotomy site, a nonunion can develop. Factors such as hardware failure, poor construct design, and patient noncompliance (premature weight-bearing) are common causes of mechanically induced nonunions.

Nonunions of mechanical etiology are most likely to be hypertrophic in nature with demonstrating exuberant bone callus (Fig. 2.9). This is indicative of a robust blood supply with poor stability at the osteotomy site. One can think of these nonunions as

Fig. 2.10 At the site of the osteotomy, there is a large gap with no bone callous present. This is indicative of an atrophic nonunion

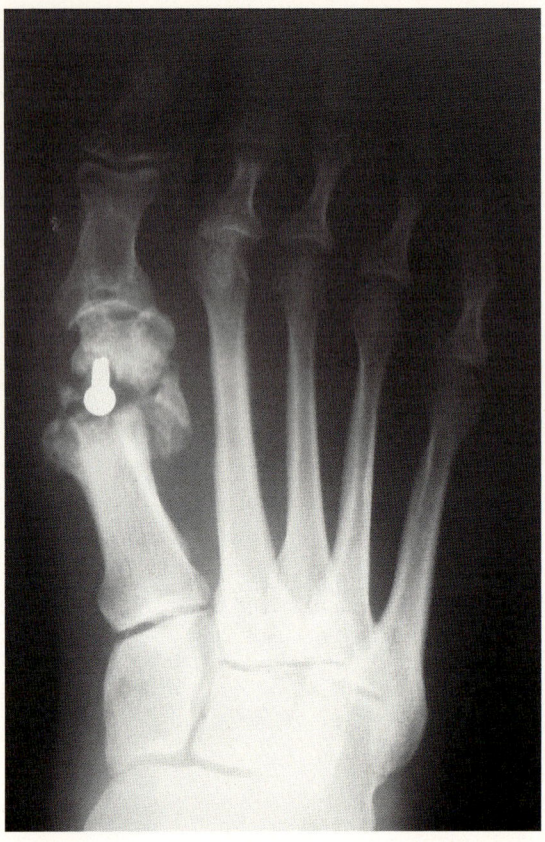

"crying out for stability." If the osteotomy position has not been compromised, often hypertrophic nonunions may be cast immobilized in order to provide stability. Revision surgery is considered only in the event that the osteotomy is malpositioned.

Biological causes of nonunions are most often the result of altered blood supply to the osteotomy site. These types of nonunions are atrophic and minimal or no bone callus is visualized (Fig. 2.10). There are many factors that may contribute to the cause of atrophic nonunions. For example, patients with advanced age have a thinner periosteum resulting in a relatively poorer periosteal blood supply.[19] Patients with hormonal imbalances, such as diabetes mellitus and hypothyroidism, are more susceptible to develop an atrophic nonunion.[19] Exogenous steroids can retard bone repair as can certain medications, such as heparin. Hypoxia caused by anemia and cigarette smoking can lead to aberrant bone healing at an osteotomy site.

The majority of nonunions are symptomatic secondary to motion at the osteotomy site. Most atrophic nonunions require surgical intervention. However, regardless of the cause, mechanical or biologic, the surgical protocol remains the same. The tenets of nonunion operative management are as follows:

1. Debridement of the nonunion
2. Bone graft osseous defect

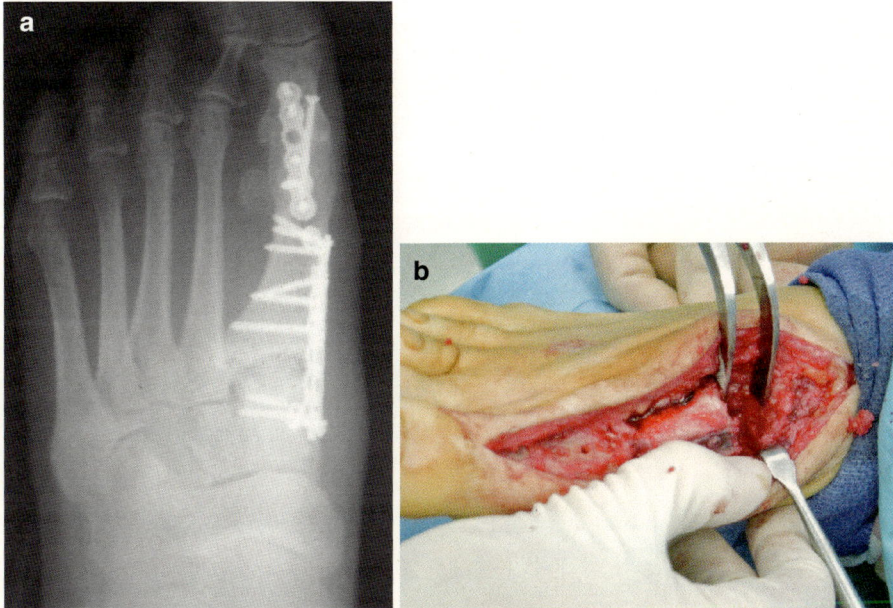

Fig. 2.11 (**a**) A nonunion is evident at the first metatarsal cuneiform joint after a failed Lapidus. Note the broken hardware in the medial cuneiform. (**b**) Aggressive debridement of the nonunion at the first metatarsal cuneiform joint is performed

3. Re-alignment of the osteotomy
4. Stable fixation
5. Consideration of adjunct bone healing enhancements (bone growth stimulator, bone morphogenic proteins, mesenchymal stem cells, etc.)

Debridement of the nonunion is the initial critical step of the revision process. Hypertrophic bone and/or fibrous tissue need to be resected from the nonunion site to obtain adequate exposure, demonstrate healthy bleeding bone margins, and allow for manipulation of the osteotomy segments (Fig. 2.11).

Following debridement, an assessment of bone graft size is required. Next, appropriate structural allogenic or autogenous bone graft is selected, measured, cut, and placed into the defect (Fig. 2.12). There are many differences between allogenic and autogenous bone grafts. Allogenic bone graft offers an advantage of ease of accessibility without volume restrictions. Autogenous bone grafts require a second surgical site and may be limited in supply but will not demonstrate histocompatibility problems. Furthermore, patients often relate prolonged donor site pain. Autogenous bone grafts were once considered to be the "gold standard" of bone grafting and thought to have a superior fusion potential. However, recent literature suggests that allogenic grafts have equivocal fusion rates when compared to autogenous bone grafts.[20]

With the graft in place, the osteotomy is realigned to restore the original intent of the initial hallux valgus procedure. Careful attention is paid to the three-dimensional

Fig. 2.12 Autogeous tricortical iliac crest bone graft is placed into the nonunion defect

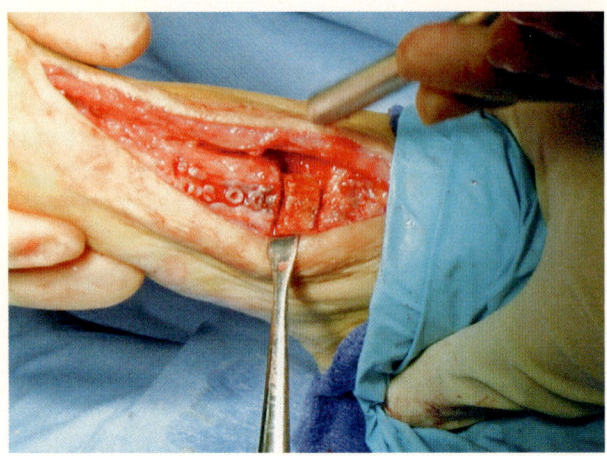

orientation of the capital segment in the three cardinal planes. Anatomic length of the first metatarsal is restored at this step.

The revision is then fixated. A combination of internal and external fixation may be considered with the ultimate goal being rigid stabilization. Internal fixation will likely require a plate and screw construct (Fig. 2.13). In recent years, anatomic plate designs specific toward foot and ankle surgery have been developed. Furthermore, locking plates have gained popularity because of their greater stability and ease of use when compared to traditional plates. The strength of a locked plate construct equals the sum of the screws and plate at the bone interface.[21] A locking plate acts as the near cortex of the bone and each screw locks into the plate at either a fixed or variable angle. Thus, the strength of the construct is distributed through all of the screws. This is inherently more stable than a traditional plate and screw construct where the strength is dependent upon only a single screw and the frictional force that occurs between the plate and the bone.[22] With a locked plate construct, all of the screws must fail for the entire construct to fail; a single screw's failure can lead to a construct's failure with traditional plate and screw fixation. Finally, if after internal fixation is applied and the stability of the construct is questioned, external fixation should be considered as adjunct fixation.

There are modalities to help promote healing after revision hallux valgus surgery.

Bone graft substitutes have been found to aid healing of bone fusions. Studies have demonstrated that ceramic-based bone graft substitutes (i.e., Vitoss) are equivalent to iliac crest graft.[23] Vitoss is a calcium phosphate bone graft substitute that, when combined with bone marrow aspirate, has osteoinductive, osteoconductive, and osteogenic properties. Cell-based bone graft substitutes (Trinity Evolution) employ mesenchymal stem cells to facilitate bone healing; Trinity Evolution also provides osteoconduction, osteoinduction, and ostegenesis to a fusion site.[24] In one study, a 91.3% rate of union was found in revision foot and ankle surgery.[25]

Bone morphogenic proteins (BMPs) are a group of growth factors and cytokines that promote formation of bone and cartilage; specifically, BMP-2,7 have been found

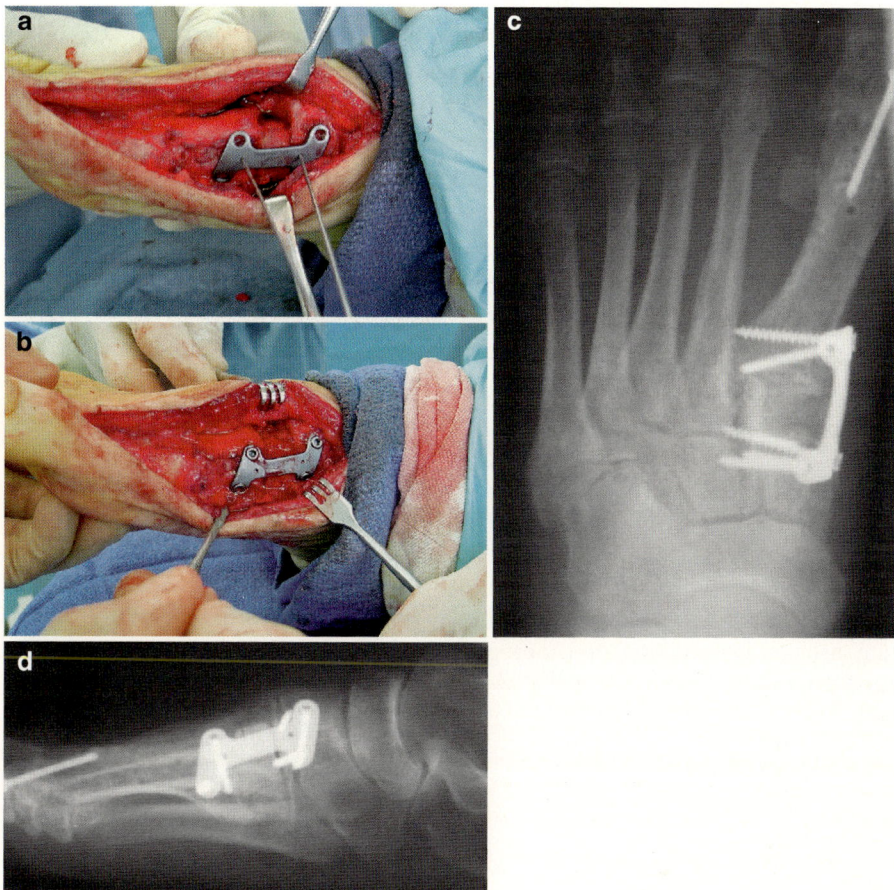

Fig. 2.13 (**a, b**) An atomically designed four-hole locking plate is applied spanning the autogenous bone graft. AP (**c**) and lateral (**d**) radiographs at 3 months postoperatively demonstrate consolidation at the graft site

to have a pivotal role in osteoblast differentiation.[25,26] There are two of these products on the market today, BPM-2 (Infuse™) and OP-1 BMP-7 (Stryker™); both have Food and Drug Administration (FDA) indications for delayed unions and nonunions.

Finally, there are many types of bone stimulation devices. There are internal and external bone stimulators; internal bone stimulators have a reported success rate in nonunions of as high as 89% but require a second surgery to remove the device[27] (Fig. 2.14). There has been a trend toward using non-implantable devices. These devices are user friendly and can be used in the patient's home. There are four types of external bone stimulators: inductive coupling, combined magnetic field, capacitative coupling, and ultrasound.[28] For example, the Exogen Ultrasound bone stimulator reports a 86% healing rate for nonunions.[29] Bone stimulators are an important adjunct to nonunion surgery.

Fig. 2.14 Lateral radiograph reveals an implantable bone growth stimulator

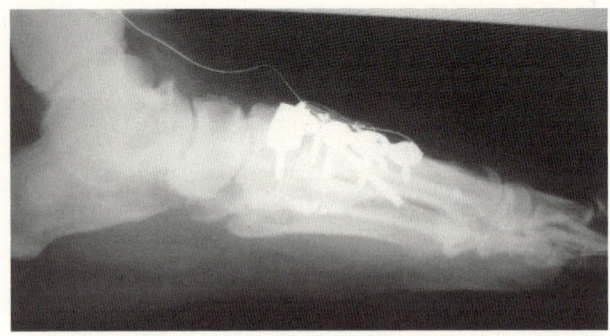

2.7 Conclusion

Hallux valgus is one of the most common elective foot and ankle procedures performed in the USA. There are potential complications that can occur that lead to revision surgery. The most common complications leading to revision hallux valgus surgery are arthrofibrosis, recurrence, hallux varus, avascular necrosis, and nonunion. Careful preoperative planning along with meticulous intraoperative dissection, osteotomy execution, and appropriate fixation are all factors to help reduce the need for revision surgery.

References

1. Scioli MW. Complications of hallux valgus surgery and subsequent treatment options. Foot Ankle Clin. 1997;2:719-39.
2. Chang TJ. Distal metaphyseal osteotomies in hallux abducto valgus surgery. In: Banks AS, Downey MS, Martin DE, Miller SJ, editors. McGlamry's comprehensive textbook of foot and ankle surgery. 3rd ed. Philadelphia: Lippincott Williams & Wilkins; 2001. p. 505-28.
3. Solan MC, Calder JD, Bendall SP. Manipulation and injection for hallux rigidus: is it worthwhile? J Bone Joint Surg Br. 2001;83:706-8.
4. Lehman DE. Salvage of complications of hallux valgus surgery. Foot Ankle Clin. 2003; 8:15-35.
5. Sammarco VJ, Acevedo J. Stability and fixation technique in first metatarsal osteotomies. Foot Ankle Clin. 2001;6:409-32.
6. Engle E, Erlick N, Krems I. A simplified metatarsus adductus angle. J Am Podiatr Med Assoc. 1983;73:620-8.
7. Alvarez R, Haddad RJ, Gould N, et al. The simple bunion: anatomy at the metatarsophalangeal joint of the great toe. Foot Ankle. 1984;24:54.
8. Yu GV, Johng B, Freireich R. Surgical management of metatarus adductus deformity. Clin Podiatr Med Surg. 1987;4:207-32.
9. Johnson KA, Cofield RH, Morrey BF. Chevron osteotomy for hallux valgus. Clin Orthop Relat Res. 1979;142:44-7.
10. Selner AJ, Selner MD, Cyr RP, Noiwangmuang W. Revisional hallux abducto valgus surgery using tricorrectional bunionectomy. J Am Podiatr Med Assoc. 2004;94:341-6.

11. Juliano PJ, Myerson MS, Cunningham BW. Biomechanical assessment of a new tenodesis for correction of hallux varus. Foot Ankle Int. 1996;17:17-20.
12. Easley ME, Kelly IP. Avascular necrosis of the hallux metatarsal head. Foot Ankle Clin North Am. 2000;5:591-608.
13. Roukis TS, Hurless JS. The hallucal interphalangeal sesamoid. J Foot Ankle Surg. 1994;4: 303-8.
14. Shereff MJ, Yang QM, Kummer FJ. Extraosseous and intraosseous arterial supply of to the first metatarsal and metatarsophalangeal joints. Foot Ankle. 1987;8:81-93.
15. Meier PJ, Kenzora JE. The risks and benefits of distal first metatarsal osteotomies. Foot Ankle. 1985;6:7-17.
16. Jones KJ, Feiwell LA, Freedman EL, Cracchiolo A. The effect of the chevron osteotomy with lateral capsule release on the blood supply to the first metatarsal head. J Bone Joint Surg. 1995;77:197-204.
17. Edwards WH. Avascular necrosis of the first metatarsal head. Foot Ankle Clin North Am. 2005;10:117-27.
18. Vora AM, Myerson MS. First metatarsal osteotomy nonunion and malunion. Foot Ankle Clin North Am. 2005;10:35-54.
19. Oloff LM. Nonunions. In: Scurran BL, editor. Foot and ankle trauma. 1st ed. New York: Churchill Livingstone Inc; 1989.p. 673-98.
20. Putzier M, Strube P, Funk JF, et al. Allogenic versus autologous cancellous bone in lumbar segmental spondylodesis: a randomized prospective study. Eur Spine J. 2009;18:687-95.
21. Greiwe RM, Archdeacon MT. Locking plate technology. J Knee Surg. 2007;20:50-5.
22. Frigg R, Appenzeller A, Christensen R. The development of the distal femur less invasive stabilization system. Injury. 2001;32(Suppl 3):SC24-31.
23. Epstein NE. Beta-tricalcium phosphate: observation of use in 100 posterolateral lumbar instrumented fusions. Spine J. 2009;8:630-8.
24. Barry FP, Murphy JM. Mesenchymal stem cells: clinical applications and biological characterization. Int J Biochem Cell Biol. 2004;36(4):568-84.
25. Rush SM, Hamilton GA, Ackerson LM. Mesenchymal stem cell allograft in revision foot and ankle surgery: a clinical and radiographic analysis. J Foot Ankle Surg. 2009;48:163-9.
26. Schuberth JM, DiDomenico LA, Mendicino RW. The utility and effectiveness of bone morphogenic protein in foot and ankle surgery. J Foot Ankle Surg. 2009;48:309-14.
27. Patterson DC, Lewis GN, Cass CA. Treatment of delayed union and nonunion with an implanted direct current stimulator. Clin Orthop Relat Res. 1980;148:117-28.
28. Downey MS, Bernstein SA. Augmentation of bone growth and healing. In: Banks AS, Downey MS, Martin DE, Miller SJ, editors. McGlamry's comprehensive textbook of foot and ankle surgery. 3rd ed. Philadelphia: Lippincott Williams & Wilkins; 2001. p.2051-64.
29. Nolte PA, van der Krans A, Patka P, Janssen IM, Ryaby JP, Albers GH. Low-intensity pulsed ultrasound in the treatment of nonunions. J Trauma. 2001;51:693-703.

Chapter 3
Insertional and Midsubstance Achilles Tendinopathy

Amol Saxena, Umile Giuseppe Longo, Vincenzo Denaro, and Nicola Maffulli

3.1 Introduction

Achilles tendinopathy is characterized by pain, impaired performance, and swelling in and around the tendon.[1] It can be categorized as insertional and noninsertional, two distinct disorders with different underlying pathophysiologies and management options.[2] Other terms used as synonymous of noninsertional tendinopathy include tendinopathy of the main body of the Achilles tendon (AT) and mid-portion Achilles tendinopathy. In this chapter, we give a detailed overview of insertional tendinopathy of the AT and tendinopathy of the main body of the AT.

3.2 Anatomy

The AT attaches to the middle and inferior aspects of the posterior calcaneus. The inferior AT fibers blend with the proximal attachment of the plantar fascia. The medial and lateral aspects of the tendon insertion have an expansion to these regions of the calcaneus. The medial aspect of the AT expansion is thicker. This expansion

A. Saxena, D.P.M. (✉)
Department of Sports Medicine, PAFMG-Palo Alto Division,
Clark Bldg., 3rd Flr, 795 El Camino Real, Palo Alto, CA 94301, USA
e-mail: heysax@aol.com

U.G. Longo, M.D. • V. Denaro, M.D.
Department of Trauma and Orthopaedic Surgery,
University Campus Bio-Medico of Rome, Rome, Italy

N. Maffulli, M.D., M.S., Ph.D., F.R.C.S (Orth).
Barts and The London School of Medicine and Dentistry,
Centre for Sports and Exercise Medicine, Mile End Hospital,
Queen Mary University of London,
London, E1 4DG, UK

A. Saxena (ed.), *Special Procedures in Foot and Ankle Surgery*,
DOI 10.1007/978-1-4471-4103-7_3, © Springer-Verlag London 2013

is important as it keeps the tendon from migrating proximally when significant surgical debridement and detachment is needed.[3,4] Calcifications of the tendon in this region arise from micro-trauma and physiological changes causing calcium to precipitate in a lower pH environment. There is an anatomically occurring retrocal-caneal bursa that is adjacent to the superior posterior calcaneus, anterior to the tendon just prior to its insertion. This upper portion of the calcaneus has smooth fibro-cartilage surface in this region. A secondary "adventitious" bursa may occur in areas with more pressure on the tendon, often from constant shoe contact. These bursae occur within the subcutaneous tissue superficial to the AT.

3.3 Insertional Achilles Tendinopathy

Ever since Haglund first described pathology with the Achilles insertion in relation to the posterior calcaneus,[5] many authors have described surgical solutions for the approximately 10% of patients with recalcitrant symptoms.[3,6-10] Nonsurgical management of posterior insertional Achilles tendinopathy such as calcific tendinopathy, retrocalcaneal exostoses, and bursitis is successful in approximately 90% of cases.[11,12] Nonsurgical management often consists of a combination of the following: rest, heel and foot inserts, physical therapy including rehabilitation exercises such as eccentric strengthening, stretching, night splints and immobilization, along with pharmacological methods though injections should be avoided and the benefits of anti-inflammatories may only be useful in acute situations and in patients with inflammatory conditions. Surgical solutions often consist of resection of the offending exostoses and calcification, degenerated tendon along with reattachment of the AT.[3,6,8,12,13]

3.3.1 Clinical Findings

Typical complaints consist of pain from the posterior aspect of the heel, within and around the AT attachment. The posterior heel may be prominent and the insertion "boggy." Swelling posterior laterally may be termed a "pump bump." Bouché and McInnes make a point of outlining the exact area of patient's pain with a "tic-tac-toe" grid so all anatomical structures potentially associated with pathology are considered. In practice, a patient may have a prominent posterolateral bursa but also have symptoms superomedially.[3] Patients may have pain on single-legged heel raise, and some may even have an avulsion due to chronic degeneration. Acute avulsion may require more immediate surgical treatment. Symptoms include pain with activity and rest, along with redness and swelling when experiencing bursitis. Laboratory investigations to rule out inflammatory arthropathies, particularly seronegative enthesopathies, are undertaken with prolonged bursitis.[14] Rheumatological consultation is obtained in patients in whom inflammatory conditions are suspected, especially if surgery is still being considered. Generally, when considering surgical intervention, symptoms are getting progressively worse with activity, despite a significant period of rest. In fact, consideration of rest for a period similar to the postoperative recovery is recommended prior to considering surgery for chronic cases.[15]

3.3.2 Diagnosis

Radiographic studies are helpful. Plain film lateral and 0°-axial radiographs are most commonly ordered[3] (Fig. 3.1). Calcaneal prominence along with tendon calcification is visible. In patients with inflammatory arthropathy, erosions of the posterior and inferior calcaneus are noted.[14] MRI examination can further reveal tendon degeneration, bursitis, and cystic changes of the calcaneus, along with ruling out stress fracture (Fig. 3.2). Diagnostic ultrasound may be helpful in identifying bursitis and tendon degeneration. Various types (cavus, planus, and rectus) of foot morphology have been found with insertional Achilles tendinopathy.[9] Decreased ankle flexibility has also been cited as a cause, but none of these associations have been scientifically validated. Surgical treatment currently has at best Level IV evidence, and primarily includes retrocalcaneal prominence resection with calcific tendon debridement, and reattachment of the AT with soft tissue anchors.[3,6,8,9,12,15] Endoscopic resection of Haglund's prominence has also been described, but indications for isolated superior calcaneal exostectomy alone are, in the authors' opinion, currently limited.[16]

3.3.3 Surgical Technique of Insertional Repair/Retrocalcaneal Exostectomy

Surgical treatment involves removal of the exostoses, pathological bursae, remodeling of the posterior heel, excision of the insertional calcification (if present), and tenodesis of the AT with soft tissue anchors. The patient is placed in the prone position. Typically local anesthesia is used, often in conjunction with intra-venous sedation, but general and spinal anesthesia may be utilized. A tourniquet is typically not used but may be placed on the thigh or on the calf.

The incision is curvilinear from superomedial adjacent to the AT just above the superior calcaneus, inferiorly, across the posterior heel, staying within skin lines as much as possible, ending infero-lateral above the plantar skin lines (Fig. 3.3). The incision is deepened, and pathological bursae and the degenerated AT is excised. An inverted "T" approach to go "through" the AT insertion is used, exposing the superior calcaneus and any insertional calcification within the tendon insertion. The insertion calcification, if present, is excised (often with an osteotome), maintaining as much as the tendon expansion as possible. The superior calcaneus is further exposed after excising the retrocalcaneal bursa. This is

Fig. 3.1 (**a**) Retrocalcaneal exostosis lateral view. (**b**) "Zero degree" axial view showing lateral calcification. (**c**) Insertional tendocalcinosis

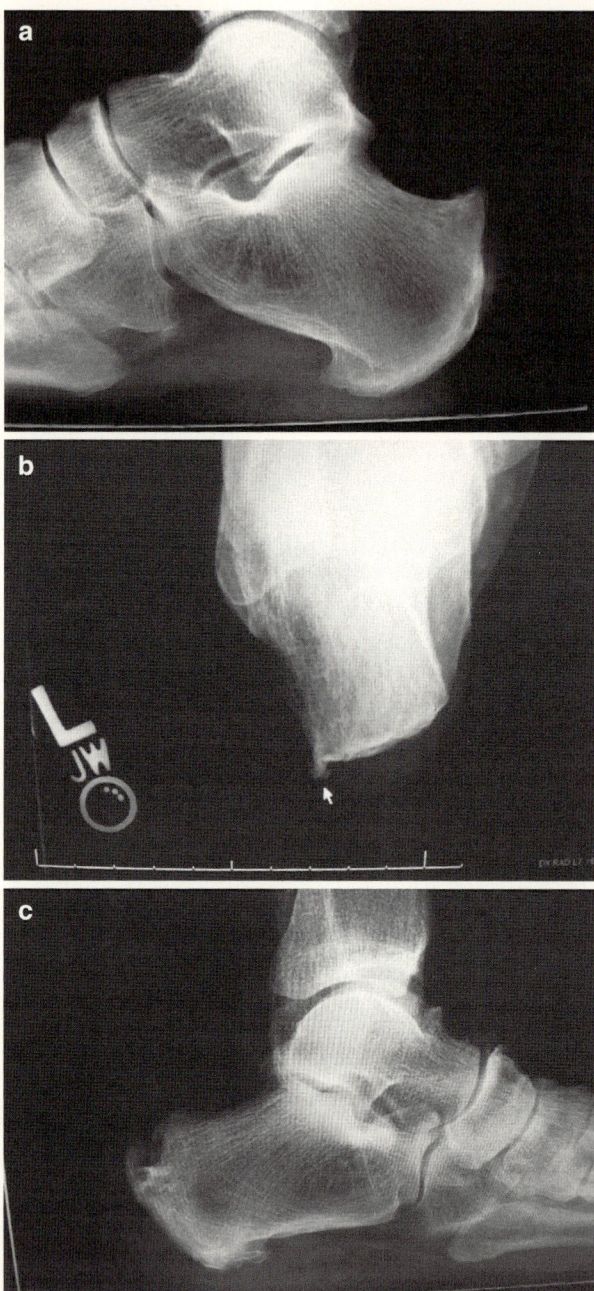

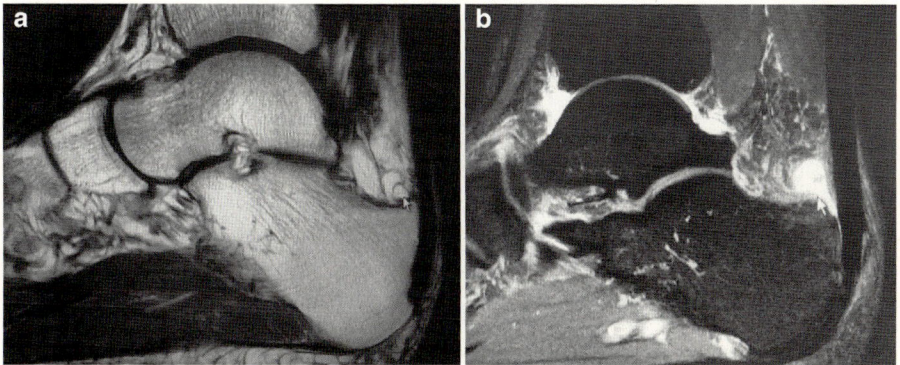

Fig. 3.2 (**a**) T1 MRI showing retrocalcaneal exostosis. (**b**) T2 MRI revealing bursitis

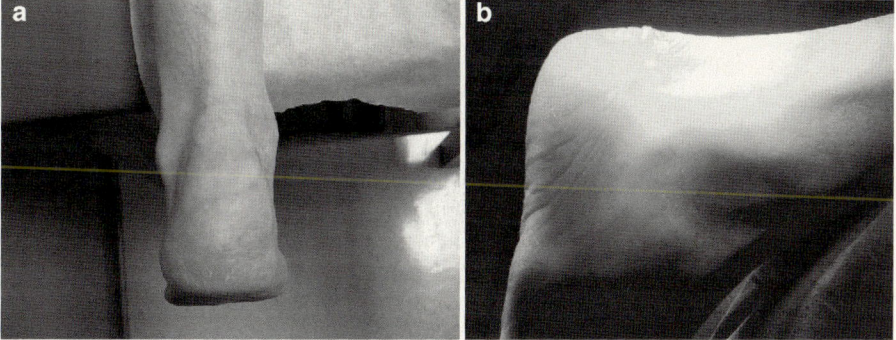

Fig. 3.3 Postoperative incisions showing (**a**) superomedial to infero-lateral approach and (**b**) transverse

resected with a curved osteotome from medial to lateral in both cases of retrocalcaneal exostoses (aka "pump bump") and insertional calcification (aka "AITC"). A reciprocating rasp is helpful in smoothing off the rough edges and making a smooth rounded remodeled calcaneus (Fig. 3.4). After copious irrigation, bone wax can be placed on the superior surfaces from medial to lateral to help prevent ectopic bone formation (though this occurs in less than 5% of patients 4 or more years postoperatively).[17]

The AT is reattached with suture anchors. Generally the number of anchors used ranges from 1 to 4[3,6,8,9] (Fig. 3.5). More anchors are used when more of the insertion needs to be reattached. Absorbable anchors superiorly may be helpful, in case re-resection is needed.[9,15] Care should be taken to place the suture knots in non-irritating regions. Irritation and granulomas from suture has recently been noted to occur in about 3% of AT surgeries in general.[13] This can occur with both absorbable and nonabsorbable materials. The tendon proximally is repaired first, particularly in cases where tendon débridement is needed. After inferior reattachment

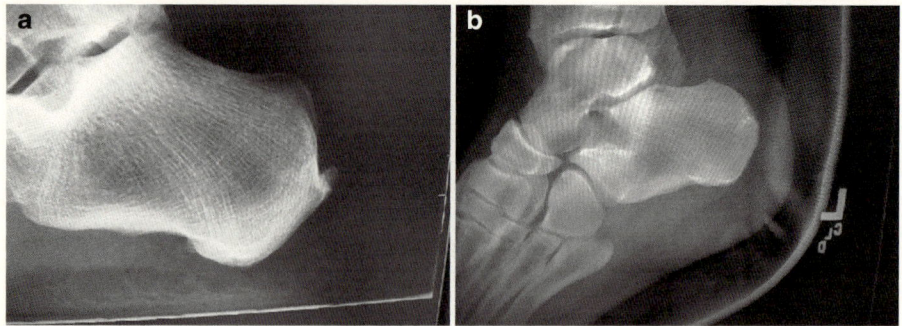

Fig. 3.4 (**a**) Preoperative and (**b**) postoperative Achilles insertional repair with retrocalcaneal exostectomy/bursectomy

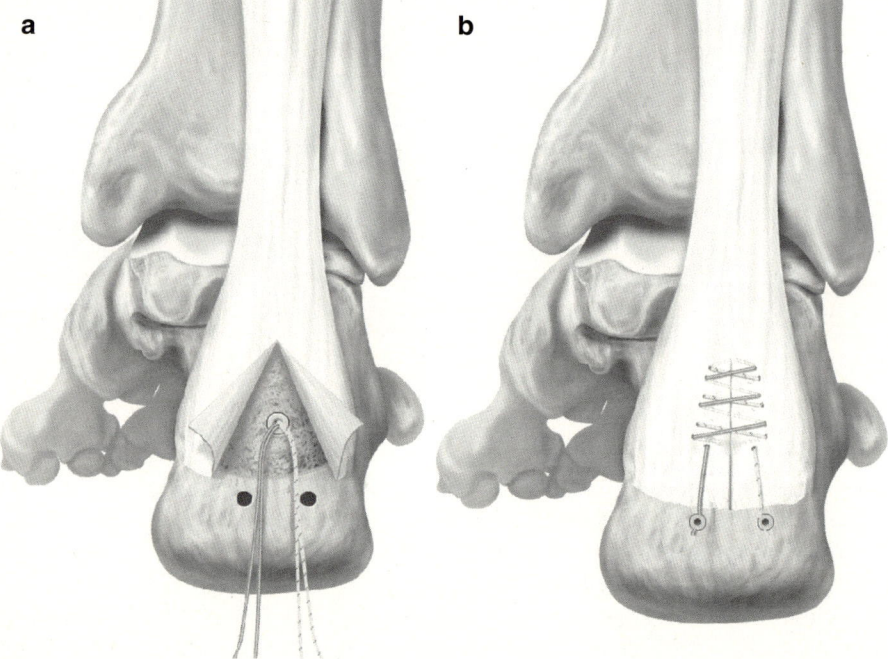

Fig. 3.5 (**a**, **b**) Suture anchors for Achilles tenodesis (Courtesy Arthrex, Inc., used with permission)

with additional locking sutures, subcutaneous sutures with absorbable material are used. The skin is re-approximated with 3–0 nylon. A sterile compression dressing is applied, and the patient is placed in a splint or below-knee cast boot in slight equinus. Patients are seen within the first postoperatively week.

3.3.4 *Postoperative Care*

Patients are usually immobilized in a below-knee cast/boot non-weight bearing, for 4 weeks, followed by a weight-bearing period for an additional 6 weeks.[3,9,15] Sutures are removed at 2 weeks. Patients are advised to take an oral anti-inflammatory (such as indomethocin 75 mg BID or naproxen sodium 500 mg BID) for 2 weeks post-surgery to prevent ectopic bone formation. Patients are advised to continue elevating and icing the limb for the entire postoperative recovery period. Active ROM is allowed at 3 weeks working on plantar flexion and inversion/eversion with a towel. Formal physical therapy is initiated around 8–10 weeks, though cross-training on a stationary bike is allowed with the boot/cast (again with the heel on the pedal) one week post-surgery while still in a cast/boot. Swimming is allowed (without flip-turns) at 6 weeks. Physical therapy includes progressive strengthening (initially with surgical tubing and/or a towel at 3 weeks) including single-legged heel raises. Return to daily activities occurs around 12 weeks; weight-bearing sport activities can take 16 or more weeks.[9,15,18] Prior to using these surgical techniques, soft tissue anchors, and recommended period of immobilization, the results of this type of surgery were not as good as currently reported.

3.3.5 *Conclusions*

Retrocalcaneal Achilles insertional pathology can be relieved by surgery. Repair of the tendon insertion after debridement and calcaneal resection with soft tissue anchors appears to improve results. Patients should be advised of variability in post-operative convalescence.

3.4 Midsubstance Achilles Tendinopathy

Although scientifically sound epidemiological data are lacking, tendinopathy of the main body of the AT is common in athletes, accounting for 6–17% of all running injuries.[19,20] However, it does present in middle-aged overweight nonathletic patients without history of increased physical activity.[21,22] To date, no data are available to establish the incidence and prevalence of Achilles tendinopathy in other populations, even though the conditions has been correlated with seronegative arthropathies (e.g., ankylosing spondylitis).[23]

The essence of tendinopathy is a failed healing response, with degeneration and haphazard proliferation of tenocytes, disruption of collagen fibers, and subsequent increase in non-collagenous matrix.[24] Tendinopathic lesions affect both collagen matrix and tenocytes. The parallel orientation of collagen fibers is lost; collagen fiber diameter and overall collagen density are decreased.

3.4.1   Diagnosis

The diagnosis of Achilles tendinopathy is mainly based on history and clinical examination. Pain is the pivotal symptom. A common symptom is morning stiffness or stiffness after a period of inactivity, and a gradual onset of pain during activity. In athletes, it occurs at the beginning and end of a training session, with a period of diminished discomfort in between. As the condition progresses, pain may occur during exercise and it may interfere with activities of daily living. In severe cases, pain occurs at rest. In the acute phase, the tendon is diffusely swollen and edematous, and tenderness is usually greatest 2–6 cm proximal to the tendon insertion. A tender, nodular swelling is usually present in chronic cases.

Clinical examination is the best diagnostic tool. Both legs are exposed from above the knees, and the patient examined while standing and prone. The AT should be palpated for tenderness, heat, thickening, nodule, and crepitation.[25] The "painful arc" sign helps to distinguish between tendon and paratenon lesions. In paratendinopathy, the area of maximum thickening and tenderness remains fixed in relation to the malleoli from full dorsiflexion to plantar flexion; lesions within the tendon move with ankle motion. There is often a discrete nodule, whose tenderness markedly decreases or disappears when the tendon is put under tension.[26] In the Royal London Hospital test, the clinician elicits local tenderness by palpating the tendon with the ankle in neutral position or slightly plantar flexed. The tenderness significantly decreases or totally disappears when the ankle is dorsiflexed.[26]

The clinical diagnosis of Achilles tendinopathy, even in experienced hands, is not straightforward, and experienced examiners may have problems in reproducing the results of clinical examination based on simple tests. If a patient presents with tendinopathy of the AT with a tender area of intratendinous swelling that moves with the tendon and whose tenderness significantly decreases or disappears when the tendon is put under tension, a clinical diagnosis of tendinopathy can be formulated, with a high positive predictive chance that the tendon will show ultrasonographic and histologic features of tendinopathy.[26] In this instance, further imaging is indicated only for confirmatory, not diagnostic, purposes, as it is unlikely to change the management of the patient.[26]

3.4.1.1   VISA-A

The Victorian Institute of Sports Assessment – Achilles (VISA-A) questionnaire specifically measures the severity of Achilles tendinopathy.[27] It covers the domains of pain, function, and activity. Scores are summed to give a total out of 100. An asymptomatic person would score 100. In clinical care, the VISA-A questionnaire provides a valid, reliable, and user-friendly index of the severity of Achilles tendinopathy. The VISA-A-S questionnaire showed good responsiveness in a randomized controlled trial (it was sensitive for clinically important changes over time with treatment, easy for the patients to fill out, and the data were easily handled).[28] It has been cross-culturally adapted to Swedish,[29] Italian,[30] and Turkish.[31]

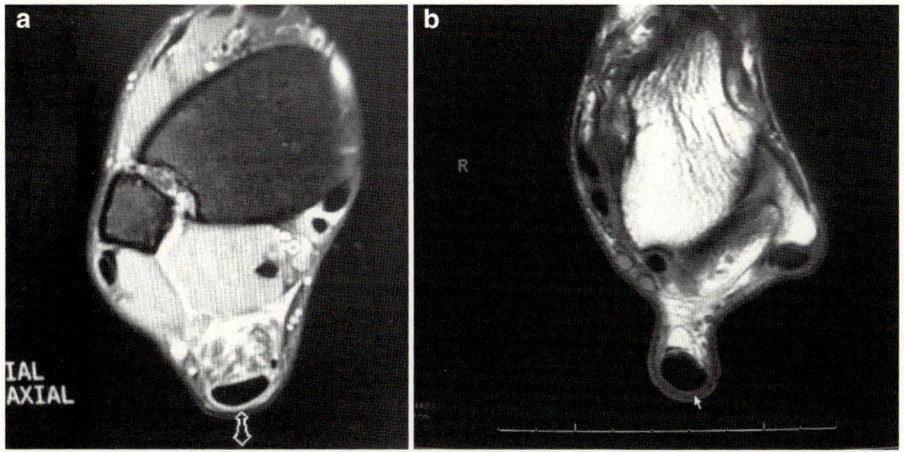

Fig. 3.6 (**a**) T2 and (**b**) T1 MRI showing paratendinosis with "halo-sign" (thickened paratenon)

3.4.1.2   Imaging

Radiographs may be useful in diagnosing associated or incidental bony abnormalities. Radiographs are routinely obtained on patients with symptoms lasting longer than six weeks to rule out bony abnormalities, and identify the possible presence of intratendinous calcific deposits and ossification.

Ultrasonography, though operator-dependent, correlates well with histopathologic finding,[32] and, especially in Europe, it is regarded as the primary imaging method. Only if ultrasonography remains unclear, MR imaging should be performed.[33] A major advantage of ultrasonography over other imaging modalities is its interactive capability.[34-36] Gray scale ultrasonography is associated with color or power Doppler to detect neovascularity.[36]

Magnetic resonance imaging (MRI) provides extensive information about the internal morphology of tendon and surrounding bone as well as other soft tissues. It allows to differentiate between paratendinopathy and tendinopathy of the main body of the tendon (Fig. 3.6). MRI is superior to ultrasound (US) in detecting incomplete tendon ruptures. However, given the high sensitivity of MRI, the data should be interpreted with caution, and correlated to the patient symptoms before making any recommendations.[37]

3.4.2   Management

The management of Achilles tendinopathy lacks evidence-based support, and tendinopathy sufferers are at risk of long-term morbidity with unpredictable clinical outcome.[38] The appropriate moment to switch from conservative to operative therapy remains unknown, as no solid data exist on the natural course of recovery. Nonoperative care should be in general a minimum of 3–6 months prior to considering surgery, since this condition has a good change of resolution. However, each patient should be evaluated independently.

3.4.2.1 Conservative Management

Several therapeutic options lack hard scientific background.[39,40]

Nonsteroidal Anti-inflammatory Drugs (NSAIDs)

Pharmacologic management strategies are essentially based on empirical evidence. Even though tendon biopsies show an absence of inflammatory cell infiltration, anti-inflammatory agents (nonsteroidal anti-inflammatory drugs and corticosteroids) are commonly used.[41] What may appear clinically as an "acute tendinopathy" is actually a well-advanced failure of a chronic healing response in which there is neither histological nor biochemical evidence of inflammation.[42] Ironically, the analgesic effect of NSAIDs[43] allows patients to ignore early symptoms, possibly imposing further damage on the affected tendon and delaying definitive healing.[44] NSAIDs appear to be effective, to some extent, for pain control. Early NSAIDs administration after an injury may have a deleterious effect on long-term tendon healing. Clearly there is a controversy on whether NSAIDs help or hinder the healing process.

Cryotherapy

Cryotherapy has been regarded as a useful intervention in the acute phase of Achilles tendinopathy, as it has an analgesic effect, reduces the metabolic rate of the tendon, and decreases the extravasation of blood and protein from new capillaries found in tendon injuries.[45] However, recent evidence in upper limb tendinopathy indicates that the addition of ice did not offer any advantage over an exercise program consisting of eccentric and static stretching exercises.[46]

Eccentric Exercise

A program of eccentric exercise has been proposed to counteract the failed healing response which apparently underlies tendinopathy, by promoting collagen fiber cross-linkage formation within the tendon, thereby facilitating tendon remodeling.[44] Although evidence of actual histological adaptations following a program of eccentric exercise is lacking, and the mechanisms by which a program of eccentric exercise may help to resolve the pain of tendinopathy remain unclear,[47] clinical results following such exercise program appear promising.[44,48] Though effective in Scandinavian population,[48,49] the results of eccentric exercises observed from other study groups[50,51] are less convincing than those reported from Scandinavia, with a 50–60% of good outcome after a regime of eccentric training both in athletic and sedentary patients. In general, the overall trend suggested a positive effect of an exercise program, with no study reporting adverse effects. Due to the lack of high-quality studies with clinically significant results, no strong conclusions can be made regarding the effectiveness of eccentric training (compared to control interventions) in relieving pain, improving function, or achieving patient satisfaction.[39,47]

In a randomized controlled trial[51] the efficacy of three protocols – a "wait-and-see" approach, repetitive low-energy shock wave therapy, and eccentric calf strengthening – for the management of chronic tendinopathy of the main body of the tendo Achillis was compared. Spontaneous recovery after more than 6 months of symptoms of tendinopathy of the main body of the tendo Achillis was unlikely in the majority of patients. The likelihood of recovery after 4 months was comparable after both eccentric loading and shock wave therapy, as applied. Success rates were in the region of 60% with either of these management modalities.

Combined management strategies (eccentric training and shock wave therapy) resulted in higher success rates compared to eccentric loading alone or shock wave therapy alone in a recent randomized controlled trial.[52] Eccentric training plus shock wave therapy should be offered to patients with chronic recalcitrant tendinopathy of the main body of the AT.[52]

Nitric Oxide

Nitric oxide is a small free radical generated by a family of enzymes, the nitric oxide synthases.[53] Recently, a prospective, randomized, double-blinded, placebo-controlled clinical trial was performed in patients with tendinopathy of the main body of the Achilles to evaluate the efficacy of nitric oxide administration via an adhesive patch.[54] Topical glyceryl trinitrate demonstrated efficacy in chronic noninsertional Achilles tendinopathy, and the treatment benefits continue at 3 years.[55] However, a recent study from England[56] failed to support the clinical benefit of topical glyceryl trinitrate patches.

3.4.2.2 Physical Modalities

The role of physical modalities in the management of tendinopathies remains unclear, and it is not possible to draw firm, evidence-based conclusions on their effectiveness.

The rationale for the clinical use of low-energy shock wave therapy to address the failed healing response of a tendon is the stimulation of soft tissue healing and the inhibition of pain receptors.[51] Low-energy shock wave therapy and eccentric training produced comparable results in a randomized controlled trial,[51] and both management modalities showed outcomes superior to the wait-and-see policy. The likelihood of recovery after 4 months was comparable after both eccentric loading and shock wave therapy, but success rates were 50–60%.

Hyperthermia induced by microwave diathermy raises the temperature of deep tissues to 41–45°C using electromagnetic power.[57] Hyperthermia induced into tissue by microwave diathermy can stimulate repair processes, increase drug activity, allow more efficient relief from pain, help removal toxic wastes, increase tendon extensibility and reduce muscle and joint stiffness.[57]

Ultrasound therapy is a widely available and frequently used electrophysical agent in sports medicine. However, systematic reviews and meta-analyses have repeatedly concluded that there is insufficient evidence to support a beneficial effect of ultrasound at dosages currently being introduced clinically. A new direction for ultrasound therapy in sports medicine has been proposed by research demonstrating that ultrasound can have clinically significant beneficial effects on injured tissue when low-intensity pulsed ultrasound is used.[58]

3.4.2.3   Intratendinous Injection

Sonographically guided intratendinous injection of hyperosmolar dextrose yielded a good clinical response in patients with chronic tendinopathy of the tendo Achillis.[59,60]

3.4.2.4   Sclerosing Injections and Neovascularization

In patients with chronic painful tendinopathy of tendo Achillis, but not in normal pain-free tendons, there is neovascularization outside and inside the ventral part of the tendinopathic area.[61,62] The good clinical effects with eccentric training may be due to the action on the neovessels and accompanying nerves. Also, local anesthetic injected in the area of neovascularization outside the tendon resulted in a pain-free tendon, indicating that this area is involved in pain generation. These are the bases for the injection of sclerosing substance polidocanol under ultrasound and color Doppler-guidance in the area with neovessels and nerves outside the tendon.

3.4.2.5   High Volume Ultrasound Guided Injections

High volume ultrasound guided injections aim to produce local mechanical effects causing neovessels to stretch, break, or occlude.[63] By occluding and possibly breaking these neovessels, the accompanying nerve supply would also be damaged either by trauma or ischemia, therefore decreasing the pain in patients with resistant Achilles tendinopathy. In a pilot study,[63] high volume image guided tendo Achillis injection of normal saline in patients with resistant Achilles tendinopathy decreased

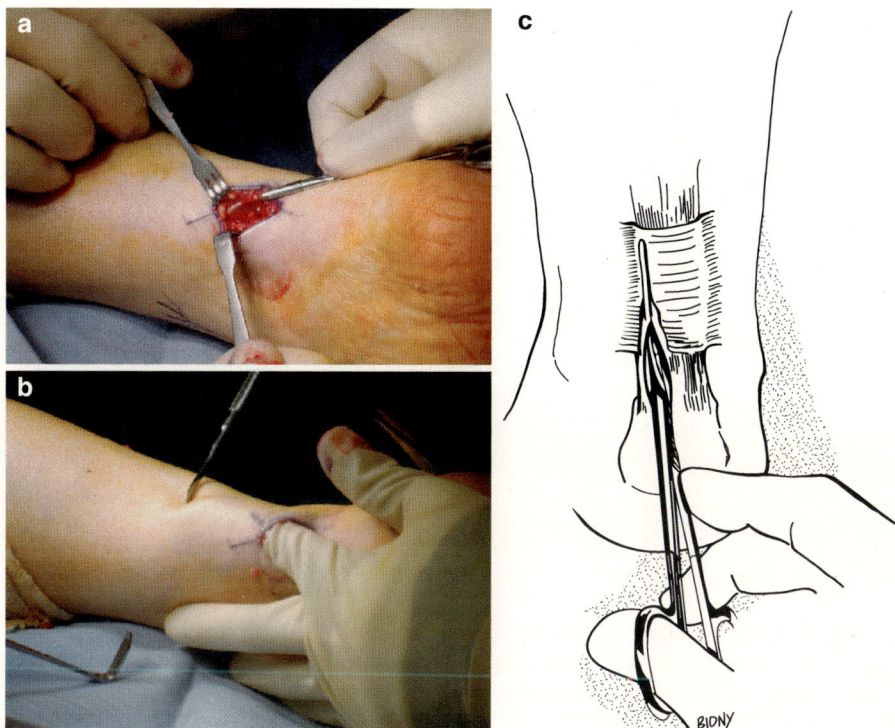

Fig. 3.7 (**a–c**) Intraoperative views and diagram of Achilles peritenolysis/decompression. Note thickened "watershed band." Key to success of the procedure is to make sure all the constricting paratenon is removed. When passively dorsiflexing the ankle, there should be no "tenting" over the Achilles tendon in the watershed region

the amount of pain perceived by patients, while at the same time improving daily functional ankle and Achilles movements in the short- and long-term.

3.4.3 Surgery

3.4.3.1 Surgical Management of Tendinopathy of the Main Body of the AT

In 24–45.5% of patients with Achilles tendinopathy, conservative management is unsuccessful, and surgery is recommended after exhausting conservative methods of management, often tried for at least 6 months.[64,65] There is a lack of trials on surgical management of Achilles tendinopathy, and therefore the high success rate needs to be interpreted with caution. Surgical options range from simple percutaneous tenotomy[66,67] (possibly ultrasound-guided[68]), to minimally invasive stripping of the tendon,[69] to open procedures (Fig. 3.7).

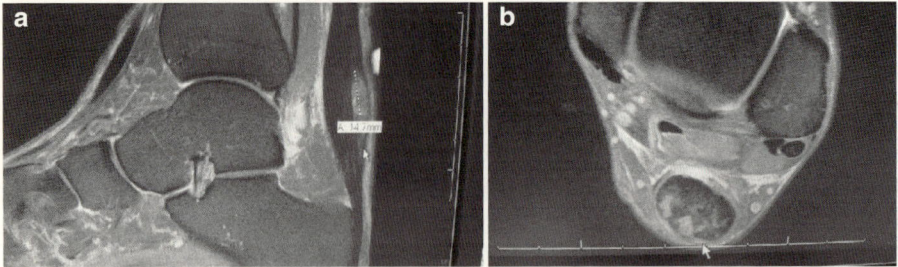

Fig. 3.8 (a) lateral T2 and (b) axial T2. Preoperative MRI showing significant longitudinal tearing of Achilles tendon in a pole-vaulter with symptoms for 2+ years

Fig. 3.9 Intraoperative view of Achilles post-débridement and longitudinal tenotomy in patient from Fig. 3.8. Because she was a high-level athlete, the tendon was repaired

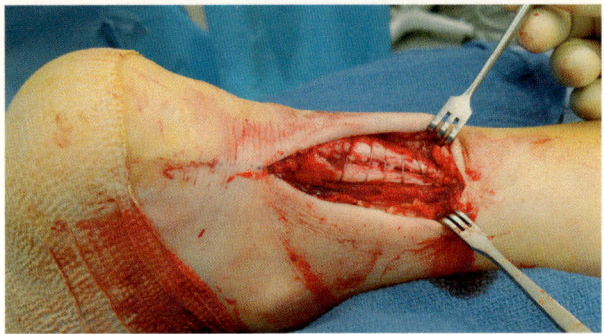

The classical aim of open surgery is to excise fibrotic adhesions, remove areas of failed healing and make multiple longitudinal incisions in the tendon to detect intratendinous lesions and to restore vascularity and possibly stimulate the remaining viable cells to initiate cell matrix response and healing[45] (Fig 3.8). However, there is no level I evidence that fibrotic adhesions should be removed, and the areas of failed healing should be excised,[66-68] at least if the pathology does not involve the paratenon. Multiple longitudinal tenotomies trigger well-ordered neoangiogenesis of the AT[70] (Fig. 3.9). This would result in improved nutrition and a more favorable environment for healing.

A more recent approach targets not the tendinous lesion itself, but the neo-innervation which accompanies the neovessels. New minimally invasive stripping techniques[69] of neovessels from the Kager's triangle of the AT for patients with tendinopathy allow to achieve safe and secure disruption of neovessels and the accompanying nerve supply, producing a denervation effect. During open procedure, if more than 50% of the tendon is debrided, consideration could be given to a tendon augmentation or transfer.[64]

3.4.3.2 Minimally Invasive Stripping

We have developed a novel management modality whereby a minimal invasive technique of stripping of neovessels from the Kager's triangle of the AT is performed.[69] This achieves safe and secure breaking of neovessels and the accompanying nerve supply.

Under local or general anesthesia, the patient is positioned prone with a calf tourniquet which is inflated to 250 mmHg after exsanguination. Four skin incisions are made. The first two incisions are 0.5-cm longitudinal incisions at the proximal origin of the AT, just medial and lateral to the origin of the tendon. The other two incisions are also 0.5-cm long and longitudinal, but 1 cm distal to the distal end of the tendon insertion on the calcaneus.

A mosquito or a tendon passer is inserted in the proximal incisions, and the AT is freed of the peritendinous adhesions. A Number 1 unmounted Ethibond (Ethicon, Somerville, NJ) suture thread is inserted proximally, passing through the two proximal incisions. The Ethibond is retrieved from the distal incisions, over the posterior aspect of the AT. Using a gentle see-saw motion, similar to using a Gigli saw, the Ethibond suture thread is made to slide posterior to the tendon, which is stripped and freed from the fat of Kager's triangle.

This minimal invasive technique reduces the risks of infection, is technically easy to master, and inexpensive. It may provide greater potential for the management of recalcitrant AT by breaking neovessels and the accompanying nerve supply to the tendon. It can be associated with other minimally invasive procedures to optimize results.

3.4.3.3 Outcome of Surgery

Most authorities anecdotally report excellent or good results in up to 85% of cases. In a systematic review,[71] most of the articles on surgical success rates reported successful results in over 70% of cases. However, this relatively high success rate is not always observed in clinical practice. The articles that reported success rates higher than 70% had poorer methods scores. Surgery appears to work better for athletes[72,73] and males.[74] There is little information on tendon transfers for chronic Achilles tendon ruptures, so one should reserve these procedures for resistant cases where there is no other viable option.[9] Even less is known about artificial tendon materials to supplement the Achilles tendon. Given that granuloma formation is common even with standard absorbable and non-absorbable suture, one should proceed with caution until longer-term studies occur.[13]

3.4.4 Postoperative Care

Rehabilitation is focused on early motion and avoidance of overloading the tendon in the initial healing phase. A period of initial splinting and crutch walking is generally used to allow pain and swelling to subside. After 14 days, patients are encouraged to start daily active and passive ankle range-of-motion exercises. The use of a removable walker boot can be helpful during this phase. Weight bearing is not limited according to the degree of debridement needed at surgery, and encourage early weight bearing. However, extensive debridements and tendon transfers may require protected weight bearing for 4–6 weeks postoperatively. After 6–8 weeks of mostly range-of-motion and light resistive exercises, initial tendon healing would have completed. More intensive strengthening exercises are started, gradually progressing to plyometrics and eventually running and jumping. Chapter 15 details typical rehabilitation post-Achilles surgery.

3.5   Conclusions

Achilles tendinopathy gives rise to significant morbidity, and, at present, only limited scientifically proven management modalities exist. The management of this condition remains a challenge, especially in athletes, in whom the physician often tries to be innovative. In many instances, this carries with it an unquantifiable risk.[75] A better understanding of tendon function and healing will allow specific management strategies to be developed.[76-78] Many interesting techniques are being pioneered.[79-82] Although these emerging technologies may develop into substantial clinical management options, their full impact needs to be evaluated critically in a scientific fashion. Soundwave/ESWT shows good promise while plasma-rich/PRP shows disappointing results in clinical studies, including randomized, prospective placebo controlled trials for Achilles tendinopathy.[83-86] Future trials should use validated functional and clinical outcomes, adequate methodology, and be sufficiently powered. Clearly, studies of high levels of evidence, for instance, large randomized trials, should be conducted to help answer many of the unsolved questions in this field.

References

1. Longo UG, Ronga M, Maffulli N. Achilles tendinopathy. Sports Med Arthrosc. 2009;17:112-26.
2. Clain MR, Baxter DE. Achilles tendinitis. Foot Ankle. 1992;13:482-7.
3. Bouché R, McInnes B. Posterior heel pain: Haglund's deformity, pump bump deformity amd Achilles insertional calcific tendonitis (AITC). In: Chang T, editor. The foot and ankle. Philadelphia: Lippincott; 2005.p.265-77.
4. Kolodziej P, Glisson RR, Nunley JA. Risk of avulsion of the Achilles tendon after partial excision for treatment of insertional tendonitis and Haglund's deformity: a biomechanical study. Foot Ankle Int. 1999;20:433-7.
5. Haglund P. Contribution to the diseased conditions of the tendo Achilles. Acta Chir Scand. 1928;63:292-4.
6. Carmont MR, Maffulli N. Management of insertional Achilles tendinopathy through a Cincinnati incision. BMC Musculoskelet Disord. 2007;8:82.
7. Leach RE, Schepsis AA, Takai H. Long-term results of surgical management of Achilles tendinitis in runners. Clin Orthop Relat Res. 1992;282:208-12.
8. Maffulli N, Testa V, Capasso G, Sullo A. Calcific insertional Achilles tendinopathy: reattachment with bone anchors. Am J Sports Med. 2004;32:174-82.
9. Saxena A, Cheung S. Surgery for chronic Achilles tendinopathy. Review of 91 procedures over 10 years. J Am Podiatr Med Assoc. 2003;93:283-91.
10. Sella EJ, Caminear DS, McLarney EA. Haglund's syndrome. J Foot Ankle Surg. 1998;37:110-4; discussion 173.

11. Johnston E, Scranton P Jr, Pfeffer GB. Chronic disorders of the Achilles tendon: results of conservative and surgical treatments. Foot Ankle Int. 1997;18:570-4.
12. Krishna Sayana M, Maffulli N. Insertional Achilles tendinopathy. Foot Ankle Clin. 2005;10:309-20.
13. Saxena A, Maffulli N, Nguyen A, Li A. Wound complications from surgeries pertaining to the Achilles tendon: an analysis of 219 surgeries. J Am Podiatr Med Assoc. 2008;98:95-101.
14. Malay S, Duggar G. Heel surgery. In: Dalton McGlamry E, editor. Comprehensive textbook of foot surgery. Baltimore: Williams & Wilkins; 1987. p. 268-83.
15. Saxena A. Results of chronic Achilles tendinopathy surgery on elite and nonelite track athletes. Foot Ankle Int. 2003;24:712-20.
16. Leitze Z, Sella EJ, Aversa JM. Endoscopic decompression of the retrocalcaneal space. J Bone Joint Surg Am. 2003;85-A:1488-96.
17. Tozun R, Pinar H, Yesiller E, Hamzaoglu A. Indomethacin for prevention of heterotopic ossification after total hip arthroplasty. J Arthroplasty. 1992;7:57-61.
18. Saxena A. Return to athletic activity after foot and ankle surgery: a preliminary report on select procedures. J Foot Ankle Surg. 2000;39:114-9.
19. Maffulli N, Binfield PM, King JB. Tendon problems in athletic individuals. J Bone Joint Surg Am. 1998;80:142-4.
20. McLauchlan GJ, Handoll HH. Interventions for treating acute and chronic Achilles tendinitis. Cochrane Database Syst Rev. 2001:CD000232.
21. Astrom M. Partial rupture in chronic Achilles tendinopathy. A retrospective analysis of 342 cases. Acta Orthop Scand. 1998;69:404-7.
22. Maffulli N, Khan KM, Puddu G. Overuse tendon conditions: time to change a confusing terminology. Arthroscopy. 1998;14:840-3.
23. Ames PR, Longo UG, Denaro V, Maffulli N. Achilles tendon problems: not just an orthopaedic issue. Disabil Rehabil. 2008;30:1646-50.
24. Maffulli N, Barrass V, Ewen SW. Light microscopic histology of Achilles tendon ruptures. A comparison with unruptured tendons. Am J Sports Med. 2000;28:857-63.
25. Teitz CC, Garrett WE Jr, Miniaci A, Lee MH, Mann RA. Tendon problems in athletic individuals. Instr Course Lect. 1997;46:569-82.
26. Maffulli N, Kenward MG, Testa V, Capasso G, Regine R, King JB. Clinical diagnosis of Achilles tendinopathy with tendinosis. Clin J Sport Med. 2003;13:11-5.
27. Robinson JM, Cook JL, Purdam C, et al. The VISA-A questionnaire: a valid and reliable index of the clinical severity of Achilles tendinopathy. Br J Sports Med. 2001;35:335-41.
28. Silbernagel KG, Thomee R, Eriksson BI, Karlsson J. Continued sports activity, using a pain-monitoring model, during rehabilitation in patients with Achilles tendinopathy: a randomized controlled study. Am J Sports Med. 2007;35:897-906.
29. Silbernagel KG, Thomee R, Karlsson J. Cross-cultural adaptation of the VISA-A questionnaire, an index of clinical severity for patients with Achilles tendinopathy, with reliability, validity and structure evaluations. BMC Musculoskelet Disord. 2005;6:12.
30. Maffulli N, Longo UG, Testa V, Oliva F, Capasso G, Denaro V. Italian translation of the VISA-A score for tendinopathy of the main body of the Achilles tendon. Disabil Rehabil. 2008;30:1635-9.
31. Dogramaci Y, Kalacy A, Kucukkubathorn N, Ynandy T, Esen E, Yanat AN, Khan K. Validation of the VISA-A questionnaire for Turkish language: the VISA-A-Tr study. Br J Sports Med. 2011;45(5):453-5.
32. Rolf C, Movin T. Etiology, histopathology, and outcome of surgery in achillodynia. Foot Ankle Int. 1997;18:565-9.
33. Neuhold A, Stiskal M, Kainberger F, Schwaighofer B. Degenerative Achilles tendon disease: assessment by magnetic resonance and ultrasonography. Eur J Radiol. 1992;14:213-20.
34. Gibbon WW. Musculoskeletal ultrasound. Baillières Clin Rheumatol. 1996;10:561-588.
35. Khan KM, Maffulli N. Tendinopathy: an Achilles' heel for athletes and clinicians. Clin J Sport Med. 1998;8:151-4.
36. Malliaras P, Richards PJ, Garau G, Maffulli N. Achilles tendon Doppler flow may be associated with mechanical load among active athletes. Am J Sports Med. 2008;36(11):2210-5.

37. Leadbetter WB. Cell-matrix response in tendon injury. Clin Sports Med. 1992;11:533-78.
38. Kader D, Saxena A, Movin T, Maffulli N. Achilles tendinopathy: some aspects of basic science and clinical management. Br J Sports Med. 2002;36:239-49.
39. Maffulli N, Longo UG. Conservative management for tendinopathy: is there enough scientific evidence? Rheumatology (Oxford). 2008;47:390-1.
40. Rompe JD, Furia JP, Maffulli N. Mid-portion achilles tendinopathy - current options for treatment. Disabil Rehabil. 2008;30(20–22):1666-76.
41. Leadbetter WB. Anti-inflammatory therapy and sports injury: the role of non-steroidal drugs and corticosteroid injection. Clin Sports Med. 1995;14:353-410.
42. Vane JR. Introduction: mechanism of action of NSAIDs. Br J Rheumatol. 1996;35:1-3.
43. Almekinders LC. The efficacy of non-steroidal anti-inflammatory drugs in the treatment of ligament injuries. Sports Med. 1990;9:137-42.
44. Mafi N, Lorentzon R, Alfredson H. Superior short-term results with eccentric calf muscle training compared to concentric training in a randomized prospective multicenter study on patients with chronic Achilles tendinosis. Knee Surg Sports Traumatol Arthrosc. 2001;9:42-7.
45. Kannus P, Jozsa L. Histopathological changes preceding spontaneous rupture of a tendon. A controlled study of 891 patients. J Bone Joint Surg Am. 1991;73-A:1507-25.
46. Manias P, Stasinopoulos D. A controlled clinical pilot trial to study the effectiveness of ice as a supplement to the exercise programme for the management of lateral elbow tendinopathy. Br J Sports Med. 2006;40:81-5.
47. Maffulli N, Longo UG. How do eccentric exercises work in tendinopathy? Rheumatology (Oxford). 2008;47:1444-45.
48. Roos EM, Engstrom M, Lagerquist A, Soderberg B. Clinical improvement after 6 weeks of eccentric exercise in patients with mid-portion Achilles tendinopathy - a randomized trial with 1-year follow-up. Scand J Med Sci Sports. 2004;14:286-95.
49. Sayana MK, Maffulli N. Eccentric calf muscle training in non-athletic patients with Achilles tendinopathy. J Sci Med Sport. 2007;10:52-8.
50. Murrell GA. Oxygen free radicals and tendon healing. J Shoulder Elbow Surg. 2007;16:S208-14.
51. Rompe JD, Nafe B, Furia JP, Maffulli N. Eccentric loading, shock-wave treatment, or a wait-and-see policy for tendinopathy of the main body of tendo Achillis: a randomized controlled trial. Am J Sports Med. 2007;35:374-83.
52. Rompe JD, Furia J, Maffulli N. Eccentric loading versus eccentric loading plus shock-wave treatment for midportion Achilles tendinopathy: a randomized controlled trial. Am J Sports Med. 2009;37:463-70.
53. Longo UG, Olivia F, Denaro V, Maffulli N. Oxygen species and overuse tendinopathy in athletes. Disabil Rehabil. 2008;30:1563-71.
54. Paoloni JA, Appleyard RC, Nelson J, Murrell GA. Topical glyceryl trinitrate treatment of chronic noninsertional Achilles tendinopathy. A randomized, double-blind, placebo-controlled trial. J Bone Joint Surg Am. 2004;86-A:916-22.
55. Paoloni JA, Murrell GA. Three-year followup study of topical glyceryl trinitrate treatment of chronic noninsertional Achilles tendinopathy. Foot Ankle Int. 2007;28:1064-8.
56. Kane TP, Ismail M, Calder JD. Topical glyceryl trinitrate and noninsertional Achilles tendinopathy: a clinical and cellular investigation. Am J Sports Med. 2008;36:1160-3.
57. Giombini A, Giovannini V, Di Cesare A, et al. Hyperthermia induced by microwave diathermy in the management of muscle and tendon injuries. Br Med Bull. 2007;83:379-96.
58. Warden SJ. A new direction for ultrasound therapy in sports medicine. Sports Med. 2003;33:95-107.
59. Hoksrud A, Ohberg L, Alfredson H, Bahr R. Ultrasound-guided sclerosis of neovessels in painful chronic patellar tendinopathy: a randomized controlled trial. Am J Sports Med. 2006;34:1738-46.
60. Maxwell NJ, Ryan MB, Taunton JE, Gillies JH, Wong AD. Sonographically guided intratendinous injection of hyperosmolar dextrose to treat chronic tendinosis of the Achilles tendon: a pilot study. AJR Am J Roentgenol. 2007;189:W215-20.

61. Knobloch K, Schreibmueller L, Longo UG, Vogt PM. Eccentric exercises for the management of tendinopathy of the main body of the achilles tendon with or without an airHeeltrade mark brace. A randomized controlled trial. B: effects of compliance. Disabil Rehabil. 2008;30(20–22): 1692-6.

62. Knobloch K, Schreibmueller L, Longo UG, Vogt PM. Eccentric exercises for the management of tendinopathy of the main body of the achilles tendon with or without the airHeeltrade mark brace. A randomized controlled trial. A: effects on pain and microcirculation. Disabil Rehabil. 2008;30(20–22):1685-91.

63. Chan O, O'Dowd D, Padhiar N, et al. High volume image guided injections in chronic Achilles tendinopathy. Disabil Rehabil. 2008;30:1697-1708.

64. Maffulli N, Kader D. Tendinopathy of tendo achillis. J Bone Joint Surg Br. 2002;84:1-8.

65. Paavola M, Kannus P, Järvinen TAH, Khan K, Józsa L, Järvinen M. Achilles tendinopathy. J Bone Joint Surg Am. 2002;84-A:2062-76.

66. Maffulli N, Testa V, Capasso G, Bifulco G, Binfield PM. Results of percutaneous longitudinal tenotomy for Achilles tendinopathy in middle- and long-distance runners. Am J Sports Med. 1997;25:835-40.

67. Testa V, Maffulli N, Capasso G, Bifulco G. Percutaneous longitudinal tenotomy in chronic Achilles tendonitis. Bull Hosp Jt Dis. 1996;54:241-4.

68. Testa V, Capasso G, Benazzo F, Maffulli N. Management of Achilles tendinopathy by ultrasound-guided percutaneous tenotomy. Med Sci Sports Exerc. 2002;34:573-80.

69. Longo UG, Ramamurthy C, Denaro V, Maffulli N. Minimally invasive stripping for chronic Achilles tendinopathy. Disabil Rehabil. 2008;30:1709-13.

70. Maffulli N. Re: etiologic factors associated with symptomatic Achilles tendinopathy. Foot Ankle Int. 2007;28:660; author reply 660-1.

71. Tallon C, Coleman BD, Khan KM, Maffulli N. Outcome of surgery for chronic Achilles tendinopathy. A critical review. Am J Sports Med. 2001;29:315-20.

72. Glaser T, Poddar S, Tweed B, Webb CW. Clinical inquiries. What's the best way to treat Achilles tendonopathy? J Fam Pract. 2008;57:261-3.

73. Maffulli N, Testa V, Capasso G, et al. Surgery for chronic Achilles tendinopathy yields worse results in nonathletic patients. Clin J Sport Med. 2006;16:123-8.

74. Maffulli N, Testa V, Capasso G, et al. Surgery for chronic Achilles tendinopathy produces worse results in women. Disabil Rehabil. 2008;30:1714-20.

75. Hamilton B, Remedios D, Loosemore M, Maffulli N. Achilles tendon rupture in an elite athlete following multiple injection therapies. J Sci Med Sport. 2008;11(6):566-8.

76. Movin T, Ryberg A, McBride DJ, Maffulli N. Acute rupture of the Achilles tendon. Foot Ankle Clin. 2005;10:331-56.

77. Sharma P, Maffulli N. Basic biology of tendon injury and healing. Surgeon. 2005;3:309-16.

78. Sharma P, Maffulli N. The future: rehabilitation, gene therapy, optimization of healing. Foot Ankle Clin. 2005;10:383-97.

79. Sharma P, Maffulli N. Biology of tendon injury: healing, modeling and remodeling. J Musculoskelet Neuronal Interact. 2006;6:181-90.

80. Sharma P, Maffulli N. Tendinopathy and tendon injury: the future. Disabil Rehabil. 2008;30(20–22): 1733-45.

81. Sharma P, Maffulli N. Tendon injury and tendinopathy: healing and repair. J Bone Joint Surg Am. 2005;87:187-202.

82. Sharma P, Maffulli N. Understanding and managing Achilles tendinopathy. Br J Hosp Med (Lond). 2006;67:64-7.

83. Rompe JD, Nafe B, Furia J, Maffulli N. Eccentric loading, shock-wave treatment or a wait-and-see policy for tendinopathy of the main body of tendo-Achillis: a randomized controlled trial. Am J Sports Med. 2007;35:374-83.

84. Saxena A, Ramdath S, O'Halloran P, Gerdesmeyer L, Gollwitzer H. Extra-corporeal pulsed-activated Therapy ("EPAT" Sound Wave) for Achilles tendinopathy: a prospective study. J Foot Ankle Surg. 2011;50(3):315-9.

85. de Vos RJ, Weir A, Tol JL, Verhaar JA, Weinans H, van Schie HT. No effects of PRP on ultra-sonographic tendon structure and neovascularisation in chronic midportion Achilles tendi-nopathy. Br J Sports Med. 2011;45(5):387-92. http://pubmed/21047840.

86. de Vos RJ, Weir A, van Schie HT, Bierma-Zeinstra SM, Verhaar JA, Weinans H, Tol JL. Platelet-rich plasma injection for chronic Achilles tendinopathy: a randomized controlled trial. JAMA. 2010;303(2):144-9. http://pubmed/20068208.

Chapter 4
Peroneal Tendinopathy

Francesco Oliva, Amol Saxena, Nicholas Antonio Ferran, and Nicola Maffulli

4.1 Surgical Techniques for Peroneal Tendons Subluxation

4.1.1 Introduction

Peroneal tendons dislocation is an uncommon sports-related injury. The first case was described by Monteggia in 1803 in a ballet dancer.[1] The injury is frequently associated with sports with cutting maneuvers such as judo, gymnastics, soccer, rugby, basketball, ice skating, skiing, water skiing, and mountaineering.[2] No specific age range is associated with the condition, but it clearly appears from the reported series that there is a relationship between dislocation of peroneal tendons and sport active people and road accidents.

Acute traumatic subluxation of the peroneal tendons is uncommon.[3] Acute injuries to the superior peroneal retinaculum can be initially managed conservatively with immobilization in a non-weight-bearing cast; this has a success rate of approx-

F. Oliva, M.D., Ph.D.
Department of Trauma and Orthopaedic Surgery,
University of Rome "Tor Vergata", Rome, Italy

A. Saxena, D.P.M. (✉)
Department of Sports Medicine, PAFMG-Palo Alto Division,
Clark Bldg., 3rd Flr, 795 El Camino Real, Palo Alto, CA 94301, USA
e-mail: heysax@aol.com

N.A. Ferran, M.B.B.S., M.R.C.S.Ed.
Department of Trauma and Orthopaedics, Lincoln County Hospital, Lincoln, Lincolnshire, UK

N. Maffulli, M.D., M.S., Ph.D., F.R.C.S (Orth).
Barts and The London School of Medicine and Dentistry, Centre for Sports and Exercise
Medicine, Mile End Hospital, Queen Mary University of London,
London, E1 4DG, UK

A. Saxena (ed.), *Special Procedures in Foot and Ankle Surgery*,
DOI 10.1007/978-1-4471-4103-7_4, © Springer-Verlag London 2013

imately 50%,[3,4] with preadolescent patients showing high rates of resolution after conservative management.[5]

In chronic subluxation, patients often report previous ankle injuries that, in some cases, may have been misdiagnosed as a sprain. An unstable ankle that gives way or is associated with a popping or snapping sensation is another common complaint. Chronic subluxation of the peroneal tendons may be traumatic or habitual and voluntary. In the latter case, congenital deficiency of the superior peroneal retinaculum (SPR) and a shallow fibular groove may play a role.[6] In traumatic chronic subluxation, there is little to be gained with conservative management, and surgical management is generally advocated.[4,6-12] Often the clinical diagnosis can be difficult, and some authors report a 60% diagnostic capability at first clinical evaluation.[13]

4.1.2   Anatomy

The peroneal muscles lie in the lateral compartment of the leg. They are innervated by the superficial peroneal nerve and supplied by the posterior peroneal artery and branches of the medial tarsal artery. The peroneus longus muscle originates from the head and upper two-thirds of the peroneal surface of the fibula, and from the intermuscular septa. In 20% of Caucasians, a sesamoid bone, the *os peroneum*, can be observed close to the calcaneocuboid joint. The peroneus brevis muscle originates from the lower two-thirds of the fibula in front of that of the peroneus longus. The two peroneal tendons enter together in a common synovial sheath 4 cm above of the lateral malleolus, going through a fibro-osseous tunnel, the retromalleolar groove. The peroneus longus tendon lies posterior and lateral to the peroneus brevis tendon.

The peroneus tertius muscle, normally absent in 10.5% of dissected limbs, arises from the distal third of the anterior aspect of the fibula. The muscle belly, usually not separated from the extensor digitorum longus muscle, ends proximal to the inferior extensor retinaculum.[14] This anatomical variant can rarely cause antero-lateral pain and snapping ankle.[15]

Another anatomical variant of the peroneal tendons is the rare peroneus quartus, which, with a number of different attachments, is present in 6.6% of the dissected legs.[16] This tendon is as important as the peroneus tertius in the differential diagnosis with peroneal tendons subluxation and posterolateral ankle pain.

The retrofibular (also called retromalleolar) groove is formed not by the concavity of the fibula itself, but by a relatively pronounced ridge of collagenous soft tissue blended with the periosteum that extends along the posterolateral lip of the distal fibula.[17,18] The other component of the retrofibular groove is the SPR posterolaterally, a fibrous band that originates from the distal lateral surface of fibula. The SPR is extremely variable in width, thickness, and insertional patterns. It normally has two bands: The superior band inserts on the Achilles tendon[19]; the inferior band inserts on the peroneal tubercle on the lateral surface of calcaneus.[20]

The peroneus longus passes between the cuboid groove and the long plantar ligament, and inserts onto the plantar surface of 1st metatarsal and the lateral face of medial cuneiform. The sural nerve lies in proximity of the peroneal groove. The sural nerve descends between the medial and lateral heads of the gastrocnemius, pierces of deep fascia proximally in the leg, and is joined by a sural communicating branch of the common peroneal nerve. It descends lateral to the Achilles tendon, near the small saphenous vein, to the region between the lateral malleolus and the calcaneus. It supplies the posterior and lateral skin of the distal third of the leg, proceeding distal to the lateral malleolus along the lateral side of the foot and little toe. It should be preserved at surgery.

The peroneal tendons receive their vascular supply from separate vincula that arise from the posterior peroneal artery and from the medial tarsal artery.[21] There are three distinct avascular zones: one in the peroneus brevis tendon when it curves around the lateral malleolus, and two in the peroneus longus.[22] The first avascular zone in the peroneus longus lies at the curve around the lateral malleolus, and the second occurs where the tendon curves around the cuboid.[22]

The peroneus brevis abducts and everts the foot, and flexes the foot plantarly. The peroneus longus plays the same functions of the peroneus brevis, but it is an important stabilizer of the medial column of the foot during stance. Together, they are dynamic stabilizers of the lateral ankle complex. Their antagonists are the flexor digitorum longus, flexor hallucis longus, and posterior and anterior tibialis.

4.1.3 Physiopathology

An acute peroneal tendons subluxation may occur when the tendons dislocate from the retrofibular groove during tendon loading. The most common mechanism is a sudden, reflexive contraction of the peroneal muscles during acute inversion of the foot with the ankle dorsiflexed, or during forced dorsiflexion of the everted foot.[20] Basset and Speer analyzed the links between the position of the foot and the type of disorders as a result of inversion ankle injuries. Ankle inversion and plantar flexion less than 15° may produce an injury of the SPR. At a plantar flexion angle greater than 25°, the peroneal tendons are protected from injury.[23]

The SPR is the primary restraint of the peroneal tendons: Its integrity is fundamental to avoid a peroneal tendon subluxation.[24] Disruption of the SPR occurs infrequently.[25] Damages of the SPR are associated with lateral ankle instability and inadequate concavity or depth of the retromalleolar groove.[26] Laxity of the SPR can result from a calcaneovalgus foot in neuromuscular diseases. Also, the rare congenital absence of the SPR must be considered as contributor to the mechanism of dislocation.[27-29]

Acute rupture of the SPR with potential subluxation of the peroneal tendons may cause longitudinal tears in the peroneus brevis tendon.[22] In the anatomical area where the peroneus brevis tendon passes through the fibular groove, the tendon is nearly avascular.[22] In cadaveric studies, disruption of the lateral collateral ankle ligaments places considerable strain on the SPR: this explains why the two conditions commonly coexist.[26]

Still poorly studied are non-traumatic subluxations of peroneal tendons, which can be caused by congenital or acquired pathological conditions. Hence, several congenital anatomical abnormalities, as a convex, flat or shallow, or, in rare cases, even absent retrofibular groove, may be present.[25,29] The absence of the SPR may also be congenital.[30] A bifid peroneus brevis has also been reported as a cause of subluxation.[31] A paralytic calcaneovalgus ankle is often associated with laxity of the retinaculum.[32] Congenital dislocation of the peroneal tendons may be associated with a calcaneovalgus foot type.[29] Acquired peroneal tendon subluxation is described in patients with neuromuscular diseases such as cerebral palsy,[3] and can also occur when the posterior surface of the lateral fibula is deformed as a consequence of osteochondritis.[33]

4.1.4 Classifications

Peroneal tendons subluxation is due mostly to a damage of the SPR. Eckert and Davis in 1976 distinguished three grades of acute tears. In grade 1, the retinaculum is separated from the collagenous lip and lateral malleolus. In grade 2, the collagenous lip is elevated with the retinaculum. In grade 3, a thin sliver of bone, visible on radiographs, is avulsed with the collagenous lip and the retinaculum.[25] Ogden in 1987 added a fourth grade, describing it as the SPR torn away from its posterior attachment on the calcaneus.[34] Clinical determination of injury grade is not possible, except for grade 3 injuries, which can be diagnosed on radiographs. Previously, some authors have described an intrasheath peroneal subluxation,[35,36] but only recently Raikin and colleagues[37] proposed as a subgroup of peroneal subluxation an intrasheath subluxation. In this instance, the peroneal tendons switch their relative positions (the longus tendon comes to lie deep and medial to the brevis tendon) within the peroneal groove. An associated tear of the peroneous brevis is described without any lesion of the superior retinaculum. The clinical signs of intrasheath subluxation are very similar to the grade 1 of Eckert and Davis classification, but ultrasonography can help to diagnose these variants. Realistically, it is hard to believe that the SPR remains intact during a switch of the positions of the peroneal tendons. Hence, probably even intrasheath peroneal dislocations should be classified as a grade I injury according to Eckert and Davis (Fig. 4.1).

Fig. 4.1 (**a**) Pre-op X-ray showing avulsed peroneal retinaculum. (**b**) MRI showing torn peroneal retinaculum. (**c**) Diagram of the classification of peroneal retinaculum tears. PLT, peroneus longus tendon; PBT, peroneus brevis tendon; SPR, superior peroneal retinaculum

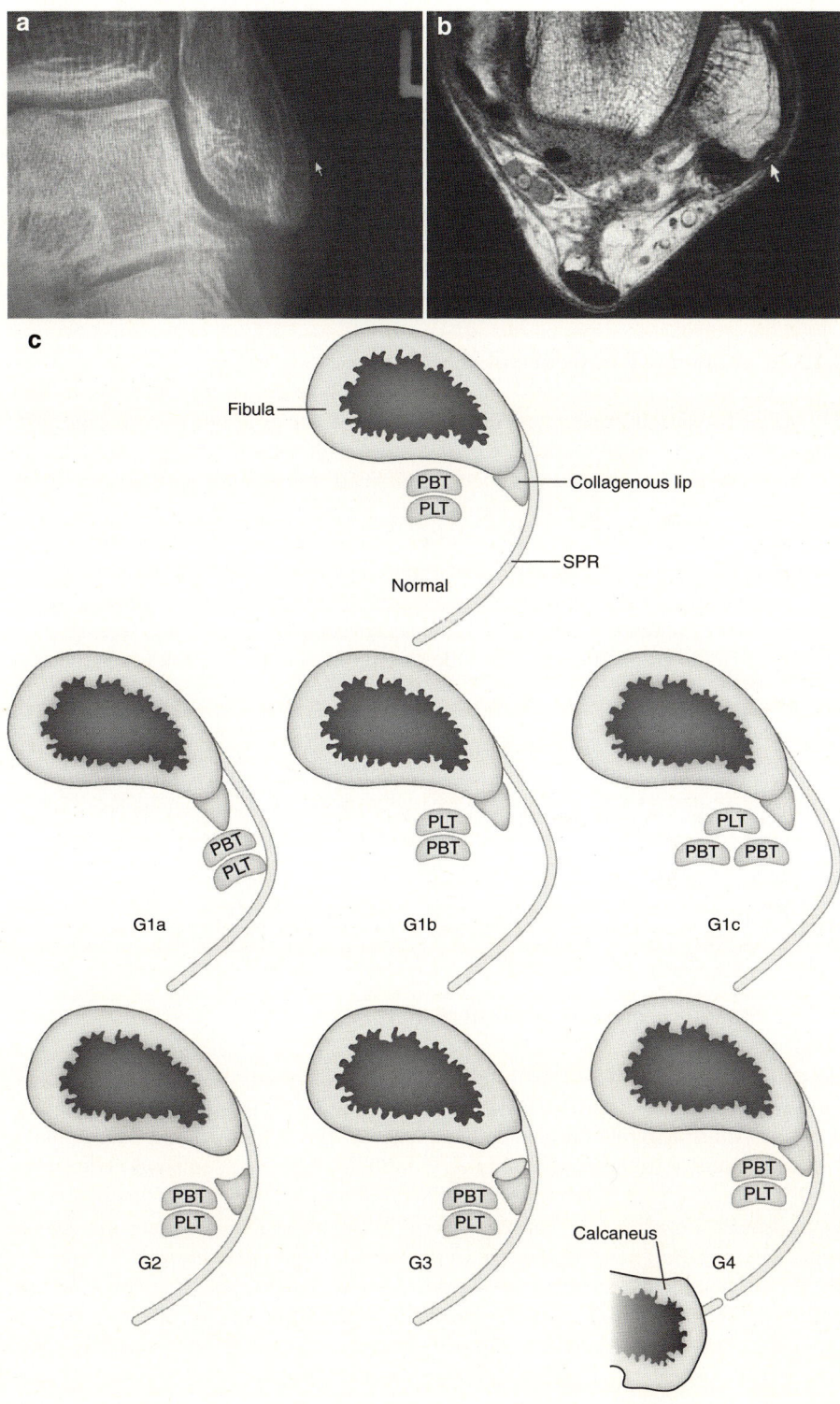

4.1.5   Surgical Techniques

Many surgical techniques limited only to case series have been described but only Level IV/Grade C evidence has been produced. No randomized studies have been conducted to determine which procedure is the most successful (Table 4.1).[38-56] Generally, five categories of surgical repair are listed: (1) Anatomic reattachment of the retinaculum; (2) Reinforcement of the superior peroneal retinaculum with local tissue transfers; (3) Rerouting the peroneal tendons behind the calcaneofibular ligament; (4) Bone block procedures; (5) Groove-deepening procedures.

4.1.5.1   Anatomic Reattachment of SPR

The aim of anatomic reattachment of the SPR is the restoration of the primary restraint of the peroneal tendons. Reattachment with sutures brought through drill holes in the distal fibula has been described by several authors.[8,25,38-40,47,48] Alternatively, Beck[6] brought the retinaculum through a slip produced in the distal fibula and fixed this with a screw, reporting on nine patients without complication. Eighteen of 21 patients treated with the "Singapore operation" at 9 years had excellent results. Three patients experienced postoperative pain and neuromas, but no recurrence was noted.[50] Karlsson and colleagues reported 13 patients with good to excellent results associating a groove deepening in conjunction with reattachment of the SPR if the posterior surface of the fibula was flat or convex.[48] Orthner et al. obtained excellent results for peroneal tendons subluxation suturing side by side the SPR in acute lesions.[43] Adachi et al. proposed retinaculoplasty, opening the false pouch through one incision, and suturing the SPR to the fibula while tensioning it. In this study, the authors reported that 15 of the 18 patients involved in sports activities returned to their previous activities without reducing their activity levels.[54] Recently, an endoscopic technique for the anatomical repair of the SPR has been described.[57] Anatomic reattachment of superior retinaculum seems to be the preferred technique in patients with acute subluxation of peroneal tendons.

4.1.5.2   Reinforcement of SPR with Soft Tissue

Several authors have described procedures to augment or reinforce an attenuated SPR with soft tissue transfer. Ellis-Jones[58] first described restraining the peroneal tendons with a strip of Achilles tendon anchored through a drill hole in the fibula. No recurrences were noted in a long-term follow-up of 15 patients who underwent the Ellis-Jones repair.[4] Thomas et al.[45] described a modification to this procedure that allowed the use of a smaller strip of Achilles tendon, reducing the risk of weakening the Achilles tendon. Use of the tendon of peroneus brevis,[39,59,60] plantaris[61,62] and peroneus quartus[63] have been described for the same purpose. Zoellner and Clancy[12] and Gould[9] used periosteal flaps to restrain the peroneal tendons in

Table 4.1 Studies and surgical techniques for the management of peroneal tendons subluxation

Authors	Year	Level of evidence	Number of cases	Procedures
Eckert and Davis[25]	1976	IV	73	Anatomical reattachment of SPR
Marti[38]	1977	IV	12	Modified Kelly
Zoellner and Clancy[12]	1979	IV	9	Groove deepening
Escalas et al.[4]	1980	IV	28	Jones procedure
Arrowsmith et al.[39]	1983	IV	6	Anatomical reattachment of SPR plus groove deepening
Poll and Duijfjes[40]	1984	IV	10	Rerouting tendon under CFL
Martens et al.[41]	1986	IV	11	Rerouting tendon under CFL
Micheli et al.[42]	1989	IV	12	Modified kelly
Orthner et al.[43]	1989	IV	23	Anatomical reattachment plus screw
Wirth[44]	1990	IV	15	Modified Viernstein and Kelly
Thomas et al. [45]	1992	IV	31	Modified Ellis-Jones
Steinböck et al.[46]	1994	IV	13	Rerouting tendon under CFL
Mason and Henderson[47]	1996	IV	11	Anatomical reattachment of SPR
Karlsson et al.[48]	1996	IV	15	Soft tissue reconstruction of superior retinaculum
Kollias and Ferkel[49]	1997	IV	12	Groove deepening
Hui et al.[50]	1998	IV	21	Anatomical reattachment of SPR
Mendicino et al.[51]	2001	IV	?	Groove deepening
Shawen et al.[52]	2004	IV	20	Groove deepening
Porter D, McCarrol J et al.[53]	2005	IV	13	Groove deepening
Adachi et al.[54]	2006	IV	20	Anatomical reattachment of SPR
Maffulli et al.[55]	2006	IV	14	Anatomical reattachment of SPR
Ogawa et al.[56]	2007	IV	15	Groove deepening

Studies which reported less than five patients are not listed

a deepened peroneal groove with satisfactory results. In patients treated with a periosteal flap from the retrofibular groove on its own or together with groove deepening, no postoperative complications were noted.[64]

4.1.5.3 Rerouting the Peroneal Tendons Behind the Calcaneofibular Ligament

This surgical technique does not address the issue of restoration of the anatomy of the SPR, but uses the calcaneofibular ligament as the natural alternative restraint. Platzgummer[65] and later Steinbock et al.[46] divided the calcaneofibular ligament, transposed the tendons behind it, and sutured the calcaneofibular ligament back together. The 13 patients operated with this technique showed good or excellent results, with no evidence of recurrence or instability. Sarmiento and Wolf divided the peroneal tendons and re-sutured them after rerouting them behind the calcaneofibular ligament[66]; 11 patients showed no evidence of recurrence or instability at follow-up, although two patients suffered a sural nerve injury. Martens et al. used the same technique of Sarmiento with excellent results at 30-month follow-up in 11 patients.[41] Both methods may potentially weaken the relevant structures. To preserve the integrity of the calcaneofibular ligament, a bone block of the ligamentous insertion on the fibula[67] or the calcaneus[40] can be mobilized, the tendons are transposed, and the bone block is reattached with a screw. Pozzo and Jackson[11] reported no complication and return to full level of activity in a case report. Poll and Duijfjes[40] reported ten patients with no recurrence or instability. Ferroudji et al. reported their experience with 19 patients, with excellent results in 17 patients. Sports activities were resumed after an average of 3.3 months.[68] This surgical technique should be preferred in patients with chronic luxation of the peroneal tendons in whom the SPR is absent.

4.1.5.4 Bone Block Procedure

These surgical procedures were developed to deepen the retrofibular groove using a bone graft as a physical restraint to the peroneal tendons. In 1920, Kelly[67] described a bone block procedure using screw fixation and later designed a wedge-shaped graft that avoided the use of screws near the ankle joint. Watson-Jones and DuVries[69,70] modified Kelly's technique. Watson-Jones[69] used an osteoperiosteal flap anchored by a soft tissue pedicle, and secured it posteriorly with sutures. DuVries[70] anchored a posteriorly displaced wedge with a screw. Other authors reported on patients with chronic subluxation operated with a modified Kelly technique with no recurrence.[38,44] In 1989, Micheli and colleagues[42] treated 12 patients with an inferiorly displaced fibula bone graft fixed with screws; one patient suffered a traumatic fracture of the graft, and two required exploration for pain; there were no recurrences of the subluxation. Adhesion of the peroneal tendons to the fresh bone wound, fractures of bone grafts, and the need for metalwork are major disadvantages of bone block procedures.[6] This surgical technique seems to be the more exposed to intraoperative and postoperative complications, and should be reserved for selected cases.

4.1.5.5 Groove Deepening

Patients presenting with a flat or convex retrofibular sulcus could be managed with this surgical technique. Zoellner and Clancy[12] elevated an osteoperiosteal flap on the posterior aspect of the distal fibula, and removed cancellous bone with a gouge. The flap was then reduced into the deepened sulcus, and the tendons replaced into this. Their nine patients had excellent results with no recurrence or instability. Hutchinson and Gustafson described a similar method in combination with SPR reattachment. Of 20 patients, three had poor results with recurrence of the subluxation, and one of these developed reflex sympathetic dystrophy.[71] Gould[9] reported a single patient in whom groove deepening was incorporated with restraint of the peroneal tendons by reflection of elevated osteoperiosteal flap. Recently, Ogawa et al. used an indirect fibular groove–deepening technique.[56] Mendicino and colleagues[51] employed intramedullary drilling and cortical impaction to achieve groove deepening. Porter et al. proposed groove deepening associated with an accelerated rehabilitation program. Eight of 13 patients returned to pre-injury sports participation.[53] The depth of the retrofibular sulcus was previously thought to play an important role in restraining the peroneal tendons.[49,52] Recently, however, the need for groove deepening has been questioned. Anatomic studies demonstrate the incidence of a flat or convex sulcus as high as 18%,[72] 28%,[58] and 30%.[73] The low incidence of peroneal tendon subluxation would suggest that the morphology of the groove is not a predisposing factor to subluxation.[72] Histologic studies demonstrating that the peroneal groove is defined by the fibrocartilagenous periosteal cushion and not by the bony sulcus add weight to this argument.

4.1.6 Preferred Surgical Technique

Under general or spinal anesthetic, the patient is placed supine on the operating table with a sandbag under the buttock of the operative side to internally rotate the affected leg. A tourniquet is applied to the thigh, the leg exsanguinated, and the cuff inflated to 250 mmHg. A 5-cm longitudinal incision is made along the course of the peroneal tendons. The incision starts posterior to the tip of the lateral malleolus and progressed proximally, staying well anterior to the sural nerve. The incision is deepened to the peroneal tendon sheath, which is incised longitudinally 3 mm posterior to the posterior border of the fibula. Normally, the SPR itself is thin and deficient, and it was detached from its posterior attachment on the calcaneus in our case series.[55] The peroneal tendons are identified by blunt dissection and protected. Attrition lesions and longitudinal tears of peroneal tendons when found are treated with a very gentle débridement or suturing with absorbable sutures.[74-76] After that, we expose the lateral aspect of the lateral malleolus, and the "pouch" formed between the bony surface of the lateral malleolus and the superior peroneal retinaculum, where the tendons subluxate, becomes visible. The SPR does not heal back to its normal attachment on the posterolateral aspect of the fibula but in an elongated fashion more anteriorly on the lateral aspect of the fibula, creating a pouch on the lateral fibula into which the tendons can subluxate. The bony surface of the lateral malleolus is roughened with a periosteal elevator to produce a bleeding surface, and three or four anchors (Mitek GII, Ethicon Ltd, Edinburgh, Scotland) with 2/0 absorbable sutures (Vicryl, polyglactin 910 braided absorbable suture, Ethicon) are inserted along the posterior border of the lower fibula (Fig. 4.2). After manual testing that the anchors cannot be dislodged, the SPR is reconstructed in a "vest over pants" fashion,[74] making sure that the pouch between the bony surface of the lateral malleolus and the SPR is totally obliterated. The ankle is kept in eversion and slight

Fig. 4.2 Anatomical
reattachment of the superior
retinaculum with anchors.
(**a**) Diagram and (**b**) X-ray
of anchor placement.
(**c**) Intraoperative view
of suture placement for
retinaculum repair

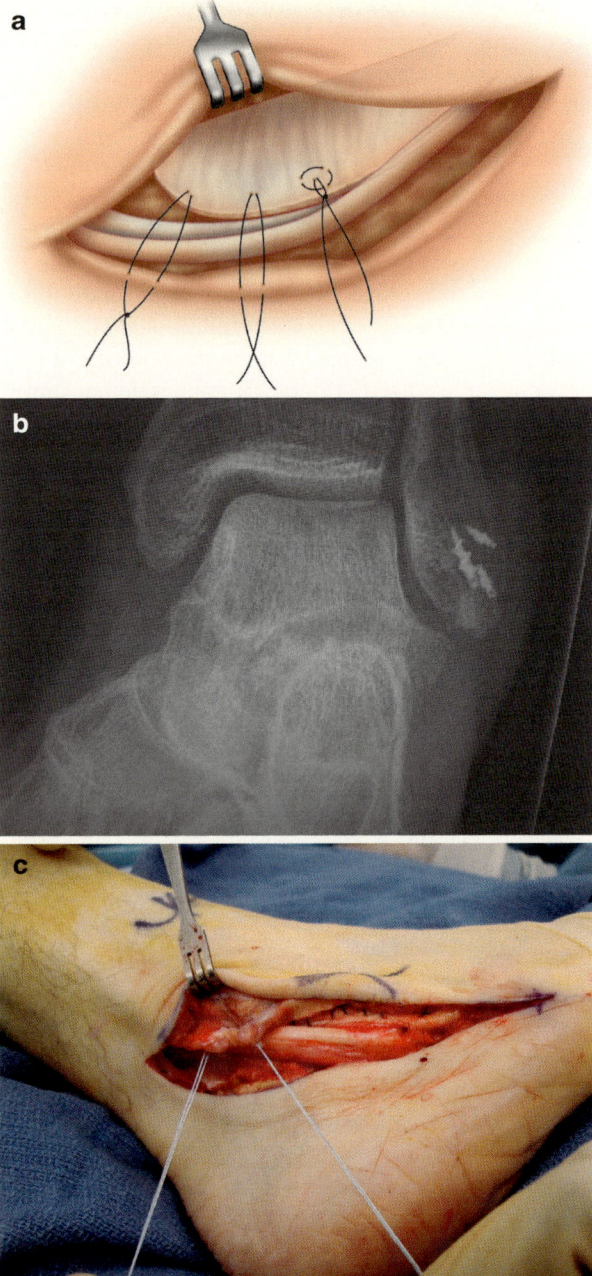

dorsiflexion so that the peroneal tendons were in the "worst possible position." The strength of the repair is tested moving the ankle through the whole range of motion. The wound is closed in layers with 2/0 Vicryl for the subcutaneous fat, un-dyed 3/0 Vicryl for subcuticular, and Steri-Strips for the skin (3M, Loughborough, United Kingdom). Dressing swabs, dressing, and crepe bandage are applied. A below-the-knee walking cast is applied with the ankle in neutral and slight eversion. Weight bearing is allowed from the day after the operation, and the cast is removed 4 weeks after the procedure, when rehabilitation is started. Gradual return to activities and to sport is allowed during the course of 3–4 months from the procedure.[55,76]

4.1.7 Postoperative Care

Patients are discharged the day after surgery, after having been taught to use crutches by an orthopedic physiotherapist. No thrombo-prophylaxis is used. Patients are allowed to bear weight on the operated leg as tolerated, but are told to keep the leg elevated as much as possible for the first 2 postoperative weeks. Patients are seen on an outpatient basis at the second postoperative week, and the cast is removed 4 weeks from the operation. Patients then mobilize the ankle with physiotherapy guidance. They are allowed to partially weight-bear, and commenced gradual stretching and strengthening exercises over 8–10 weeks after surgery. Cycling and swimming are started 2 weeks after removal of the cast. Patients are allowed to return to their sport on the fifth postoperative month.[55,75,76]

4.2 Surgical Techniques for Peroneal Tendon Tears

4.2.1 Introduction

Peroneal tendon tears were thought to be uncommon and a relatively new entity when reported by Evans in 1966. Peroneal tendon tears were seldom described until the early 1990s, when numerous case reports and moderately sized case series were published.[23,77-89] Peroneal tendon tears are thought to occur from both acute trauma and chronic instability, with and without subluxation. Peroneal retinaculum insufficiency is described in the preceding section. Chronic retinaculum insufficiency has been associated with peroneal tendon tears.[80-82,90,91] As with peroneal retinaculum pathology, tendon tears can often be difficult to recognize immediately. Diagnostic tests and clinical exam are paramount. Sobel and Mizel describe the proximal injuries as "Zone I" and the distal injuries associated with the Os Peroneum as "Zone II." Zone I injuries generally involve tears and dislocations of the tendon of peroneus brevis, while Zone II injuries involve Peroneus Longus pathology often with an Os Peroneum. They coined this condition POPS, Painful Os Peroneum

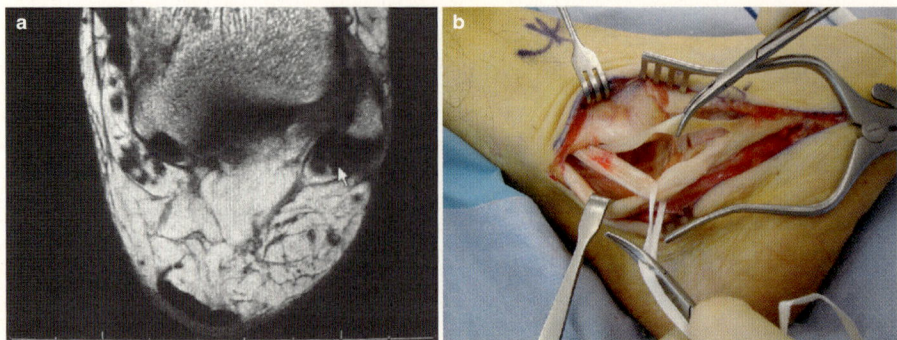

Fig. 4.3 (**a**) MRI showing accessory peroneal (quartus) tendon and peroneal brevis tear. (**b**) Intra-op view showing accessory peroneal (quartus) tendon and peroneal brevis tear

Syndrome.[81] Surgical treatment for both regions is often effective; the current treatment recommendations are based on Level IV & V Evidence.[80]

4.2.2 Anatomy

Much of the pertinent anatomy has been described in the previous section. In addition, the incidence of the Os Peroneum and its association with lateral foot pain should be considered.[79,81] The Os Peroneum is present in 4–26% of individuals, depending on race and ethnicity.[79,92-94] A low-lying muscle from Peroneus Brevis or an anomalous Peroneus Quartus has also been associated with peroneal tendon tears (Fig. 4.3).[16,95,96] Peroneal tubercle hypertrophy has also been noted with peroneal tendon tears.[78-81,89]

4.2.3 Clinical Findings

Patients with peroneal tendon tears complain of lateral ankle and foot pain. Acute onset of pain can occur with inversion injuries. Patients may state they felt a "pop" and have ankle weakness. Ankle instability was noted as early as 1979 with peroneal tears.[97] Clinically, patients may have noticeable pain with active resistance to the Peronei, and with single-legged weight bearing. Proprioception is altered. Swelling is often present along the peroneal tendons. Cavo-varus foot structure may be present causing a supinated foot structure, thereby putting more strain on the Peroneals. A Coleman block test should be performed to evaluate for a rigidly plantarflexed first ray causing hindfoot varus, versus a calcaneus varus (Fig. 4.4).[80] Weight-bearing plain radiographs should identify ankle varus, degenerative arthritis, accessory ossicles, and exostoses (Fig. 4.5). An Os Peroneum is often present

Fig. 4.4 (**a**) Patient with right-sided peroneus longus tear, with previous repair on left. Note plantarflexed 1st metatarsal. (**b**) Coleman block test showing varus rearfoot when forefoot is on the ground. (**c**) With forefoot suspended off the ground, the rearfoot moves to neutral. This demonstrates that the patient's rearfoot varus deformity is due to the plantarflexed 1st metatarsal

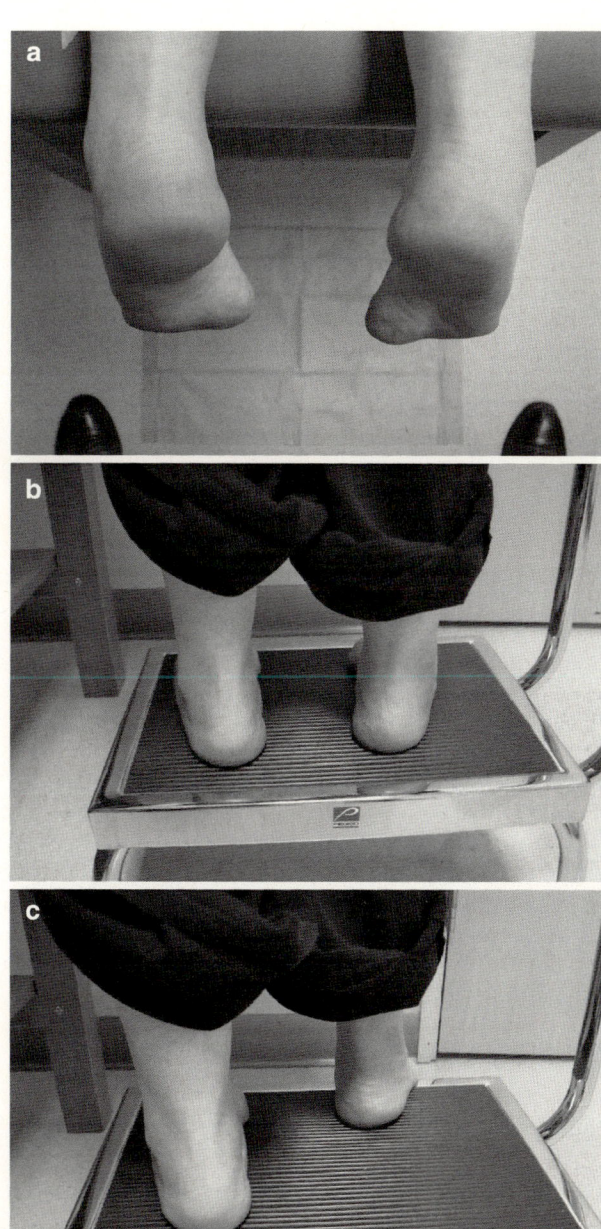

Fig. 4.5 Prominent peroneal
tubercle

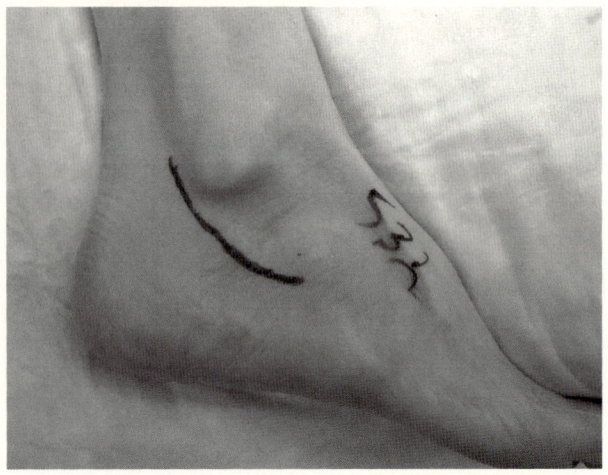

within the Peroneus Longus tendon in either a bony or cartilaginous form. A proximally migrated Os Peroneum indicates rupture of the Peroneus Longus
(Fig. 4.6).[80-82,86,88,89,94] Other bony structures can be associated with peroneal tendinopathy. A hypertrophied peroneal tubercle on the lateral calcaneus can often be
associated with fraying and even laceration of the adjacent tendons, which is best
visualized on MRI (Fig. 4.7).[80-82,86] Subluxation of the Peronei from posterior to
the fibula may result in tearing of the Peroneus Brevis in particular, more commonly in older patients (Fig. 4.8). This may be due to long-standing insufficiency.[80,98]
Inspection of shoe gear, inserts, and orthoses should also be performed. History of
inflammatory arthritis such as rheumatoid arthritis, Gout and Reiter's syndrome,
and subsequent testing when indicated should be considered.[99]

Radiographic tests for peroneal tendinopathy also include tenograms and MRI
examinations. Tenograms are useful for diagnosing stenosing tenosynovitis
(Fig. 4.9). MRI can also indentify this, particularly since fluid is often evident in
pathological states of tendons.[27,90] Ultrasound may be used as it shows fluid within
the tendon sheath and has high specificity for dislocations and tears, but osteochondral and transchondral defects and accessory ossicles may not be seen with ultrasound.[37,80] Fluid in the peroneal sheath may be indicative of a longitudinal tear,
particularly with MRI (Fig. 4.10).[80,86,88,90] MRI has a fairly high sensitivity and
specificity rate, and has become the "gold standard," though false-positives occur
very commonly.[80,86,90] The fact that many patients have asymptomatic tears noted on
MRI exams points to the critical importance of the clinical exam.

To conclude a patient may have a peroneal tendon tear when suggested on MRI,
and it is important in this instance to document peroneal weakness and pain.
A diagnostic injection within the peroneal sheath (from proximal to the retinaculum
with approximately 2 mL of local anesthetic) providing relief can confirm the diagnosis, and is recommended in less clear-cut cases.[81] Care should be taken not to
anesthetize the local nerves and infiltrate into the ankle or subtalar joint, which can

Fig. 4.6 Proximally migrated os peroneum indicating peroneus longus rupture

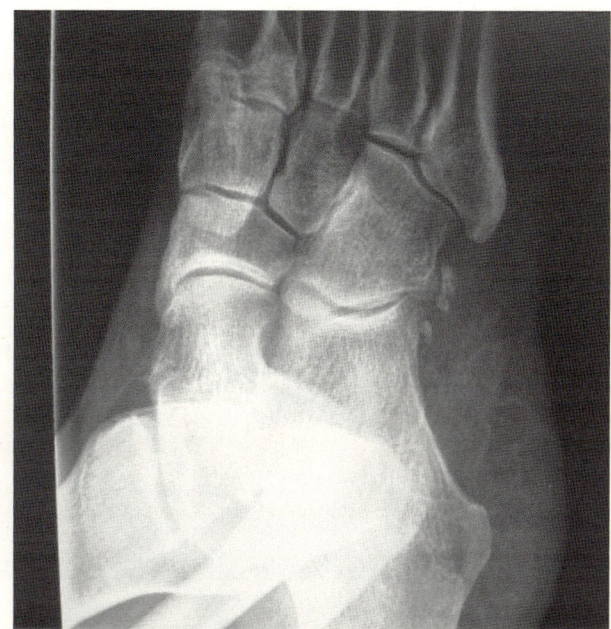

Fig. 4.7 MRI showing hypertrophic peroneal tubercle causing fraying of peroneals

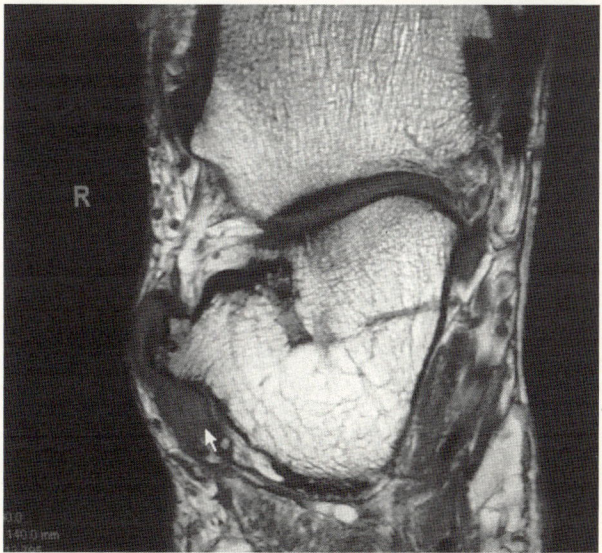

give false relief of symptoms from injecting the wrong structures. Generally, peroneal tenosynovitis without tendon tear responds to nonsurgical treatment. (In fact, the local anesthestic injection, if performed, can produce a volume adhesiotomy and further relieve symptoms.) Typical nonsurgical treatment of peroneal tendinopathy includes bracing, inserts including custom orthoses and/or shoes with lateral

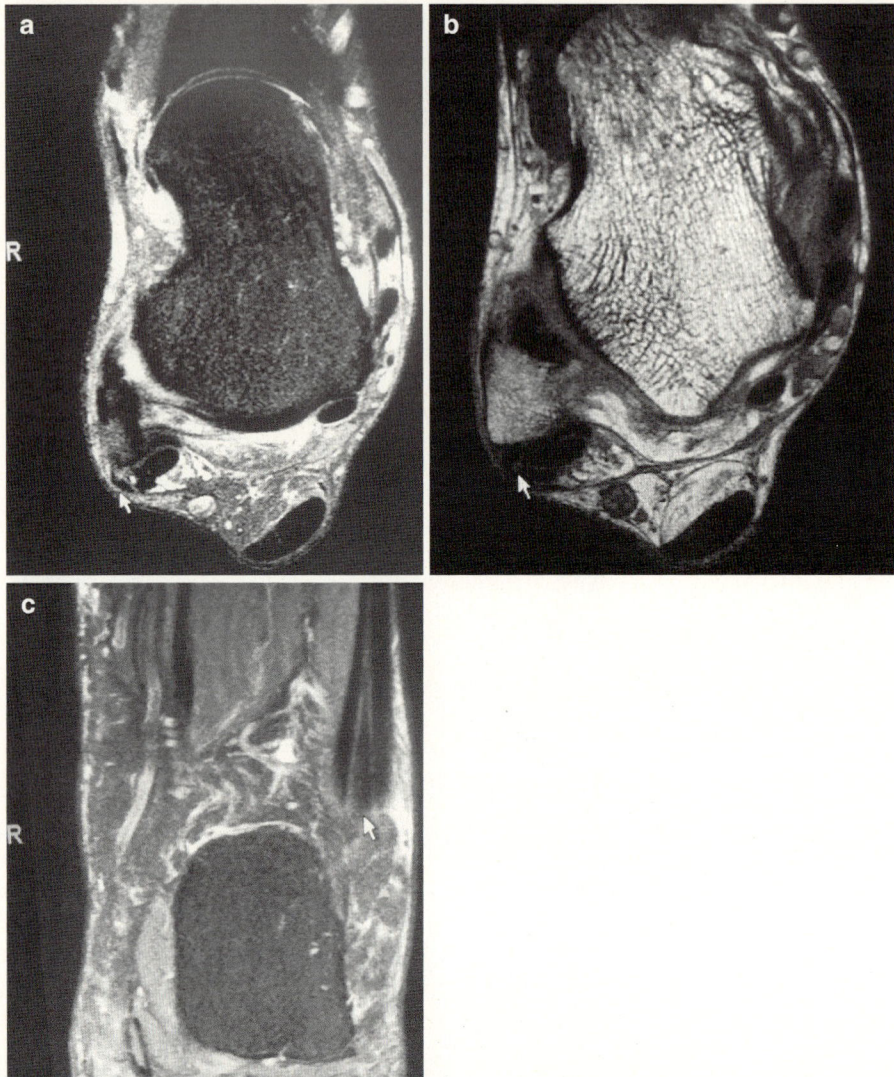

Fig. 4.8 MRI showing avulsed peroneal collangenous lip (**a**), split peroneus brevis (**b**), absent peroneus brevis with empty sheath (**c**)

Fig. 4.9 Tenogram of stenosing tenosynovitis

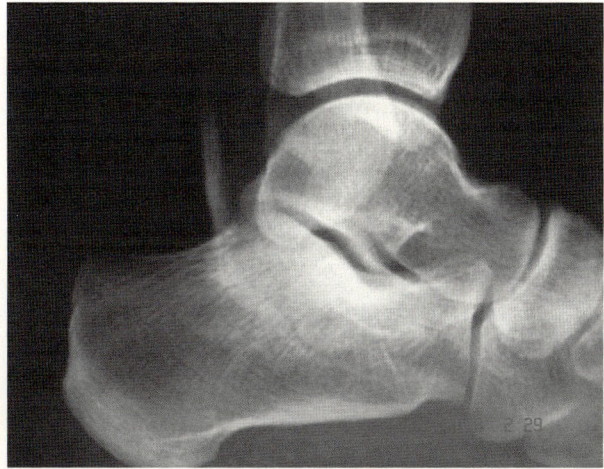

(valgus) wedging, physical therapy and immobilization in a below-knee boot or cast, though the long-term results of this can be unsatisfactory. If patients report worsening of symptoms with physical therapy, it is likely due to a peroneal tendon tear becoming aggravated with increased activity. At this point, one should consider surgical intervention. Results of surgical treatment of peroneal tendon tears have been well-documented in case series with good success. Many authors report significant improvement of patients' activity levels and functional scores post-surgery even in the long-term.[13,27,80,82-87,89,91,98,99]

4.2.4 Surgical Technique

Surgical treatment typically involves repair of the torn tendon(s). General anesthesia is typically preferred with a pneumatic thigh tourniquet. Spinal or regional anesthesia may be used. The patient is generally placed in the lateral position on a "bean bag," unless other procedures such as ankle arthroscopy need to be performed. During the surgical portion of the tendon repair, the bean bag is inflated to help lateralize the patient if adequate internal rotation of the lower limb is available. Otherwise, the patient is re-positioned lateral intraoperatively, and re-prepping and draping is performed. It is helpful to mark the proposed lateral incision sites prior to distending the ankle joint with arthroscopy, if being performed prior to tendon repair.

A lateral incision is typically made along the course of the peronei tendons, in the region of the patient's pain and pathology. The incision may be extended proximally if a retinaculum repair or a more proximal rupture needs to be addressed. The distal portion of the incision can be directed more dorsally for concomitant ankle stabilization. The common peroneal sheath is incised, the tendons inspected, together with the adjacent bony structures (Fig. 4.11). The tendons can be

Fig. 4.10 Fluid in peroneal
sheath on MRI with torn
peroneals frontal (**a**) and
axial (**b**) views

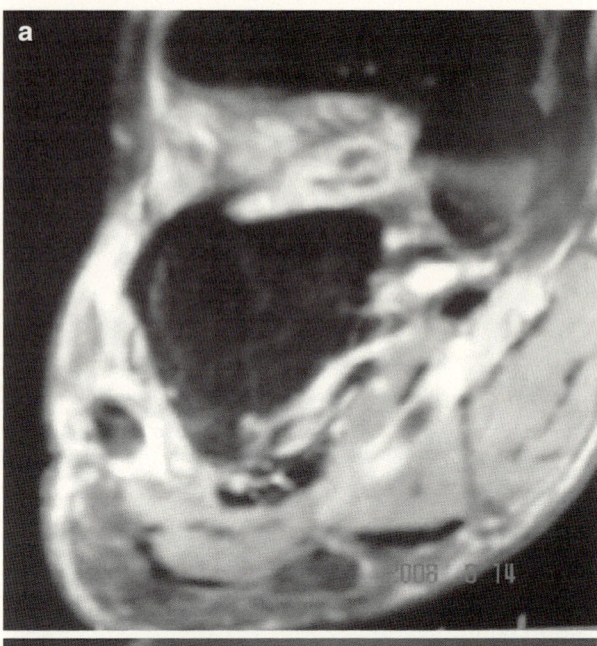

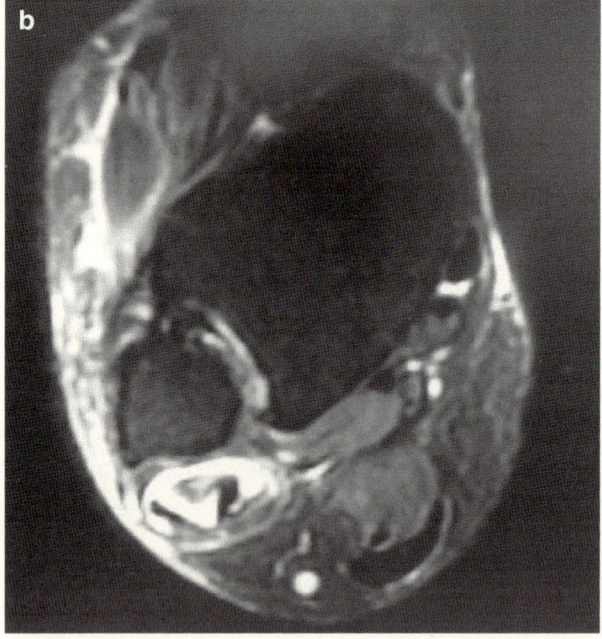

Fig. 4.11 (**a**) Peroneal sheath opened showing torn peroneus longus. (**b**) Peroneal sheath opened showing torn peroneus brevis. Note exostoses adjacent to tear (**c**)

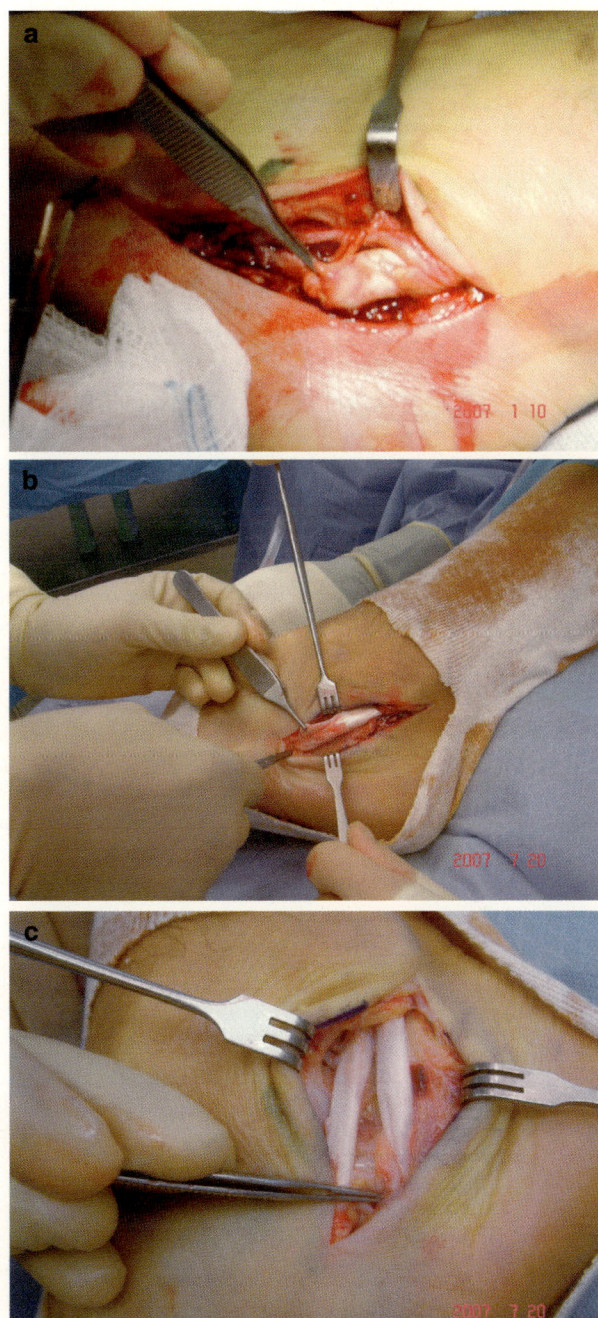

Fig. 4.12 Repaired tendon

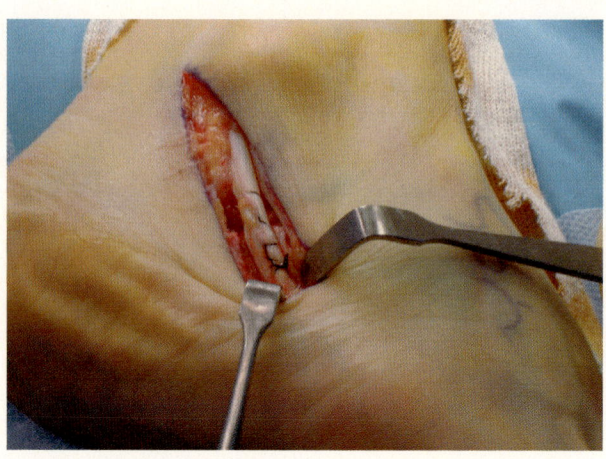

manipulated with moistened umbilical tape. When an Os Peroneum is excised, the distal and proximal aspects of the Peroneus Longus tendon are tenodesed to the Peroneus Brevis with 2–0 or 3–0 monofilament suture. In North America, nonabsorbable sutures are more commonly used, while in Europe, absorbable sutures are preferred.[75,76,83-89] In patients with chronically degenerated and frayed tendons, excision of the abnormal tendon is performed. Delayed primary repair is commonly performed by tubularizing the torn tendon with nonabsorbable monofilament suture, though other materials have been utilized. (Fig. 4.12) If there is a large gap after débridement of nonviable tissue, the tendon is tenodesed to the adjacent tendon. Some authors recommend tenodesis when greater than 50% of the tendon girth or 2 cm of the length is damaged.[80,82,85,86] Tendon "substitutes" being utilized for tendon repair have been promoted, but no long-term studies exist to date. Often, in chronic cases when both tendons are torn, the Peroneus Longus has retracted proximally, and the distal aspect of the Peroneus Brevis is intact. In such cases, the tendon of peroneus Longus is tenodesed to the base of the 5th metatarsal to maintain eversion of the foot.[81,86] The surgical wound is closed in layers.

If both tendons are severely damaged and not reconstructable, a free tendon graft may be used, such as doubled Plantaris tendon or a transfer of either the Flexor Hallucis or Digitorum Longus can be performed. An interim procedure of inserting a Hunter's Rod as a temporary conduit has been described prior to delayed repair.[80,91,100] A second procedure involving tendon transfer for peroneal reconstruction is performed 3 months later.[27,100]

Surgically, other structural issues may need addressing. Exostoses from the peroneal tubercle or distal fibula should be reduced.[80,81,86] Bone wax can be applied. The surgeon should be prepared in older patients to apply supplemental bone graft/substitute when the peroneal tubercle is resected as often the underlying calcaneus is cystic, particularly in females. Subluxations are surgically corrected with ligament repair, accessory muscle resection, and groove deepening if needed, as described in the section above. Severe rearfoot varus deformity (>10°) generally should be addressed at the time of surgery, though, in highly athletic patients, this may be

Fig. 4.13 Lateral displacement calcaneal osteotomy in a patient with severe calcaneal varus and both peroneal tendons ruptured, oblique (**a**) and lateral (**b**) X-rays

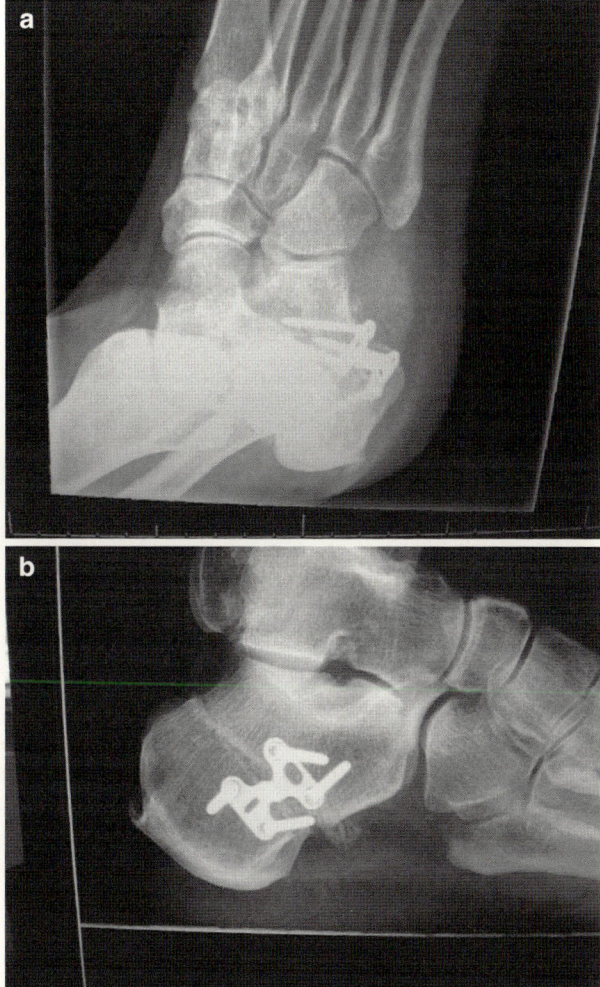

deferred.[27,86] For calcaneal varus deformity, a combined lateral displacement and varus reducing osteotomy is performed with either plate or screw fixation (Fig. 4.13). With patients that have a rigidly plantarflexed 1st metatarsal, an osteotomy of the base is performed to elevate it to the level of the 2nd metatarsal. Care should be taken to avoid creating a transfer lesion to the 2nd metatarsal, but this is essentially unavoidable with a short 1st metatarsal. Consideration of prophylactic shortening of an elongated 2nd metatarsal should be done if elevating a short plantarflexed 1st metatarsal. Plate or screw fixation is also used on the 1st metatarsal (Fig. 4.14). Other surgical considerations for severe instability are subtalar arthrodesis (for absent Peroneus Brevis) or calcaneal-cuboid arthrodesis (for absent Peroneus Longus).[27,81] Postoperative complications from peroneal tendon repair can include

Fig. 4.14 Elevating 1st
metatarsal osteotomy in a
patient with torn peroneus
brevis and plantarflexed 1st
metatarsal lateral (**a**) and AP
(**b**) X-rays

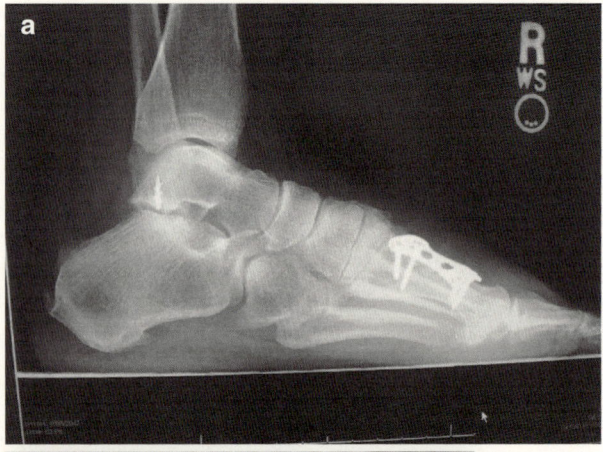

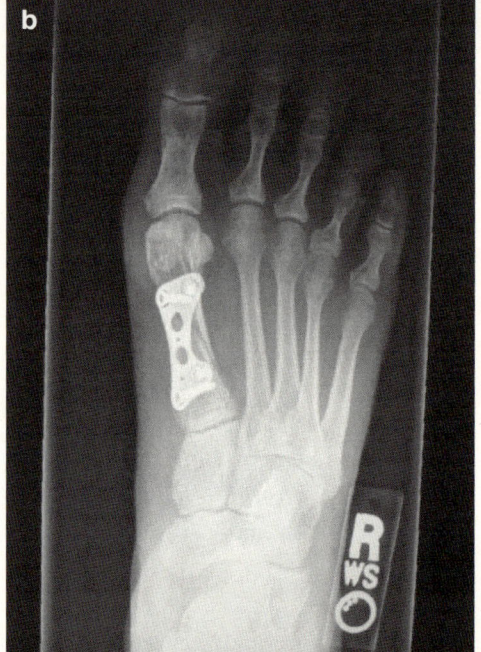

continued symptoms with activity limitations, re-rupture (particularly if structural
deformity is not addressed), and neurovascular compromise.[27,80,85,86]

4.2.5   Postoperative Care

Postoperatively patients with peroneal tendon repair alone are kept non-weight
bearing for 3 weeks, generally with a below-knee cast or boot. Stationary biking
with the heel on the pedal is permitted with a boot or cast once edema and pain

subsides, and swimming is allowed after 4 weeks. Ankle range-of-motion exercises can be begun at 3 weeks. If a calcaneal or 1st metatarsal osteotomy is performed, patients are kept non-weight bearing for 4–6 weeks, depending on bony consolidation. Patients wear a below-knee cast boot for 6–10 weeks until pain-free (the longer time frame is used for patients with osteotomies). Physical therapy is initiated between 5 and 10 weeks. Return to regular activities including sports takes 3–6 months. Consideration of ankle support or taping, and possibly foot orthoses for the first year postoperative should be assessed. Most athletic patients use ankle brace or tape for the first sport season after the surgery.

4.3 Conclusion

Recurrent peroneal tendon subluxation is an uncommon sports- and road-related injury. It occurs when the acute injury is misdiagnosed or not adequately managed. The primary pathology is the damage of the Superior Peroneal Retinaculum, which is the main restraint to the peroneal tendons. Diagnosis relies on clinical suspicion and clinical examination. There is no standardized method to report the severity of the condition, and therefore, it is difficult to compare the various case series. Many surgical techniques have been described, but it is hard to understand from the relatively small series which procedure is the gold standard. In our experience, if an anatomic approach is used, reattachment of the SPR is a most appropriate technique. Rarely, the retinaculum in recurrent cases may not be robust enough to withstand repair, and a different approach to the problem may be required. Randomized controlled trials may be the way forward in determining the best surgical procedure for subluxing peroneals. Repair of torn Peroneal tendons appears more straightforward with tubularization of the tendons involved. Tenodesis to the adjacent peroneal tendon is needed in cases of excision of an Os Peroneum, and where >50% of the tendon girth is lost or more than 2 cm of tendon length is damaged. FHL transfer may be indicated in special cases where reconstruction is not possible. Surgeons should consider other forms of structural pathology such as ankle instability, exostoses, calcaneal varus, and plantarflexed 1st metatarsal; these should be addressed appropriately as described in Chap. 7.

References

1. Monteggia GB. Instituzini chirurgiche, part III. Stamperia Pirotta Maspero, Milan;1803:336-41.
2. Mizel MS. Orthopedic knowledge update. Foot and ankle 2. Rosemont: American Academy of Orthopedic Surgeons; 1998.
3. Stover CN, Bryan DR. Traumatic dislocation of the peroneal tendons. Am J Surg. 1962;103:180-6.
4. Escalas F, Figueras JM, Merino JA. Dislocation of the peroneal tendons. J Bone Joint Surg. 1980;62:451-3.
5. Kojima Y, Kataoka Y, Suzuki SJ, Akagi M. Dislocation of the peroneal tendons in neonates and infants. Clin Orthop Relat Res. 1991;266:180.

6. Beck E. Operative treatment of recurrent dislocation of the peroneal tendons. Arch Orthop Trauma Surg. 1981;98:247-50.

7. Alm A, Lamke L, Liljedahl S. Surgical treatment of dislocation of the peroneal tendons. Injury. 1975;7:14-9.

8. Das DS, Balasubramaniam P. A repair operation for recurrent dislocation of peroneal tendons. J Bone Joint Surg Br. 1985;67:585-7.

9. Gould N. Technique tips: footings, repair of dislocating peroneal tendons. Foot Ankle. 1986;6:208-13.

10. Jones E. Operative treatment of chronic dislocation of the peroneal tendons. J Bone Joint Surg. 1932;4:574-6.

11. Pozzo J, Jackson A. A rerouting operation for dislocation of peroneal tendons: operative technique and case report. Foot Ankle. 1984;5:42-4.

12. Zoellner G, Clancy WJ. Recurrent dislocation of the peroneal tendon. J Bone Joint Surg. 1979;61:292-4.

13. Dombek MF, Lamm BM, Saltrick K, Mendicino RW, Catanzariti AR. Peroneal tendon tears: a retrospective review. J Foot Ankle Surg. 2003;42:250-8.

14. Joshi SD, Joshi SS, Athavale SA. Morphology of peroneus tertius muscle. Clin Anat. 2006;19:611-4.

15. Sammarco GJ, Henning C. Peroneus tertius muscle as a cause of snapping and ankle pain: a case report. Am J Sports Med. 2007;35:1377-9.

16. Zammit J, Singh D. The peroneus quartus muscle. Anatomy and clinical relevance. J Bone Joint Surg Br. 2003;85:1134-7.

17. Molloy R, Tisdel C. Failed treatment of peroneal tendon injuries. Foot Ankle Clin. 2003;8: 115-29.

18. Brage ME, Hansen ST Jr. Traumatic subluxation/dislocation of the peroneal tendons. Foot Ankle. 1992;13:423-31.

19. Davis WH, Sobel M, Deland J, Bohne WH, Patel MB. The superior peroneal retinaculum: an anatomic study. Foot Ankle Int. 1994;15:271-5.

20. Kumai T, Benjamin M. The histological structure of the malleolar groove of the fibula in man: its direct bearing on the displacement of peroneal tendons and their surgical repair. J Anat. 2003;203:257-62.

21. Sobel M, Geppert MJ, Hannafin JA, Bohne WH, Arnoczky SP. Microvascular anatomy of the peroneal tendons. Foot Ankle. 1992;13:469-72.

22. Petersen W, Bobka T, Stein V, Tillmann B. Blood supply of the peroneal tendons: injection and immunohistochemical studies of cadaver tendons. Acta Orthop Scand. 2000;71:168-74.

23. Bassett FH 3rd, Speer KP. Longitudinal rupture of the peroneal tendons. Am J Sports Med. 1993;21:354-7.

24. Safran MR, O'Malley D Jr, Fu FH. Peroneal tendon subluxation in athletes: new exam technique, case reports, and review. Med Sci Sports Exerc. 1999;31:487-92.

25. Eckert WR, Davis EA. Acute rupture of the peroneal retinaculum. J Bone Joint Surg. 1976;58A:670-3.

26. Geppert MJ, Sobel M, Bohne WH. Lateral ankle instability as a cause of superior peroneal retinacular laxity: an anatomic and biomechanical study of cadaveric feet. Foot Ankle. 1993;14: 330-4.

27. Selmani E, Gjata V, Gjika E. Current concepts review: peroneal tendon disorders. Foot Ankle Int. 2006;27:221-8.

28. Bonnin M, Tavernier T, Bouysset M. Split lesions of the peroneus brevis tendon in chronic ankle laxity. Am J Sports Med. 1997;25:699-703.

29. Purnell ML, Drummond DS, Engber WD, Breed AL. Congenital dislocation of the peroneal tendons in the calcaneovalgus foot. J Bone Joint Surg Br. 1983;65:316-9.

30. Bonnin JG. Injuries of the ankle. Darien: Hafner Publishing Co; 1970. p.32.

31. Hammerschlag WA, Goldner JL. Chronic peroneal tendon subluxation produced by an anomalous peroneus brevis: case report and literature review. Foot Ankle. 1989;10:45-7.

32. Estor A, Aimes A. La luxation congenitale des tendons des muscles peroniers lateraux. Rev Orthop. 1923;10:1.
33. Harper MC. Subluxation of the peroneal tendons within the peroneal groove: a report of two cases. Foot Ankle Int. 1997;18:369-70.
34. Oden RR. Tendon injuries about the ankle resulting from skiing. Clin Orthop Relat Res. 1987;216:63-9.
35. McConkey JP, Favero KJ. Subluxation of the peroneal tendons within the peroneal tendon sheath. A case report. Am J Sports Med. 1987;15:511-3.
36. Stukenborg-Colsman C, Wirth CJ. Resection of the tendon of the peroneal brevis muscle in "clicking" peroneal tendons – a report of 3 cases. Z Orthop Ihre Grenzgeb. 2000;138:265-8.
37. Raikin SM, Elias I, Nazarian LN. Intrasheath subluxation of the peroneal tendons. J Bone Joint Surg Am. 2008;90:992-9.
38. Marti R. Dislocation of the peroneal tendons. Am J Sports Med. 1977;5:19-22.
39. Arrowsmith SR, Fleming LL, Allman FL. Traumatic dislocations of the peroneal tendons. Am J Sports Med. 1983;11:142-6.
40. Poll RG, Duijfjes F. The treatment of recurrent dislocation of the peroneal tendons. J Bone Joint Surg Br. 1984;66:98-100.
41. Martens MA, Noyez JF, Mulier JC. Recurrent dislocation of the peroneal tendons. Results of rerouting the tendons under the calcaneofibular ligament. Am J Sports Med. 1986;14:148-50.
42. Micheli LJ, Waters PM, Sanders DP. Sliding fibular graft repair for chronic dislocation of the peroneal tendons. Am J Sports Med. 1989;17:68-71.
43. Orthner E, Polcik J, Schabus R. Dislocation of peroneal tendons. Unfallchirurg. 1989;92: 589-94.
44. Wirth CJ. A modified Vierstein and Kelly surgical technique for correcting chronic peroneal tendon dislocation. Z Orthop Ihre Grenzgeb. 1990;128:170-3.
45. Thomas JL, Sheridan L, Graviet S. A modification of the Ellis Jones procedure for chronic peroneal subluxation. J Foot Surg. 1992;31:454-8.
46. Steinböck G, Pinsger M. Treatment of peroneal tendon dislocation by transposition under the calcaneofibular ligament. Foot Ankle Int. 1994;15:107-11.
47. Mason RB, Henderson JP. Traumatic peroneal tendon instability. Am J Sports Med. 1996;24:652-8.
48. Karlsson J, Eriksson BI, Sward L. Recurrent dislocation of the peroneal tendons. Scand J Med Sci Sports. 1996;6:242-6.
49. Kollias SL, Ferkel RD. Fibular grooving for recurrent peroneal tendon subluxation. Am J Sports Med. 1997;25:329-35.
50. Hui JH, De Das S, Balasubramaniam P. The Singapore operation for recurrent dislocation of peroneal tendons: long-term results. J Bone Joint Surg Br. 1998;80:325-7.
51. Mendicino RW, Orsini RC, Whitman SE, et al. Fibular groove deepening for recurrent peroneal subluxation. J Foot Ankle Surg. 2001;40:252-63.
52. Shawen SB, Anderson RB. Indirect groove deepening in the management of chronic peroneal tendon dislocation. Tech Foot Ankle Surg. 2004;3:118-25.
53. Porter D, McCarroll J, Knapp E, Torma J. Peroneal tendon subluxation in athletes: fibular groove deepening and retinacular reconstruction. Foot Ankle Int. 2005;26:436-41.
54. Adachi N, Fukuhara K, Tanaka H, Nakasa T, Ochi M. Superior retinaculoplasty for recurrent dislocation of peroneal tendons. Foot Ankle Int. 2006;27:1074-8.
55. Maffulli N, Ferran NA, Oliva F, Testa V. Recurrent subluxation of the peroneal tendons. Am J Sports Med. 2006;34:986-92.
56. Ogawa BK, Thordarson DB, Zalavras C. Peroneal tendon subluxation repair with an indirect fibular groove deepening technique. Foot Ankle Int. 2007;28:1194-7.
57. Lui TH. Endoscopic peroneal retinaculum reconstruction. Knee Surg Sports Traumatol Arthrosc. 2006;14:478-81.
58. Jones E. Operative treatment of chronic dislocation of the peroneal tendons. Bone Joint Surg. 1932;14:574-6.

59. Smith TF, Vito GR. Subluxing peroneal tendons. An anatomic approach. Clin Podiatr Med Surg. 1991;8:555-77.
60. Gurevitz SL. Surgical correction of subluxing peroneal tendons with a case report. J Am Podiatr Assoc. 1979;69:357-63.
61. Miller JW. Dislocation of peroneal tendons, a new operative procedure. A case report. Am J Orthop. 1967;9:136-7.
62. Hansen BH. Reconstruction of the peroneal retinaculum using the plantaris tendon: a case report. Scand J Med Sci Sports. 1996;6:355-8.
63. Mick CA, Lynch F. Reconstruction of the peroneal retinaculum using the peroneus quartus. A case report. J Bone Joint Surg Am. 1987;69:296-7.
64. Lin S, Tan V, Okereke E. Subluxating peroneal tendon: repair of superior peroneal retinaculum using a retrofibular periosteal flap. Tech Foot Ankle Surg. 2003;2:262-7.
65. Platzgummer H. Uber ein einfaches Verfahren zur operativen Behandlung der habituellen Peronaeussehnenluxation. Arch Orthop Unfallchir. 1967;61:144-50.
66. Sarmiento A, Wolf M. Subluxation of peroneal tendons. Case treated by rerouting tendons under calcaneofibular ligament. J Bone Joint Surg Am. 1975;57:115-6.
67. Kelly RE. An operation for the chronic dislocation of the peroneal tendons. Br J Surg. 1920;7:502.
68. Ferroudji M, Spaas F, Martens M. Rerouting operation for recurrent dislocation of the peroneal tendons by the Pöll and Duijfjes procedure. Foot Ankle Surg. 2003;9:103-8.
69. Watson-Jones R. Fractures and joint injuries. 4th ed. Baltimore: Williams &Wilkins; 1956.
70. DuVries HL. Surgery of the foot. 4th ed. St. Louis: C.V. Mosby Co.; 1978.
71. Hutchinson BL, Gustafson LS. Chronic peroneal tendon subluxation. New surgical technique and retrospective analysis. J Am Podiatr Med Assoc. 1994;84:511-7.
72. Edwards ME. The relation of the peroneal tendons to the fibula, calcaneus and cuboideum. Am J Anat. 1928;42:213-53.
73. Mabit C, Salanne PH, Blanchard F, Boncoeur-Martel F. Fiorenza. The retromalleolar groove of the fibula: a radioanatomical study. Foot Ankle Surg. 1999;5:179-86.
74. Oliva F, Ferran N, Maffulli N. Peroneal retinaculoplasty with anchors for peroneal tendon subluxation. Bull Hosp Jt Dis. 2006;63:113-6.
75. Ferran NA, Oliva F, Maffulli N. Recurrent subluxation of the peroneal tendons. Sports Med. 2006;36:839-46.
76. Ferran NA, Oliva F, Maffulli N. Management of recurrent subluxation of the peroneal tendons. Foot Ankle Clin. 2006;11:465-74.
77. Evans JD. Subcutaneous rupture of the tendon of peroneus longus: report of a case. J Bone Joint Surg Br. 1966;48:507-9.
78. Sammarco GJ. Peroneal tendon injuries. Orthop Clin North Am. 1994;25:135-45.
79. Sobel M, Geppert M, Olson E, Bohne W, Arnoczky S. The dynamics of peroneous brevis splits: a proposed mechanism, technique of diagnosis, and classification of injury. Foot Ankle. 1992;13:413-22.
80. Heckman DS, Reddy S, Pedowitz D, Wapner KL, Parekh SG. Operative treatment for peroneal tendon disorders. J Bone Joint Surg Am. 2008;90(2):404-18.
81. Sobel M, Mizel M. Peroneal tendon injury in current practice in foot and ankle surgery, vol. 1. New York: Mc-Graw Hill, Inc; 1993:30-56.
82. Squires N, Myerson MS, Gamba C. Surgical treatment of peroneal tendon tears. Foot Ankle Clin. 2007;12(4):675-95.
83. Slater HK. Acute peroneal tendon tears. Foot Ankle Clin. 2007;12(4):659-74.
84. Steel MW, DeOrio JK. Peroneal tendon tears: return to sports after operative treatment. Foot Ankle Int. 2007;28(1):49-54.
85. Redfern D, Myerson M. The management of concomitant tears of the peroneus longus and brevis tendons. Foot Ankle Int. 2004;25(10):695-707.
86. Saxena A, Cassidy A. Peroneal tendon injuries: an evaluation of 49 tears in 41 patients. J Foot Ankle Surg. 2003;42(4):215-20.

87. Cooper ME, Selesnick FH, Murphy BJ. Partial peroneus longus tendon rupture in professional basketball players: a report of 2 cases. Am J Orthop. 2002;31(12):691-4.
88. Brandes C, Smith R. Characterization of patients with primary peroneus longus tendonopathy. Foot Ankle Int. 2000;21:462-8.
89. Saxena A, Pham B. Longitudinal peroneal tendon tears. J Foot Ankle Surg. 1997;36(3):173-9.
90. Kuwada GT. Surgical correlation of preoperative MRI findings of trauma to tendons and ligaments of the foot and ankle. J Am Podiatr Med Assoc. 2008;98(5):370-3.
91. Borton DC, Lucas P, Jomha NM, Cross MJ, Slater K. Operative reconstruction after transverse rupture of the tendons of both peroneus longus and brevis. Surgical reconstruction by transfer of the flexor digitorum longus tendon. J Bone Joint Surg Br. 1998;80(5):781-4.
92. LeMinor JM. Comparative anatomy and significance of the sesamoid bone of the peroneus longus muscle (os peroneum). J Anat. 1987;15:85-99.
93. Muehleman C. Os peroneum: a case of mistaken identity. Clin Anat. 2008;21:741.
94. Sobel M, Pavlov H, Geppert M, Thompson F, DiCarlo E, Davis W. Painful os peroneum syndrome: a spectrum of conditions responsible for plantar lateral foot pain. Foot Ankle Int. 1994;15:112-24.
95. Geller J, Lin S, Cordas D, Vierira P. Relationship of a low-lying muscle belly to tears of the peroneus brevis tendon. Am J Orthop. 2003;32:541-4.
96. Sobel M, Levy M, Bohne W. Congenital variations of the peroneus quartus muscle: an anatomic study. Foot Ankle. 1990;11:81-90.
97. Abraham E, Stimaman J. Neglected rupture of the peroneal tendons causing recurrent sprains of the ankle: case report. J Bone Joint Surg Am. 1979;61:1247-8.
98. Saxena A, Ewen B. Peroneal retinaculum tears: surgical results in 31 athletic patients. Submitted to J Foot Ankle Surg. 2010;49(3):238-41.
99. Lagoutaris E, Adams H, DiDomenico L, Rothenberg R. Longitudinal tears of both peroneal tendons associated with tophaceous gouty infiltration: a case report. J Foot Ankle Surg. 2005;44:222-4.
100. Wapner K, Taras J, Lin S, Chao W. Staged reconstruction for chronic rupture of both peroneal tendons using hunter rod and flexor hallucis longus tendon transfer: a long-term follow-up study. Foot Ankle Int. 2006;27:591-7.

Chapter 5
Osteochondral Lesions of the Talus

Amol Saxena

Talar lesions are extremely common with all types of ankle injuries including sprains and fractures. Some report that in up to 50% of ankle fractures and severe sprains, some type of talar lesion will occur. These are common sports injuries and are found with all types of ankle sprains and fracture/dislocations.[1-3] When talar lesions occur acutely, they are typically operated on immediately post-injury if there is a significantly displaced fragment. Most lesions are dealt with sub-acutely or chronically.

The term "osteochondral lesion" of the talus is often used for all lesions of the talus, whether they are transchondral or truly osteochondral. Further confusing the terminology is the use of the term "osteochondritis dissecans," which should be used for pediatric aseptic necrosis of the talus which is not usually traumatically induced. These erroneous terms are misleading and may be responsible for the variability in the results of treatments. In essence, one needs to compare "apples to apples."

Transchondral lesions are essentially "scuffs," de-laminations, or tears of talar articular cartilage that generally do not involve bone (Fig. 5.1).[3-5] Full-thickness tears can yield bare exposed subchondral bone. There are various classifications of these lesions. The main differentiation should be: If the lesion involves bone loss, it is a true osteochondral lesion. The classic Berndt and Hardy talar dome classification system is a hybrid of these two pathologies, as Type I lesions just involve cartilage, whereas Types II–IV involve cartilage and bone.[4] Other classification schemes involve describing progressive degradation of articular cartilage.[6]

A. Saxena, D.P.M.
Department of Sports Medicine, PAFMG-Palo Alto Division,
Clark Bldg., 3rd Flr, 795 El Camino Real,
Palo Alto, CA 94301, USA
e-mail: heysax@aol.com

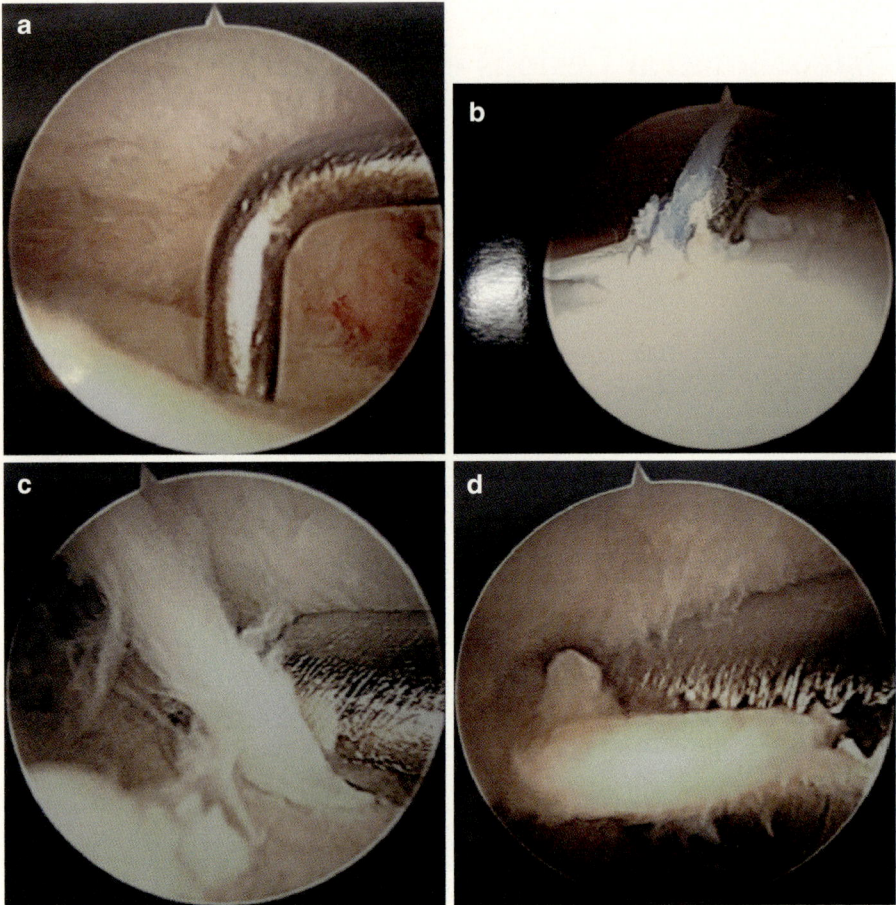

Fig. 5.1 Transchondral lesion "flap" softened cartilage being probed (**a**), separating flap (**b**), excising flap with shaver (**c**), and removing flap with grasper (**d**)

Osteochondral lesions are also classified with other various systems. Often radiographic findings are used to assess lesions. Hepple et al described their magnetic resonance imaging (MRI) staging system of talar dome injury. Stages 1–4 consist of progressively worse injury to the chondral surface. Specifically Stage 1 is a lesion only within the articular cartilage. Stage 2 injuries represent bony trabecular compression with (2A) or without (2B) surrounding bony edema. Stages 3 and 4 describe increasing degrees of osteochondral fragment separation (Fig. 5.2). These injuries can be treated with microfracture. Stage 5 indicates subchondral cysts and avascular bone (Fig. 5.3). These type of lesions are often treated with bone grafting, either autogenous or allograft.[7]

Other classification systems have been described often to help base treatment. Scranton and McDermott added a fifth stage to Berndt and Hardy's system for lesions having an intact cartilage cap, but cystic underlying bone. "Bone bruises" occur with ankle injuries and are visible via MRI in up to 39% of cases. Asymptomatic lesions can occasionally be seen, but may not require treatment, though the incidence of this is not well studied. Chondral injuries are visible arthroscopically in 66% of acutely arthroscoped ankles.[8] Ferkel and Cheng created a specific arthroscopic classification system for chondral injuries having six grades (A-F) ranging from smooth cartilage (A), rough (B), fibrillated/fissured (C), flap or exposed bone (D), loose undisplaced fragment (E), or displaced fragment (F).[6]

The talo-tibial articulation is very critical. It has less room for derangement as 1 mm of displacement can create load imbalance due to toss of talar contact of 30–40%. This subsequent malalignment leads to premature wear, and is common with lateral ankle sprains. This can induce chondral and osteochondral injury.[9]

Recent literature has increased significantly in the past decade as to the results of treatment of talar lesions. Nonsurgical treatment can be attempted and may be successful for early chondral injuries and true "bone bruises" (i.e., micro-trabecular fractures), which generally consists of a period of non-weightbearing and immobilization. There is no uniform nonsurgical treatment regimen for talar injuries, partly due to variability in classification. Unfortunately, just as the preoperative classification and nomenclature vary, so does the postoperative assessment scoring systems. When dealing with athletic patients, one has to take into consideration "down-time" and return to activity (RTA) time frames. In general, treatment of osteochondral lesions has a longer RTA than chondral lesions.[3]

Surgical treatment is recommended for most talar articular lesions that are deep, large, involve bony defects, and/or are displaced. Osteotomy may be required in

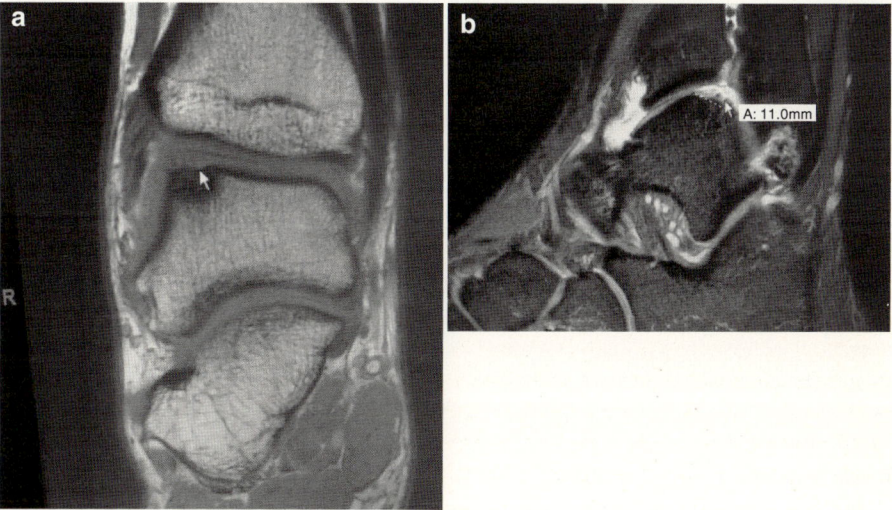

Fig. 5.2 AP T1 MRI (**a**) and lateral T2 (**b**) showing lateral transchondral lesion. Debridement of same lateral transchondral lesion (**c**), after debridement (**d**), introduction of microfracture pick (**e**), placement of microfracture pick (**f**), after performing microfracture: note bleeding (**g**)

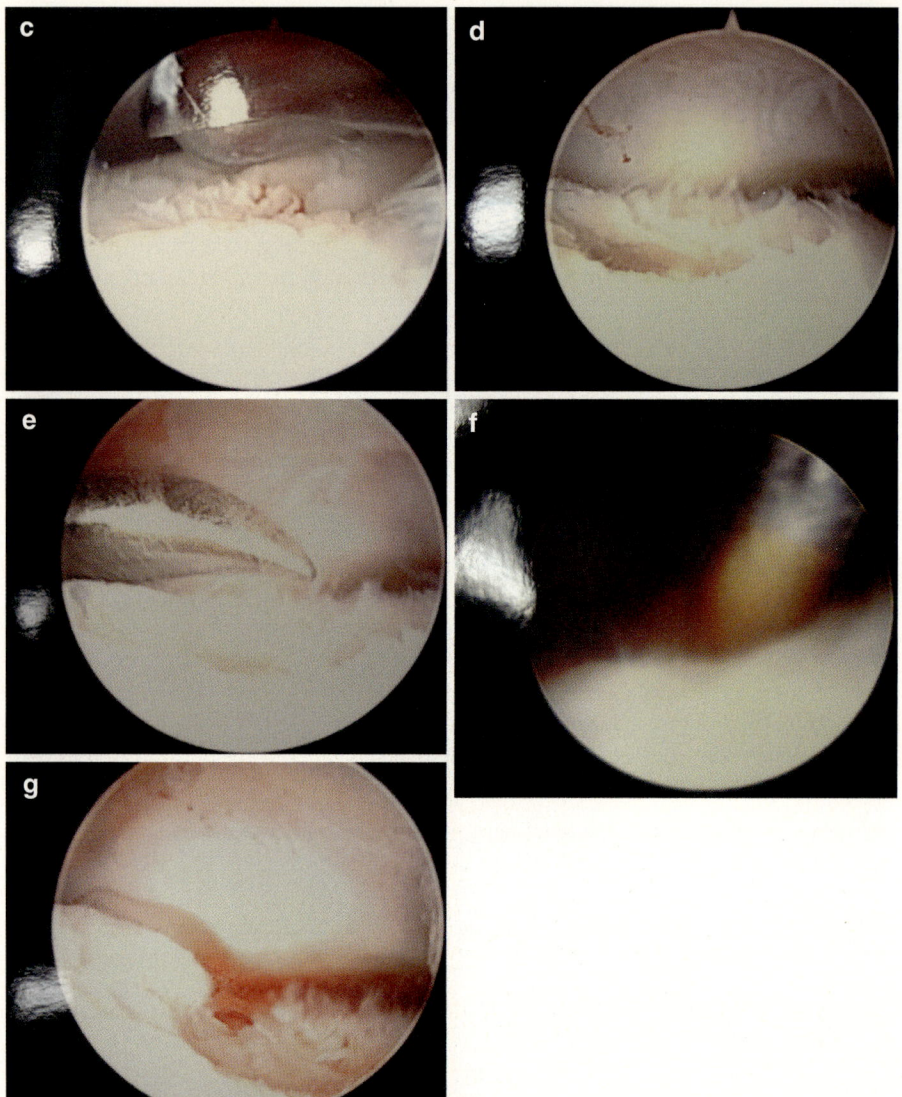

Fig. 5.2 (continued)

Fig. 5.3 Osteochondral lesions with cystic and avascular bone. AP T1 (**a**) and lateral T1 (**b**)

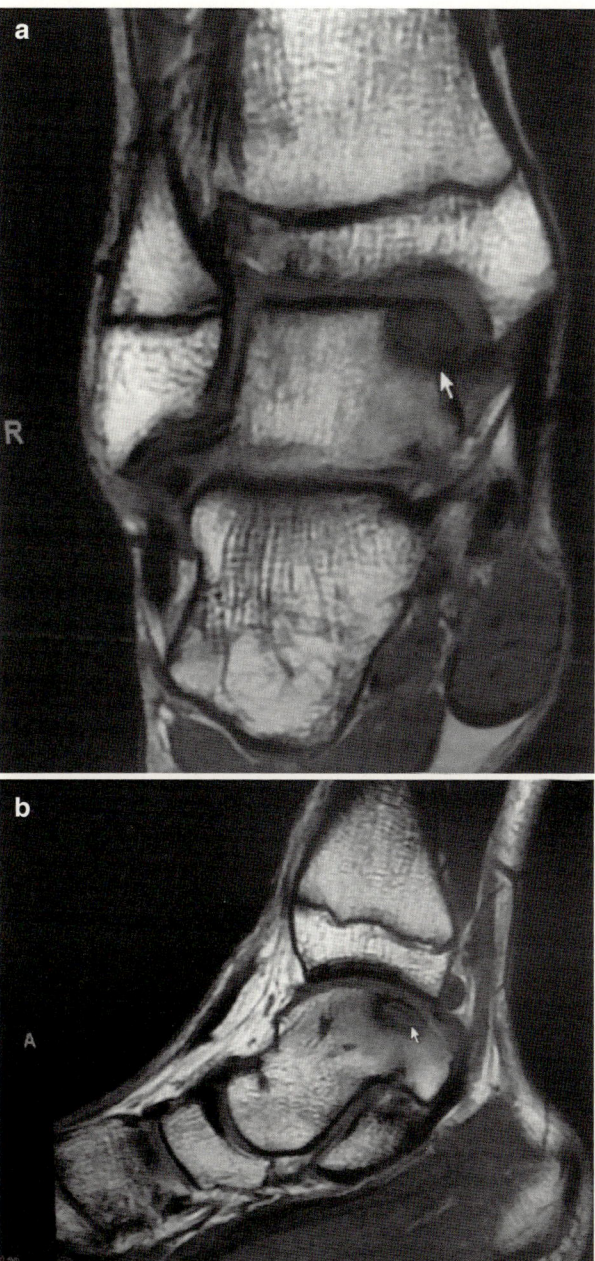

many cases to gain access to talar lesions. In fact, recent studies have shown accessibility of talar osteochondral lesions can be limited, and which osteotomies may be needed.[10-13] Lesion location traditionally has been classified as antero-lateral and poster-medial on the talar dome. This recently has been refuted by studies. Central lateral and medial locations are actually the most common, whereas the classic locations are actually less common. Elias et al reviewed 428 MRI studies of ankle with talar dome injuries. Mid-medial lesions were the most common occurring 227 times (53%) while true posterior medial lesions only occurred 58 times (14%). Central lateral defects were the second most common lesion, making up 26% of the cohort.[14] Osteotomy may be needed to gain access to central lesions. In addition to medial malleolar and fibular osteotomies to gain access to medial and lateral lesions respectively, other oblique osteotomies may be preferred (Fig. 5.4).[10-15] Recent study of

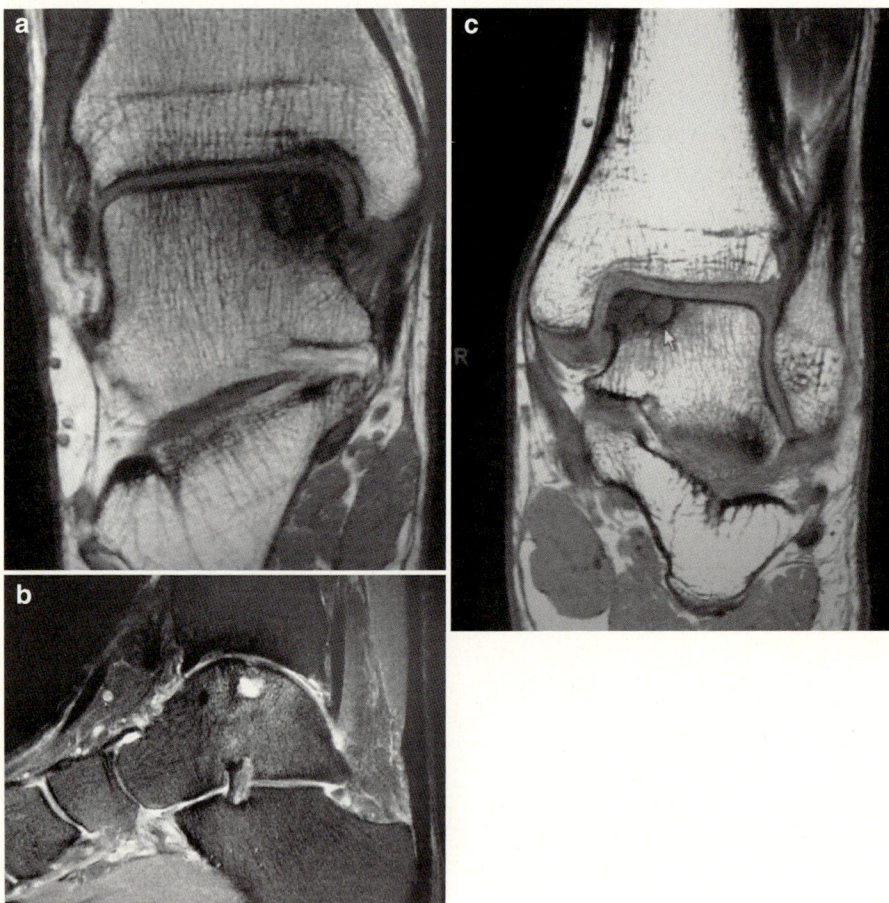

Fig. 5.4 OCDs requiring osteotomies. Medial malleolar (**a–c**), central pyramidal (**d**) and lateral malleolar (**e, f**)

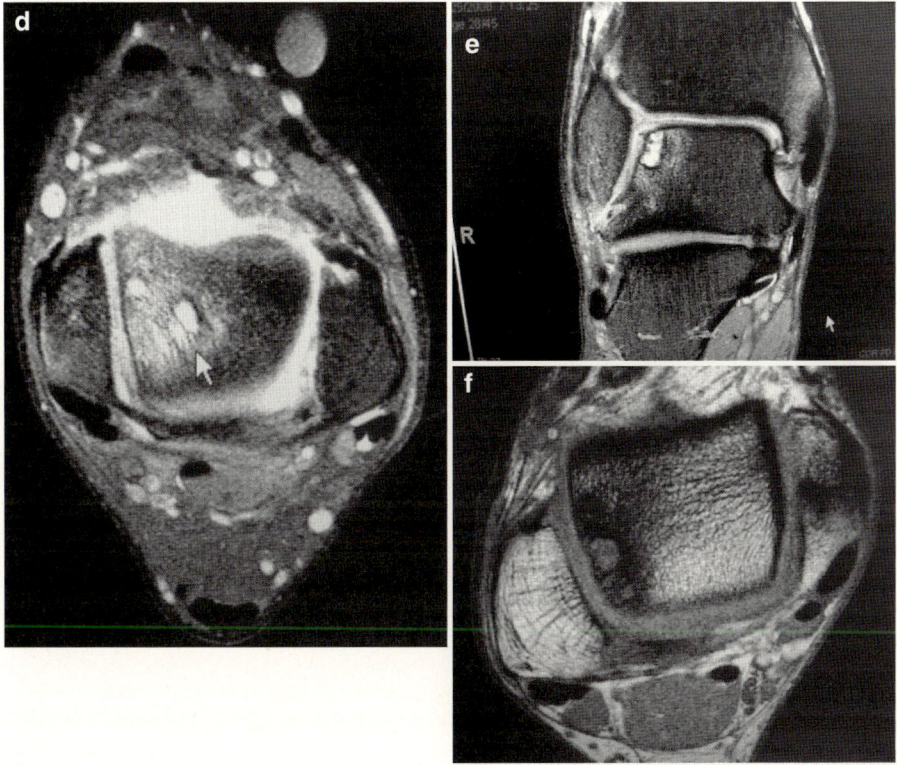

Fig. 5.4 (continued)

postero-lateral lesion access has shown fibular osteotomy gives significantly increased access.[10] Another study on accessibility showed a unique anterior tibial wedge osteotomy gives good access for central and medial lesions.[11]

Procedures for large osteochondral deficits could also require either fresh allograft or a second surgery for articular cartilage re-implantation, which has even longer RTA.[15-17] Microfracture and drilling are typical first-line treatment for chondral defects and smaller osteochondral lesions.[18-22] Furthermore, long-term evaluation of the traditional debridement and drilling of "osteochondral" lesions has shown that 35% of patients note deterioration over time.[23] This gives credence to bone grafting procedures for true osteochondral defects. Authors have shown favorable results from autogenous bone graft without cartilage transfer.[3,24] Retrograde drilling with insertion of bone graft for lesions with intact articular cartilage has shown favorable results as well.[20,25] Other treatment methods such as cartilage re-implantation and osteochondral allograft have been studied, but due to increased morbidity and cost are not recommended as first-line treatment.[15-18]

Fig. 5.5 Microfracture pick for a transchondral lesion

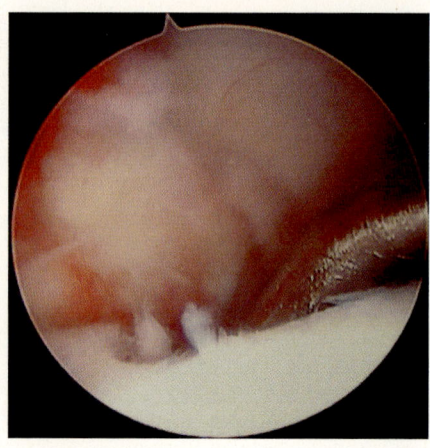

5.1 Treatment Protocols

Based on current research outcomes and RTA, the author recommends the following protocols.

5.1.1 *Transchondral Talar Lesions*

Typical treatment of transchondral talar lesions (TLTs) involves debridement and microfracture of the lesion when there is full-thickness cartilage loss (Fig. 5.5). Generally this is done arthroscopically visualizing with either a 2.7- or 4.0-mm 30° arthroscope. Standard antero-lateral and antero-media portals are created. Other accessory portals are used as needed. Transmalleolar drilling can be performed either with image-guidance or directly through visualization of an osteochondral trephine hole opposite the lesion for medial defects.[26] Details of this procedure are found elsewhere in this text. If the cartilage lesion is a large viable flap, fixation to the talus can be performed. This is often performed with bio-fixatives. In cases where the cartilage appears to be grossly intact under direct inspection, retrograde drilling can be performed. This is done under image and arthroscopic control (Fig. 5.6). Newer arthroscopic equipment allows for easier performance of these techniques in the ankle (Fig. 5.7). Postoperatively, patients are kept non-weightbearing for a minimum of three to six weeks, using a below-knee cast boot unless an osteotomy was performed. In those cases, patients are kept non-weightbearing for six weeks, with the first three weeks in a cast. After weightbearing is initiated, patients are maintained in the boot until 6–12 weeks post-surgery. (The longer time frame is for those undergoing osteotomy.) Physical therapy is initiated at 6–10 weeks post-surgery. Return to sports typically takes three or more months.

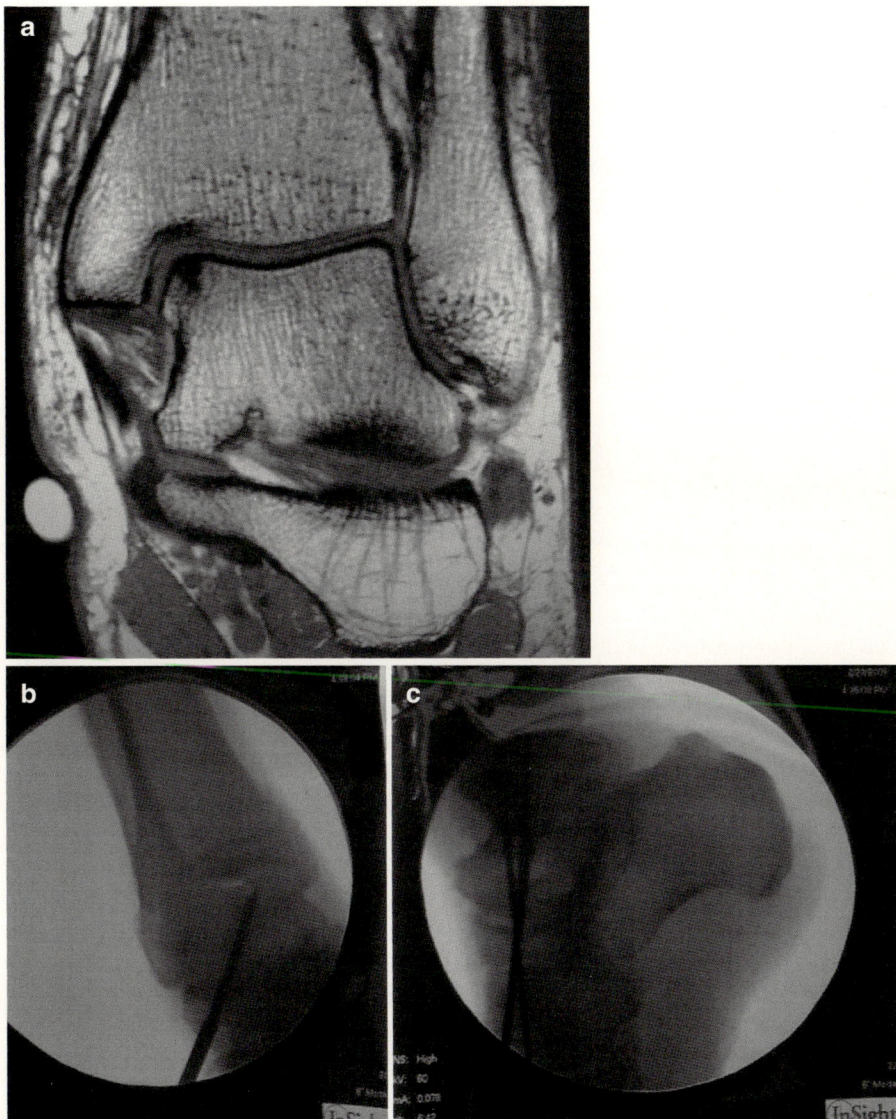

Fig. 5.6 MRI of a lesion (**a**) requiring retrograde drilling via image (**b**, **c**)

Difficult TLT cases are those lesions that involve a large portion of the talar surface area, bipolar lesions and corner lesions. Initial treatment can include above
proposed methods. However, if lesions do not yield asymptomatic relief, other
options described below may be needed.

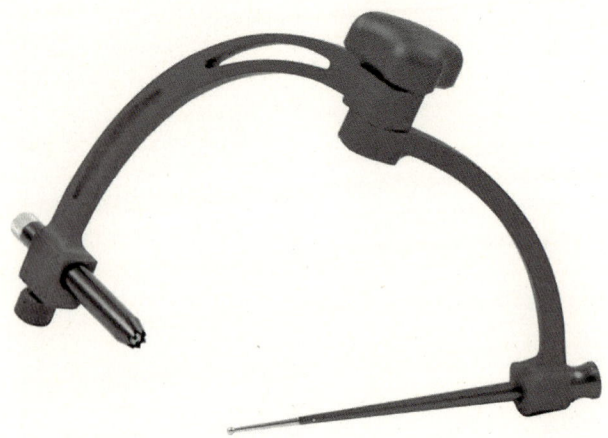

Fig. 5.7 Radiolucent guide (Arthrex, Inc., Naples, FL USA) to assist with retrograde drilling and bone grafting (Courtesy Arthrex, Inc., used with permission)

5.1.2 Osteochondral Lesions of the Talus

True osteochondral lesions of the talus involve bone loss. The supporting surface of the talus is stressed more due to this loss of structure. Research supports the theory that replacing the bone both with (i.e., OATS or osteochondral autologous/allograft transfer) and without cartilage provides good relief.[3,25] Based on Ferkel et al's long-term study which showed drilling and currettement alone of osteochondral lesions yields favorable results only 72% of the time, supports the need for bone replacement.[24] The author prefers to perform autologous morselized bone graft to these defects. Osteotomy may be needed to gain access, along with metallic fixation for postoperative stabilization. (Ideally titanium screws and plates are used so as to allow for additional MRI evaluation.) After curettage of the lesion, often via open arthrotomy, autogenous bone is harvested from the medial malleolus (for medial lesions), lateral calcaneus (lateral lesions), or ipsilateral iliac crest (large lesions), and tamped into the defect (Fig. 5.8). In some cases, retrograde drilling and bone grafting can be performed. Bone can be tamped into place when articular cartilage is intact but bone void exists (Fig. 5.6). Longer-term study is needed of these techniques but short-term results of retrograde drilling for talar osteochondral defects (OCDs) appear promising and have the benefit of preserving the cartilage surface.[27]

Though the autogenous OATS procedure shows reasonable results in the talus, donor site morbidity from the knee leaves patients with significant deficits; in some studies, more than 50% of patients complained of significant knee pain.[28-32] Allograft OATS adds to the cost of the procedure and given that 30% of the cartilage cells may not be viable 24 h after implantation, harvesting from the knee may be an unnecessary step. One study described autogenous bone graft from a non-weight-bearing portion of the talus with favorable results, which may be a better option in some situations since the cartilage thickness is similar.[31,33]

The author does utilize osteochondral allograft for corner or edge lesions, failed microfracture cases and sub-total ankle arthroplasty for large lesions (Figs. 5.9 and 5.10). Fresh talar allograft requires side matching and sizing. Recent studies show

Fig. 5.8 Postoperative bone graft (patient in Fig. 5.4a, b)

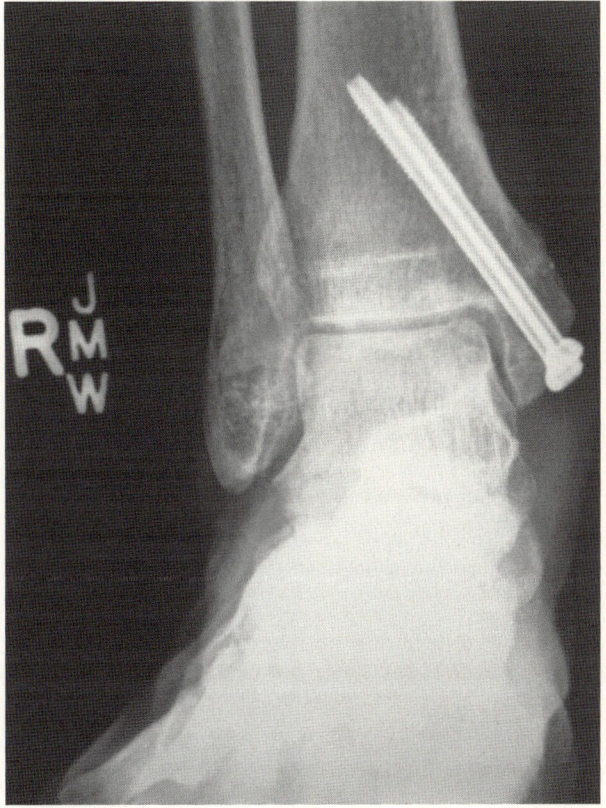

good results. The technique with fresh allografts involves matching the excised portion of the talus. Intraoperative imaging may show a "step-off" due to the difference in donor subchondral plate thickness. Therefore, clinical intraoperative inspection is mandatory on all sides of the donor placement. Fixation is generally with bio-screws or pins. Raikin recently reported on 15 cases with average defect size of over 6,000 mm³ with good results.[16] He found graft stability and viability were maintained both structurally and functionally after mean follow-up 4.5 years post-implantation. He used metallic fixation and average patient age was 41.9 years. Metallic screws make subsequent re-imaging with MRI difficult. "Second-look" arthroscopies can show viable articular cartilage, but few studies relate this.[3,16,24,34]

5.2   Postoperative Management

Postoperative management of osteochondral lesion repair is typically six weeks non-weightbearing in a cast or boot, and then an additional 10–12 weeks in the boot until pain-free, or if an osteotomy was performed, bony healing has been achieved. Allograft incorporation could take several weeks longer (than 12 weeks). X-rays of

Fig. 5.9 X-ray (**a**) and MRI
(**b**, **c**) of a patient undergoing fresh osteochondral
allograft (**d**)

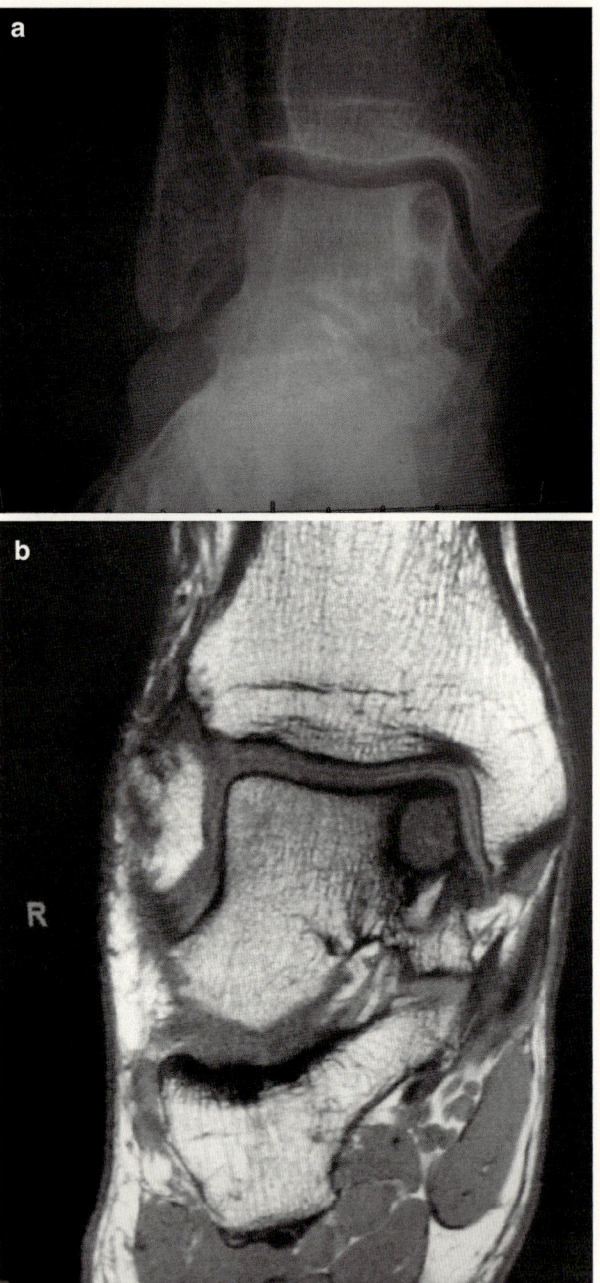

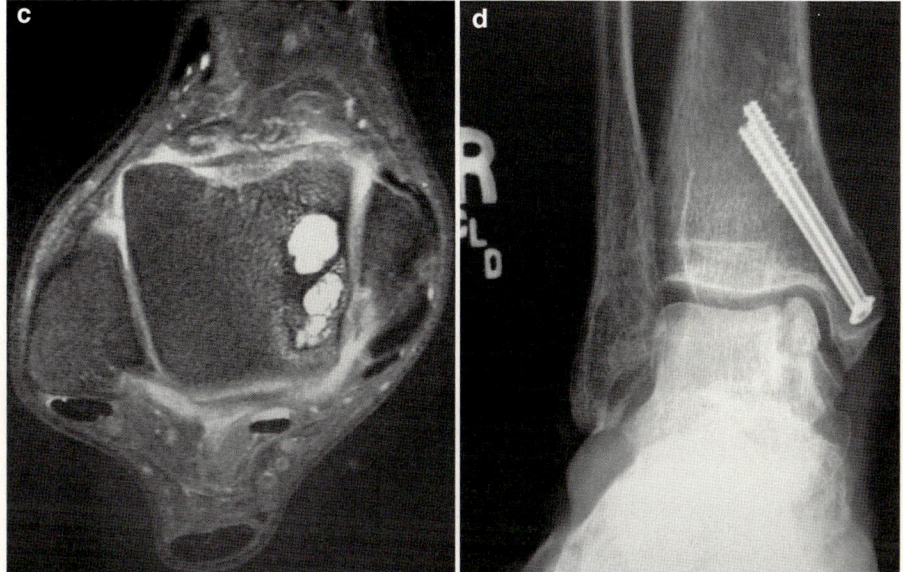

Fig. 5.9 (continued)

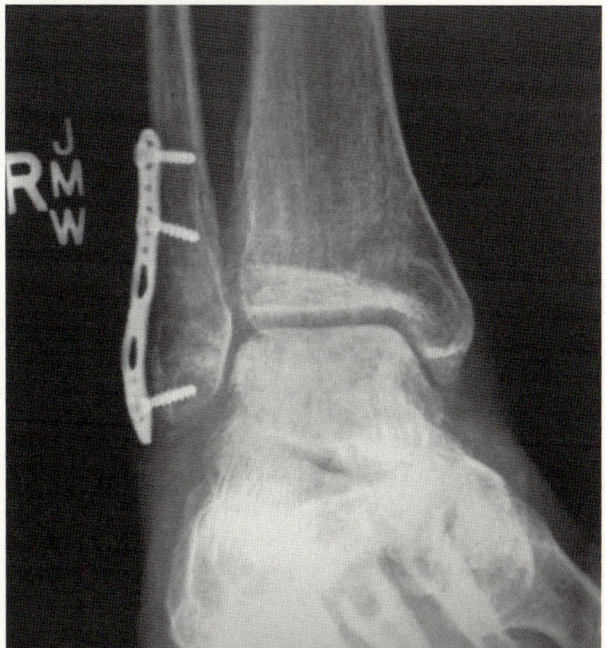

Fig. 5.10 Osteochondral allograft for lateral corner OCD (patient in Fig. 5.4e, f)

Fig. 5.11 Antero-pyramidal osteotomy for autogenous bone graft of a central-medial OCD (patient in Fig. 5.4c, d). Note lucency in distal tibia from bioresorbable screw used to fixate osteotomy immediate (**a**) and three month post-op X-rays (**b**)

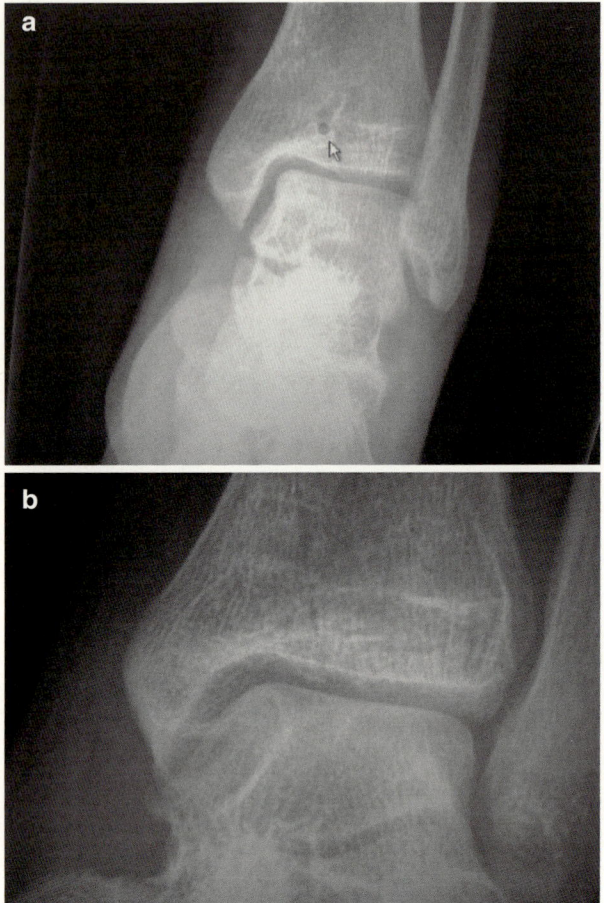

bone graft incorporation and of the osteotomy if performed are obtained. Osteotomies that are fixed with resorbable screws may have persistent lucencies within the screw "tracks" (Fig. 5.11). Formal physical therapy starts at 10 weeks. Impact activities and sport resumption take approximately six months or even longer, especially for allograft patients. Most patients use an ankle brace or tape for sports postoperatively. One should note that similar treatments can be employed for chondral and osteochondral lesions of the tibial plafond and malleolar articular portions of the ankle as well. A treatment algorithm based on current literature and the author's experience is presented in Fig. 5.12. Treatment for failed OCDs can include ankle arthrodiastasis, realignment osteotomies, total ankle arthroplasty, and arthrodesis, discussed elsewhere in this text.

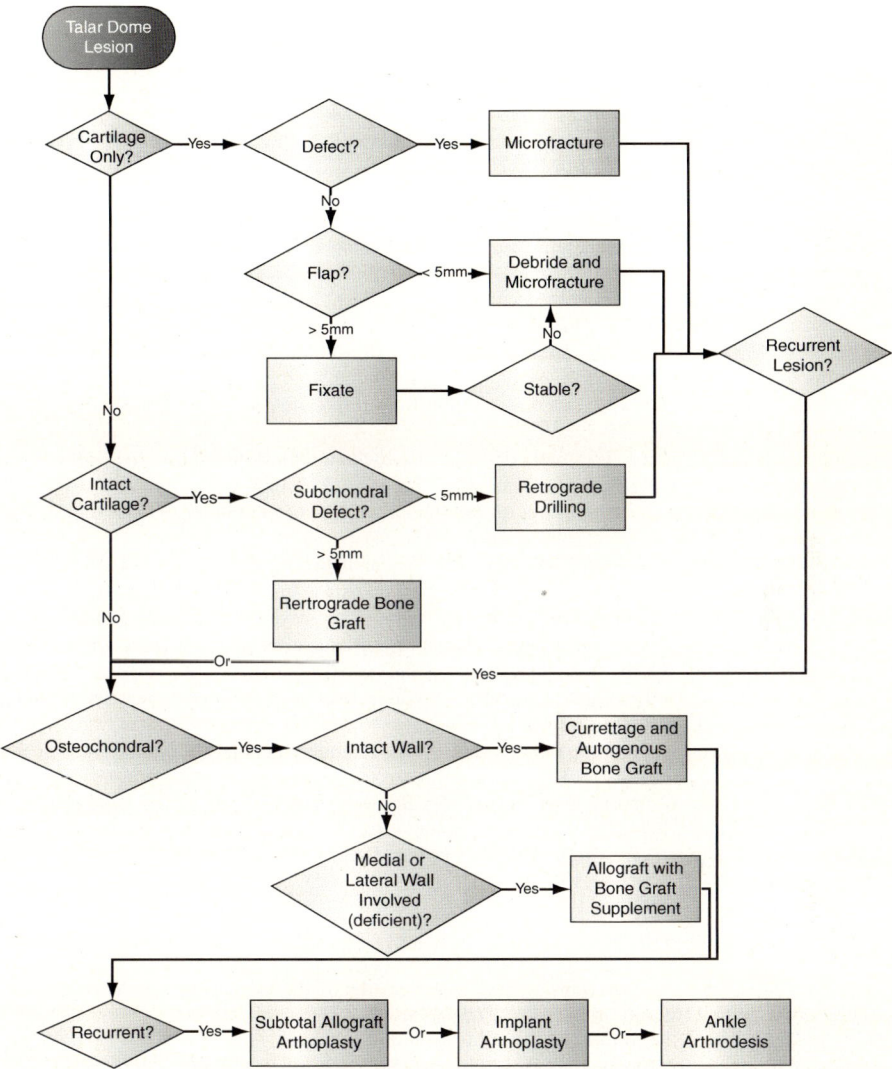

Fig. 5.12 Algorithm for Treatment of Talar Dome Lesions. Note: Most microfracture and retrograde drilling procedures are performed arthroscopically while autogenous bone grafting is performed via open arthrotomy. 5 mm refers to the diameter of the lesion measured intraoperatively. In addition, lesion location determines if an osteotomy is necessary with a lateral fibular, anterior tibial (pyramidal), or medial malleolar (inverted chevron) approach

References

1. DeLee JC. Fractures and dislocations of the foot. In: Mann RA, Coughlin MJ, eds. Surgery of the foot and ankle. 6th editors St. Louis: Mosby; 1991:1465-518.
2. Ferkel RD. Arthoscopy of the ankle and foot. In: Mann RA, Coughlin MJ, editors Surgery of the foot and ankle. St. Louis: Mosby; 1993:1277-312.
3. Saxena A, Eakin C. Articular talar injuries in athletes: results of microfracture and autogenous bone graft. Am J Sports Med. 2007;35:1680-7.
4. Berndt AL, Harty M. Transchondral fractures (osteochondritis dissecans) of the talus. J Bone Joint Surg Am. 1959;4:988-1020.
5. Labovitz J, Scweitzer M. Osseous occult injuries after ankle sprains: incidence, location, pattern, and age. Foot Ankle Int. 1998;19:661-7.
6. Ferkel R, Cheng J. Ankle and subtalar arthroscopy. In: Kelikian A, editor Operative treatment of the foot and ankle. New York: Appleton-Croft; 1999:321.
7. Hepple S, Winson I, Glew D. Osteochondral lesions of the talus; a revised classification. Foot Ankle Int. 2000;21(12):789-793.
8. Scranton P, McDermott J. Treatment of type V osteochondral lesions of the talus with ipsilateral knee osteochondral autografts. Foot Ankle Int. 2001;22:380-4.
9. Caputo AM, Lee JY, Spritzer CE, et al. In vivo kinematics of the tibiotalar joint after lateral ankle instability. Am J Sports Med. 2009;37(11):2241-8.
10. Garras DN, Santangelo JA, Wang DW, Easley ME. A quantitative comparison of surgical approaches for posterolateral osteochondral lesions of the talus. Foot Ankle Int. 2008;29(4):415-20.
11. Kreuz P, Steinwachs M, Erggelet C, Lahm A, Henle P, Niemeyer P. Mosiacplasty with autogenous talar autograft for osteochondral lesions of the talus after failed primary arthroscopic management. Am J Sports Med. 2006;34(1):55-63.
12. Muir D, Saltzman C, Tochigi Y, Amendola N. Talar dome access for osteochondral lesions. Am J Sports Med. 2006;34:1457-63.
13. Navid DO, Myerson MS. Approach alternatives for treatment of osteochondral lesions of the talus. Foot Ankle Clin. 2002;7(3):635-50.
14. Elias I, Zoga AC, Morrison WB, Besser MP, Schweitzer ME, Raikin SM. Osteochondral lesions of the talus: localization and morphologic data from 424 patients using a novel anatomical grid scheme. Foot Ankle Int. 2007;28(2):154-61.
15. Zengerink M, Szerb I, Hangody L, Dopirak RM, Ferkel RD, van Dijk CN. Current concepts: treatment of osteochondral ankle defects. Foot Ankle Clin. 2006;11(2):331-59.
16. Raikin S. Fresh osteochondral allografts for large volume cystic osteochondral defects of the talus. J Bone Joint Surg. 2009;91-A(12):2818-26.
17. Whittaker JP, Smith G, Makwana N, et al. Early results of autologous chondrocyte implantation in the talus. J Bone Joint Surg Br. 2005;87(2):179-83.
18. Giannini S, Buda R, Vannini F, DiCaprio F, Grigolo B. Arthroscopic autologous chondrocyte implantation in osteochondral lesions of the talus: surgical technique and results. Am J Sports Med. 2008;36:873-80.
19. Becher C, Thermann H. Results of microfracture in the treatment of articular defects of the talus. Foot Ankle Int. 2005;26(8):583-9.
20. Kono M, Takao M, Naito K, Uchio Y, Ochi M. Retrograde drilling for osteochondral lesions of the talar dome. Am J Sports Med. 2006;34:1450-6.
21. Tol J, Struijs P, Bossuiyt P, Verhagen R, van Dijk C. Treatment strategies in osteochondral defects of the talar dome: a systematic review. Foot Ankle Int. 2000;21:119-26.
22. Van Dijk C, Verhagen R, Struijs P. Systematic review of treatment strategies for osteochondral defects of the talar dome. Foot Ankle Clin. 2003;2:233-42.
23. Ferkel RD, Zanotti RM, Komenda GA, et al. Arthroscopic treatment of chronic osteochondral lesions of the talus: long-term results. Am J Sports Med. 2008;36(9):1750-62.
24. Draper S, Fallet L. Autogenous bone grafting for the treatment of talar dome lesions. J Foot Ankle Surg. 2000;39(1):15-23.

25. Taranow W, Bisignani G, Towers J. Retrograde drilling of osteochondral lesions of the medial talar dome. Foot Ankle Int. 1999;20(8):474-80.
26. Grady J, Hughes D. Arthroscopic management of talar dome lesions using a transmalleolar approach. J Am Podiatr Med Assoc. 2006;96(3):260-3.
27. Gobbi A, Francisco R, Lubowitz J, Allegra F, Canata G. Osteochondral lesions of the talus: randomized controlled trial comparing chondroplasty, microfracture and osteochondral autograft transplantation. J Arthos Rel Surg. 2006;2210:1085-92.
28. Baltzer AW, Arnold JP. Bone-cartilage transplantation from the ipsilateral knee for chondral lesions of the talus. Arthroscopy. 2005;21(2):159-66.
29. Hangody L, Fules P. Autologous osteochondral mosaicplasty for the treatment of full-thickness defects of weight-bearing joints: ten years of experimental and clinical experience. J Bone Joint Surg Am. 2003;85:25-32.
30. Kreuz PC, Steinwachs M, Edlich M, et al. The anterior approach for the treatment of posterior osteochondral lesions of the talus: comparison of different surgical techniques. Arch Orthop Trauma Surg. 2005;5:1-6.
31. Reddy S, Pedowitz D, Parekh S, Sennett B, Okereke E. The morbidity associated with osteochondral harvest from asymptomatic knees for the treatment of osteochondral lesions of the talus. Am J Sports Med. 2007;35:80-5.
32. Valderabano V, Leumann A, Rasch H, Egelhof T, Hintermann B, Pagenstert G. Knee-to-ankle mosaicolasty for the treatment of osteochondral lesions of the ankle joint. Am J Sports Med. 2009;37(Supp 1):105S-11.
33. Kreuz PC, Steinwachs M, Erggelet C, Lahm A, Henle P, Niemeyer P. Mosaicplasty with autogenous talar autograft for osteochondral lesions of the talus after failed primary arthroscopic management: a prospective study with a 4-year follow-up. Am J Sports Med. 2006;34(1):55-63.
34. Lee B, Bai L, Yoon T, Jung S, Seon J. Second-look arthroscopic findings and clinical outcomes after microfracture for osteochondral lesions of the talus. Am J Sports Med. 2009;37(Supp 1): 63S-70.

Chapter 6
Acquired Adult Flatfoot Deformity

Joseph S. Park and Lew C. Schon

Acquired adult flatfoot deformity (AAFD), also referred to as posterior tibialis insufficiency, is a clinical entity which has only been recently recognized in the literature. First described in 1953,[1] the progression of dysfunction and eventual deformity has only recently been better understood by physicians treating this complex disorder. Early recognition and treatment of this disorder enable surgeons to utilize techniques which can maximize foot function and preserve joint range of motion. Recognition of the early stages of the disorder and the interplay between tendon degeneration and predisposing anatomic or physiologic factors allows for the institution of both nonoperative and operative management. Delayed treatment of acquired adult flatfoot deformity can result in rigid, painful deformities which may require triple arthrodesis. As literature has shown, the natural history of triple arthrodesis can lead to progression of adjacent joint arthrosis, including the ankle and adjacent midfoot/forefoot joints.[2-4] Through the use of tendon transfers, calcaneal and midfoot osteotomies, and ligament reconstructions, the surgeon can avoid the associated long-term morbidity associated with fusion procedures.

6.1 Etiology/Anatomy

Although recent literature has focused on the dysfunction of the posterior tibialis tendon, progression of adult flatfoot involves complex changes in foot architecture including attenuation of capsular structures and intrinsic ligaments.[5] While the

J.S. Park, M.D.
Department of Orthopaedic Surgery,
Union Memorial Hospital, Baltimore, MD, USA

L.C. Schon, M.D. (✉)
Department of Orthopaedics, Union Memorial Hospital,
3333 N. Calvert St. #400, Baltimore, MD 21218, USA
e-mail: lewschon@comcast.net

A. Saxena (ed.), *Special Procedures in Foot and Ankle Surgery*,
DOI 10.1007/978-1-4471-4103-7_6, © Springer-Verlag London 2013

posterior tibialis is the crucial dynamic stabilizer, static stability is afforded by the bony anatomy and soft tissue structures including the spring ligament, talonavicular capsule, plantar fascia, and deltoid ligament.[6,7]

The posterior tibialis muscle, enervated by the tibial nerve, originates from the posterior aspect of the tibia, interosseous membrane, and fibula from the proximal third of the leg. As it courses toward the posterior aspect of the medial malleolus, it becomes tendinous at the junction of the middle and distal one third of the leg. The flexor retinaculum binds the tendon within a shallow groove in the tibia as it takes an abrupt curve anteriorly toward the navicular tuberosity. By passing medial to the axis of the subtalar joint, it acts as the principal inverter of the foot. In addition to its main insertion on the naviculum, it has lesser insertions on the sustentaculum, all three cuneiforms, the cuboid, and second, third, and fourth metatarsal bases.[8]

Thought to be an overuse or age-related phenomenon, degeneration of the posterior tibialis tendon usually occurs in the portion that is subjected to the most biomechanical forces. As the posterior tibialis tendon courses posterior to the medial malleolus, it is subjected to frictional and compressive forces which can result in fraying and degeneration of the tendon. In the normal tendon, there is an increase in fibrocartilage in the portion which courses behind the malleolus. This fibrocartilage has been shown to degenerate with advanced age.[9] In addition, this area of increased stress coincides with the region of relative hypovascularity,[10] further compromising tendon-healing capability in this zone. Furthermore, tendon injury initiates the inflammatory cascade (IL-1 and IL-6) and an increase in metalloproteinase activity, leading to further tendon destruction.[11]

There are many causes of pediatric flatfoot deformity, including tarsal coalition, os navicular syndrome, Koehler's disease, and congenital vertical talus.[12] While these are beyond the scope of this chapter, they are important considerations when evaluating the adolescent who presents with a painful flatfoot disorder. Unrecognized coalition patients, for example, may require more extensive reconstructive procedures to correct their deformities.

In the general population, congenital pes planus is often asymptomatic, even into late adulthood. Preexisting alignment issues may make the posterior tibialis tendon more vulnerable to inflammation and associated degenerative changes. An acute increase in pain or sudden onset of inversion weakness may represent posterior tibialis rupture in a previously asymptomatic patient with pes planus.

Similarly, medical comorbidities including obesity, systemic steroid use, diabetes mellitus, floroquinolone antibiotic use, and inflammatory conditions including rheumatoid arthritis[13] can result in tendon rupture or dysfunction.[14] A thorough medical history and workup is critical in the care of these patients, especially with preoperative and postoperative management.

6.2   Diagnosis/Evaluation

The examination of a patient with suspected posterior tibialis dysfunction begins with observation of the patient. By viewing both feet from multiple angles as the patient stands, the examiner can assess height of the midfoot arch, abduction through

Fig. 6.1 Clinical appearance of Stage III AAFD with marked hindfoot valgus, collapse of the medial longitudinal arch, and midfoot abduction; the "too many toes" sign

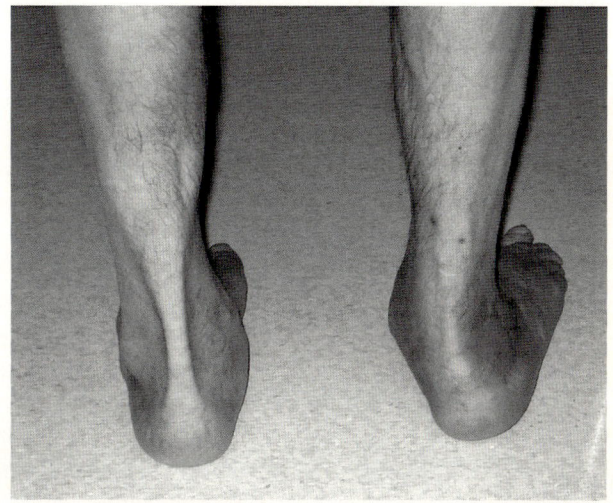

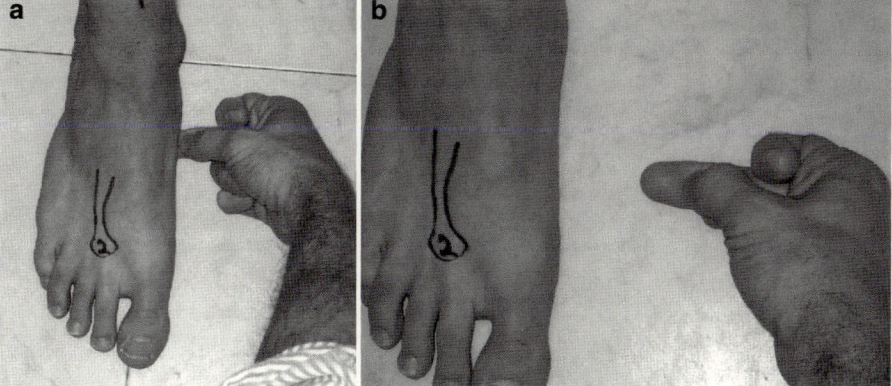

Fig. 6.2 Illustration of the "fingometer" for documentation of maintenance or collapse of the medial longitudinal arch. (**a**) Inserting finger under arch, (**b**) noting measurement on finger

the midfoot, and heel alignment. In addition, this allows for direct comparison of the symptomatic extremity to the contralateral side. Talar head prominence, indicative of midfoot abduction and talonavicular uncoverage, should also be noted. This abduction can be appreciated when viewing the foot from behind, the "too many toes sign" (Fig. 6.1).[15] The presence of callosities or ulcers on the plantar aspect of the foot could be indicative of alteration in alignment and aberrant load distribution.

For each exam, it is also our practice to document maintenance of the arch through use of the "fingometer" (Fig. 6.2). The examiner inserts his middle finger into the space beneath the highest aspect of the midfoot arch. This maximal distance is then measured and also compared to the contralateral value. Decrease in this "fingometer" value can indicate interval collapse of the arch while a stable measurement implies maintenance of the arch, despite posterior tibialis weakness or pain. Advanced mid-foot arthritis and collapse, which can also result in pes planus, can easily be mistaken for posterior tibialis dysfunction. Viewing the hindfoot from behind the patient can help to distinguish between these two entities. Pes planus from midfoot arthritis is often associated with maintained heel alignment, while with posterior tibialis dys-function, it is the valgus hindfoot alignment which dictates the midfoot and forefoot deformities.

Watching the patient walk barefoot in the hallway can allow the examiner to observe their overall limb alignment, cadence of their gait, condition of the arch of the foot, presence or absence of heel inversion on heel rise, and can give a general sense of the physical conditioning of the patient. Complex deformities, including concurrent genu valgum, may need to be treated in conjunction with an adult recon-structive surgeon. In deciding which deformity should be addressed first, the level of impairment from each should be considered. For example, if a patient will require a triple arthrodesis to correct his distal deformity, it may be prudent to pursue knee realignment first. The lack of accommodation and fixed alignment of the fused hindfoot may necessitate correction of the proximal deformity in order to determine the optimal position for fusion. In contrast, a mild, asymptomatic genu valgum should be left alone if a non-fusion reconstructive alternative is being considered. However, if such alignment issues are a concern, standing long-leg radiographs are a prerequisite for optimal treatment.

Assessment of neurovascular function is standard as for every foot and ankle patient. General testing for sensibility in peripheral nerve distributions, motor func-tion of specific muscle/tendon complexes, and palpation of dorsalis pedis and pos-terior tibial arteries should be performed and documented for every patient. Additional tests, including Semmes-Weinstein filament testing and toe-perfusion pressures, should be performed or ordered for patients with any evidence of sensory or vascular impairment.

In addition to a general orthopedic exam, including evaluation for spine, hip, and knee pathology, a focused exam for evaluation for posterior tibialis dysfunction should be performed. With the patient seated, the posterior tibialis tendon should be palpated along its course, especially behind the medial malleolus and distally toward its main insertion onto the naviculum. Swelling, bogginess, or a frank defect in the tendon should all be documented. Lateral tenderness can also be present, especially with subfibular impingement or with fibular stress fracture. Next, range of motion of the ankle and hindfoot should be measured. Beginning with the foot in a fully abducted and everted position, passive range of motion to the fully inverted position can be measured. It is our practice to describe the range of motion as an angle defined by the second metatarsal shaft compared to the axis of the tibial shaft (Fig. 6.3). It is again important to compare the affected extremity to the contralateral as a baseline. Limitation in passive subtalar range of motion may represent advanced degenerative changes which would not be benefited by tendon transfer or calcaneal osteotomy. Passive ankle dorsiflexion and plantar flexion should also be measured, both with the knee flexed 90° and fully extended. If the deformity is flexible,

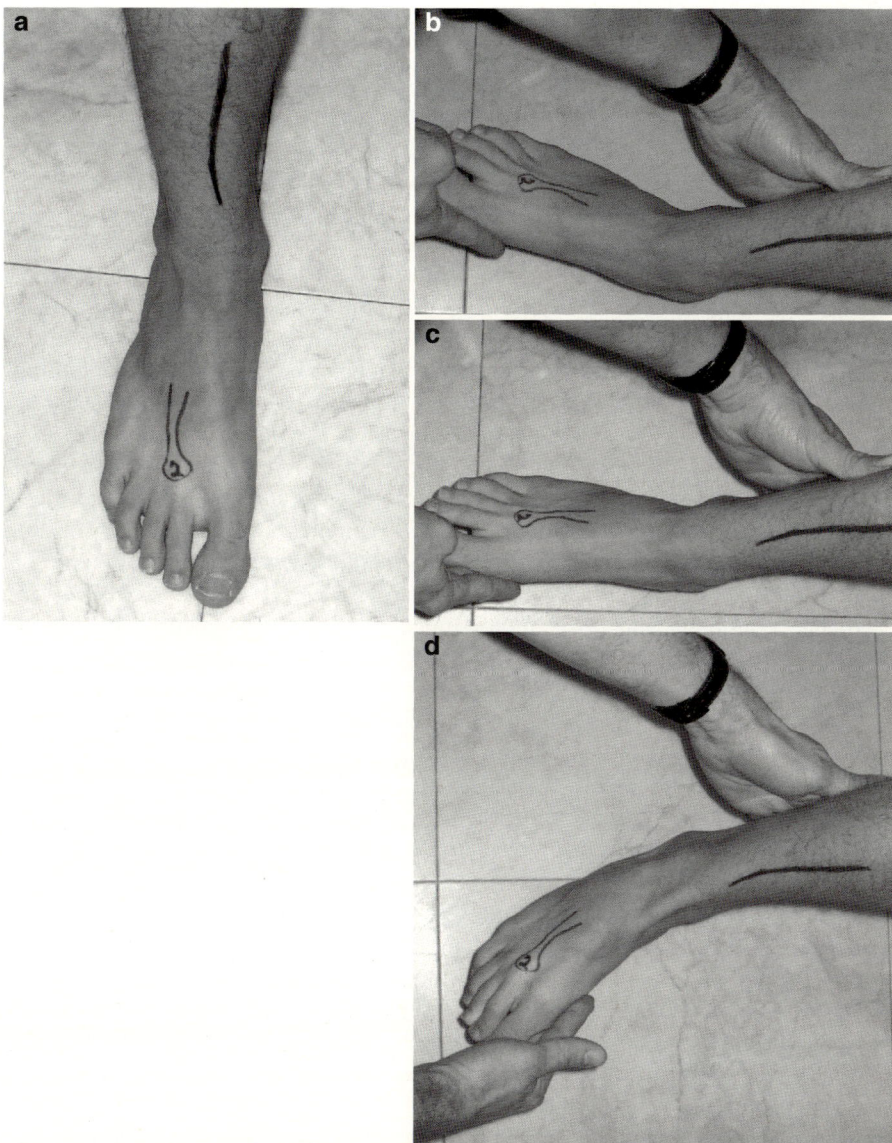

Fig. 6.3 Clinical exam for posterior tibialis tendon function. (**a**) range of motion is described in degrees by comparing the second metatarsal shaft to the tibial shaft axis as a reference. Inversion strength is tested in (**b**) the fully abducted/everted position, (**c**) neutral position, and (**d**) in the fully adducted and inverted position

measurement should take place with the hindfoot corrected to neutral coronal alignment. True assessment of equinus contracture is impossible unless the hindfoot is corrected out of valgus.[16] Limitation of dorsiflexion with the knee extended, but not in the flexed position, suggests isolated gastrocnemius contracture. As discussed previously, any evidence of midfoot arthritis, including crepitance with range of motion, warmth, or dorsal prominence, should be documented and evaluated as a possible cause of pes planus deformity.

The exam should now proceed to assessing the function of the posterior tibialis tendon. The traditional single stance heel rise test is useful to assess posterior tibialis function. The ability of the patient to invert the hindfoot with single stance heel rise does not necessarily rule out dysfunction. Difficulty with repetitive heel rises may uncover early dysfunction or attenuation, and repeat examination after extended walking can similarly diagnose more subtle involvement. False-positives for failure to single stance heel rise can also be present. Poor balance, generalized weakness, Achilles tendon dysfunction, painful midfoot arthritis, or rigid hindfoot deformity can result in difficulty interpreting this physical exam finding. In addition, as painful synovitis can prevent the patient from even attempting a single stance heel rise, a more systematic and precise motor exam is also required.

Tendon continuity and intact motor function can be confirmed by having the patient invert the foot against resistance (Fig. 6.3). As recruitment of the tibialis anterior can provide inversion function, the examiner should place the foot in a maximally plantarflexed position to isolate the posterior tibialis. The foot should then be placed in the maximally inverted position to determine if there is an inversion lag, a difference in passive versus active range of motion. Inversion lag, or the inability to maintain the maximal inverted position against resistance, may represent attenuation or stretching of the posterior tibialis tendon. Resisted inversion should then be performed from the neutral position, as well as the fully abducted position to assess tendon power along the entire range of tendon excursion. As motor function is graded with respect to full range of motion, the presence of inversion lag, even if power is full within that range, is defined as 4/5. We further classify this group of patients as 4−, 4, or 4+ depending on the tendon power. This enables us to document an overall estimate of the motor function, despite the loss of active terminal inversion. From our own experience, patients who have well-maintained inversion power to 20° beyond neutral (4+/5 strength) have demonstrated improved responses to both bracing and less invasive surgical procedures (for example, isolated flexor digitorum longus [FDL] transfer). If range of motion is full, as compared to the passive arc of motion, we define the grade as 5− or 5, depending on the amount of resistance the patient is able to overcome. Testing the tendon power throughout the entire arc of motion is important, as the inability to power the foot beyond neutral when starting in a fully abducted position could indicate tenosynovitis or focal tendon fraying which can lead to mechanical or pain-related impairment in motor strength. Clear, consistent documentation of exam findings enables us to follow interval improvement or deterioration of tendon function with different treatment modalities and on serial office visits.

6.3   Radiographic Evaluation

Every patient with a symptomatic flatfoot deformity should be evaluated with standing anteroposterior (AP), lateral, and oblique views of the foot and ankle. As many patients can actively prevent the midfoot collapse present when observing their gait, they should be instructed to relax their foot and ankle musculature during weight-bearing views. Radiographic angles can also be measured and documented. On the AP, an increased talus-first metatarsal angle and percentage of talar head uncoverage can indicate abduction of the midfoot. The talonavicular joint can also be visualized clearly on the oblique view. The lateral x-ray can demonstrate loss of calcaneal pitch, decrease in talocalcaneal angle, elevation of the medial column, and extension of the first metatarsal with respect to the talus. However, as radiographic angles can vary greatly depending on technique, we do not have absolute numerical criteria for operative treatment. In addition to overall alignment, any ankle, hindfoot, or adjacent joint arthritis should be documented as these factors may necessitate concurrent arthrodesis of affected joints along with flatfoot reconstruction. Finally, as stated previously, the patient with a proximal deformity of the hip or knee should be assessed with standing full-length extremity radiographs.

While many patients present to our office with magnetic resonance imaging (MRI) studies, the findings do not dictate our treatment algorithm. For example, a patient with 3/5 posterior tibialis strength and progressive hindfoot valgus would still be treated operatively, even if there was no evidence of frank tendinopathy on MRI. Therefore, we do not routinely order MRI for all patients. However, MRI can be useful in demonstrating the extent of tendon or muscle involvement and can help diagnose preexisting hindfoot or adjacent joint arthrosis. In addition, findings consistent with attenuation of the deltoid ligament or spring ligament, plantar fascia rupture, FDL, or peroneal tendon involvement can alter the operative plan for these patients.

As clinical deformity is often more significant than radiographs may suggest, actual photographs often further emphasize ongoing deformation of the affected foot and ankle. We routinely obtain standing clinical photographs, and often a video of the patient walking to get a better overall sense and to document the patient's condition and impairment in gait.

6.4   Classification

Johnson and Strom first described the first three stages of posterior tibialis dysfunction in 1989.[17] Patients with Stage I dysfunction typically present with posterior tibialis pain without obvious progressive planovalgus deformity. Although able to perform an isolated single stance heel rise, repetitive stresses may uncover weakness in a side-to-side comparison. Their posterior tibialis motor power is typically 5/5, although synovitis may limit their function to 5-/5. These patients do not

Fig. 6.4 Severe talonavicular uncoverage (>50%). This patient required a medial displacement calcaneal osteotomy plus lateral column lengthening using the Hintermann modification

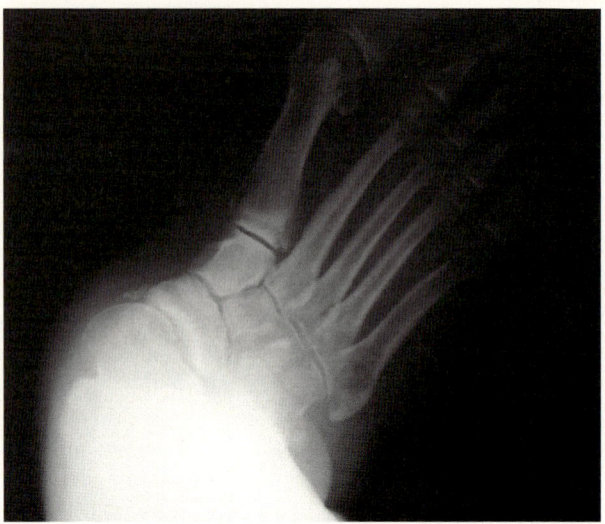

normally have an inversion lag as Stage I represents tenosynovitis without significant stretch or attenuation of the tendon.

Stage II is defined as a flexible planovalgus deformity with evidence of tendon elongation but represents a broad spectrum of pathology. Clinically, these patients are typically not able to perform a single stance heel rise, and have evidence of inversion lag on physical exam. In addition, they may have lateral pain as a result of subfibular impingement. It is essential that their deformity is correctable to their baseline alignment, although a tight gastroc–soleus complex may prevent full correction. Stage II has subsequently been subdivided into various categories by multiple authors.[18,19] In our practice, we differentiate these subgroups into three types using 40% as a cutoff. Type IIa is defined as less than 40% uncoverage, IIb as 40–50% uncoverage. We further add Type IIc with talonavicular uncoverage of more than 50% which may signify the need for fusion procedure for optimal correction (Fig. 6.4).

As Stage III posterior tibialis tendon dysfunction represents rigid deformity due to longstanding rupture of the tendon, these patients will typically require more significant reconstructive procedures involving arthrodeses. Clinically, they will have a rigid valgus hindfoot alignment, severe abduction of the midfoot, a compensatory supination of the forefoot, and functional loss of posterior tibialis power. The most important clinical finding is that the hindfoot valgus and midfoot abduction cannot be corrected to neutral, even under general anesthesia. The presence of forefoot varus does not dictate classification of the dysfunction as Stage III as it may be present in all stages. It must be assessed independently as it may be due to multiple etiologies including instability or degenerative changes at the first metatarso-cuneiform, naviculo-medial cuneiform joints, or deficient medial column (congenital), or as a compensatory adaptation to the hindfoot deformity.

Stage IV dysfunction, as described by Myerson in 1997, represents progression of the hindfoot deformity to include valgus of the ankle with lateral talar tilt.[20]

Fig. 6.5 Stage V AAFD with valgus talar tilt within the mortise, and fibular stress fracture

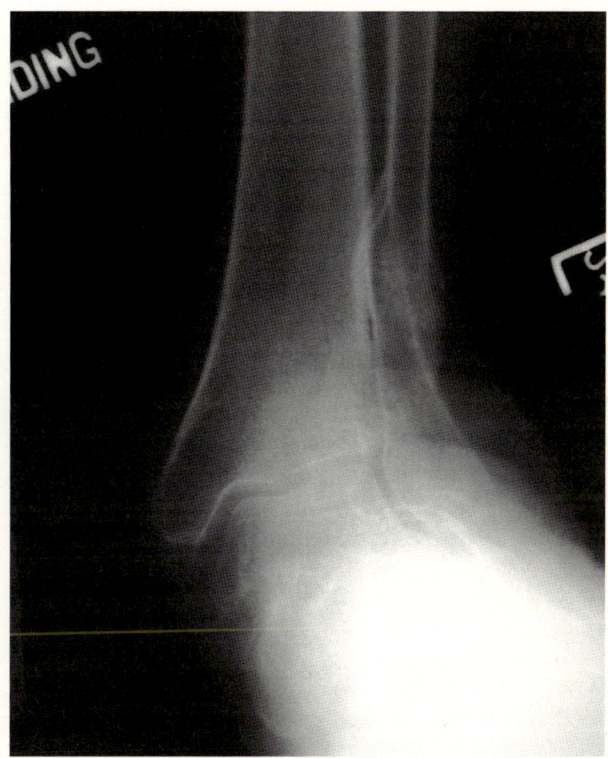

Further categorized into IVa and IVb depending on whether the foot deformity is flexible or fixed respectively, these patients also require treatment of their ankle deformity with deltoid reconstruction, osteotomy, arthroplasty, or arthrodesis. The clinical presentation is similar to either Stage II or III, depending on rigidity of the associated foot deformities. Associated ankle valgus is often difficult to diagnose clinically and is often made on weight-bearing radiographs of the ankle.

Finally, Stage V, defined as end-stage deformity involving a stress fracture of the fibula, was described in 2002 by Schon and Chiodo in unpublished data (Fig. 6.5). This group of patients normally requires corrective ankle osteotomies and/or arthrodesis for treatment of their deformities. Clinically, these are often severely impaired patients whose diagnosis or treatment has been delayed for a variety of reasons, including lack of medical attention, multiple comorbidities including neuropathy, or lack of compliance.

6.5 Management

Earlier recognition of this clinical entity has allowed for successful management with either conservative nonoperative measures alone or in conjunction with joint-sparing reconstructive procedures. Therefore, most patients can be managed without triple arthrodesis and the long-term complications associated with this procedure.

Fig. 6.6 Airlift™ Brace, (DonJoy orthopedics, Vista, CA) designed by the senior author (LS) to limit eversion through use of semirigid plastic shells oriented to match the malleolar axis, a Velcro support strap designed to lift the medial arch, and an adjustable air-bladder for additional arch support and improved fit

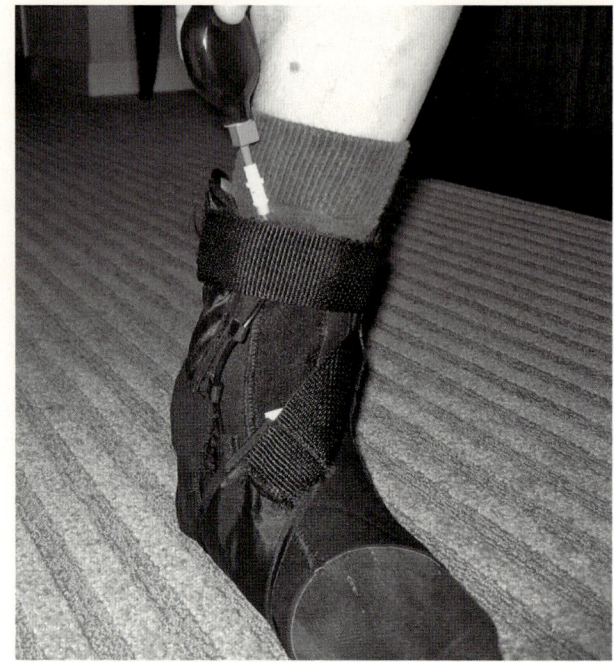

6.5.1 Stage I

For patients who present with Stage I disease, conservative management – including bracing or shoe modification, decrease in intensity or duration of activity, and sometimes physical therapy – can lead to resolution of their symptoms. In our practice, we prescribe an off-the-shelf brace (Airlift™, DonJoy Orthopedics, Vista, CA) which was specifically designed by the senior author (LS) for posterior tibialis tendon dysfunction (Fig. 6.6). The brace limits eversion through use of semirigid plastic shells oriented to match the malleolar axis, a Velcro support strap designed to lift the medial arch, and an adjustable air-bladder for additional arch support and improved fit. Additionally, a camboot can be worn in conjunction with the Airlift™ brace for more strenuous activities. Alternatively, an Arizona brace, articulated ankle foot orthosis, stirrup brace, or standard lace-up brace have all been utilized for treatment of early tendon dysfunction.[21,22] Some patients may obtain relief with a custom foot orthosis designed with a medial longitudinal arch support and posting of the medial heel. In general, however, shoe modification or insoles are not sufficient to alleviate symptoms for patients with advanced tendinopathy.

We typically allow 6 weeks in the brace to assess for clinical improvement. If patients demonstrate resolution of their pain without evidence of hindfoot or midfoot deformity, we continue brace treatment for an additional 6 weeks before gradually weaning them from bracing.

Physical therapy can be initiated once the acute inflammatory phase begins to subside. Goals include reduction of inflammation, and strengthening of the posterior tibialis, FDL, flexor hallucis longus, and gastroc–soleus complex. In addition, if a tight heel-cord is present, Achilles stretching exercises should be instituted to maximize range of motion of the ankle and subtalar joints. Multiple authors have demonstrated good results and high patient satisfaction with a combination of physical therapy and orthoses.[23,24]

For some patients, medial pain persists, despite maintained tendon power and alignment. After 6–12 weeks of conservative management, we consider shock-wave therapy or platelet-rich plasma (PRP) injections for this subgroup of patients. Shock-wave therapy has been demonstrated to induce tenocyte division and activity in vitro[11] and PRP has been shown to be beneficial to tenocytes in in vitro studies via cytokine response (unpublished data). Approximately 70% of our patients demonstrate clinical improvement after PRP injection, thereby avoiding surgical intervention (unpublished data). However, as we have noted a transient increase in pain after PRP injection which normally resolves after 2–6 weeks, we routinely utilize post-injection bracing.

Isolated tenosynovectomy and FDL transfer has been described for operative treatment of these patients. However, literature has demonstrated a significant rate of failure for tendon procedures without correction of preexisting flatfoot deformity.[25] It is our preference to use an adjunctive corrective procedure such as arthroereisis and/or Cotton procedure if a midfoot varus deformity exists. In the rare patient with symmetric bilateral hindfoot valgus, a calcaneal osteotomy may also be necessary. A symptomatic os naviculum may also be addressed with a modified Kidner procedure to advance the posterior tibialis tendon. Concurrent correction of alignment issues allows for the greatest chance of success from tendon transfer.

6.5.2 Stage II

As most operative candidates have Stage II tendon dysfunction, our treatment algorithm and specific considerations reflect the various options available to address the spectrum of deformity within this broad category. Specific surgical protocol is selected after evaluating the patient with regard to several decision-making factors. These factors are listed in Table 6.1, arranged in order of magnitude of importance.

Clinical presentation, the most important factor, involves assessment of pain and swelling of the ankle and medial arch, collapse of the medial longitudinal arch (as documented by "fingometer"), hindfoot valgus, midfoot abduction, and evaluation of posterior tibialis tendon motor function. For example, a patient with severe hindfoot valgus and significant abduction through the midfoot may require lateral column lengthening or double calcaneal osteotomy (medial displacement osteotomy plus lateral column lengthening). Pronounced supination of the midfoot when the hindfoot is corrected to neutral can signify the need for first metatarso-cuneiform fusion, Cotton osteotomy, or rarely naviculo-medial cuneiform fusion for optimal

Table 6.1 Treatment protocol for AAFD – decision-making factors

Factor	Specific examples
Clinical presentation	Location of pain, degree of collapse of medial longitudinal arch, hindfoot valgus, baseline alignment (contralateral), midfoot abduction, posterior tibialis tendon function, rigidity of deformity, range of motion
Radiographic features	*AP*: % of Talonavicular uncoverage, talus-1st MT angle
	Lateral: Talus – 1st MT angle, height of medial column (distance beneath medial cuneiform)
	Documentation of degenerative changes
Special considerations	Obesity, patient compliance, systemic healing factors/ medications
Intraoperative findings	Tendon condition ("springiness"), spring ligament, deltoid ligament, gastroc–soleus contracture, forefoot supination, joint instability/degenerative changes
Surgeon's preference	Comfort with specific procedures, choice of implants, review of outcomes

MT metatarsal

correction. A Strayer procedure versus tendo-Achilles lengthening (TAL) may also be required, depending on exam of the gastroc–soleus complex. Typically, we use a Strayer if the magnitude of equinus contracture is 15° or less. More significant contracture is treated with percutaneous TAL via the Hoke triple cut technique.

Radiographic evaluation, including weight-bearing x-rays and MRI, when indicated, also affects surgical decision-making. Degenerative changes at specific joints, ligamentous involvement or additional tendon dysfunction can dictate isolated arthrodesis or soft tissue procedures. For instance, a patient with medial pain, attenuation of the deltoid ligament on MRI plus lateral tilting of the talus on stress radiographs may be benefited by imbrication of the deltoid ligament as an adjunctive procedure. Talonavicular uncoverage greater than 40% on AP x-ray may signal the need for lateral column lengthening procedure or even talonavicular fusion.

Special considerations include such issues as obesity, patient compliance, and systemic factors which affect healing and soft tissue quality. Diabetes, steroid use, and disease modifying anti-rheumatoid drugs are several indications for which we would alter our treatment regimen. As an example, a morbidly obese, diabetic patient with isolated posterior tibialis dysfunction without deformity may benefit from subtalar arthroereisis in addition to FDL transfer, which may be sufficient to treat a less high-risk patient. Similarly, a patient who may have difficulty complying with weight-bearing restrictions as a result of balance issues or poor physical conditioning may require additional fixation for osteotomies or tendon transfers. PRP obtained from bone marrow aspirate from the iliac crest or calcaneus can also be added for this high-risk patient population. The effect of these factors highlights the importance of having an extensive discussion with each patient regarding risks, potential complications, and expected outcome for each procedure. In some salvage cases, issues such as vascular insufficiency, previous infection, or multiple medical comorbidities may have lead to prolonged nonoperative management until arthrodesis remains as the only treatment option to correct painful, progressive deformity. Each patient should be assessed individually, and such decisions require the input of the patient, their family, and primary care physicians.

Intraoperative findings may also alter the choice of appropriate surgical procedure. Examples of such findings include posterior tibialis tendon quality ("springiness"), condition of the deltoid ligament or spring ligament, equinus contracture or forefoot supination (varus) after correction of hindfoot alignment. In the rare patient with 4+ or 5−/5 tendon strength with minimal deformity, intraoperative confirmation of a "springy," or resilient and non-degenerative posterior tibialis tendon may be treated with debridement and advancement via suture anchor fixation. Attenuation of the deltoid or spring ligament can also be treated with imbrication or advancement with suture anchor placement. Residual equinus contracture can be addressed with TAL or Strayer, depending on the magnitude of the contracture. Finally, supination of the forefoot after hindfoot realignment may require medial column fusion or Cotton osteotomy to correct extension deformity of the first ray.

Surgeon preference represents the last major factor regarding surgical rationale. Familiarity and success with certain procedures, as well as modifications to these procedures will inevitably alter the decision-making process regarding operative treatment. However, it should be emphasized that the treating physician must be able to address all aspects of the deformity to obtain optimal outcomes. Inadequate correction or selection of inappropriate procedure may negatively impact the clinical results from surgery and may increase the likelihood of subsequent salvage procedures including arthrodesis. For instance, isolated FDL transfer without correction of hindfoot malalignment will limit the success of the procedure, thereby limiting available options for subsequent treatment. Our specific preferences, with clinical and radiographic criteria are listed in Table 6.2.

6.5.2.1 Surgical Procedures

As there are an unlimited number of procedures that are used for treatment of flexible flatfoot deformity, only our preferred operative procedures are briefly described below. Surgery is performed under general anesthesia versus intravenous (IV) sedation plus local anesthesia. A thigh tourniquet is applied and preoperative cefazolin or clindamycin is administered prior to incision. We typically begin with the patient in a semi-lateral position with a beanbag, allowing for access to the lateral aspect of the calcaneus for osteotomy, as well as to the ipsilateral iliac crest if bone marrow aspirate is to be performed. Following osteotomy, we release the bean bag, allowing access to the medial aspect of the ankle with external rotation of the operative extremity. We then proceed with FDL transfer and examine the foot for residual supination or equinus. To correct forefoot supination, our preference is to perform a Cotton osteotomy, thereby plantarflexing the first ray. Equinus is addressed with Strayer or TAL, depending on magnitude of deformity and nature of contracture (gastrocnemius alone versus entire gastroc–soleus complex). Arthroereisis may also be performed, depending on the operative indications and specific considerations discussed previously.

Table 6.2 Operative protocol with radiographic and clinical criteria

Operative procedures	AP X-ray criteria		Lateral X-ray criteria	Clinical heel valgus clinical exam
	T-N uncoverage (%)	AT1MTA	LT1MTA	
Isolated FDL transfer	<20	<15°	<10°	<5° valgus, <5° side-to-side difference, able to invert 20° beyond midline
FDL Tx, subtalar arthroereisis	20–30	<20°	<10°	<5° valgus, able to invert 20° beyond midline, obesity or other systemic factor
FDL Tx, MDCO	20–40	<35°	<20°	<20° valgus, <10° side-to-side difference, unable to invert beyond midline
FDL Tx, MDCO, subtalar arthroereisis	<40	<40°	<25°	<20° valgus, <10° side-to-side difference, obesity, or other systemic factor
FDL Tx, Evans' LCL	40–50	<50°	<25°	>20° valgus, unable to invert beyond midline
FDL Tx, Calcaneo-cuboid LCL	>50	>50°	>25°	>20° valgus, unable to invert beyond midline
FDL Tx, MDCO, Evans' LCL[a]	>50	>50°	>25°	>20° valgus, unable to invert beyond midline

T-N Talonavicular, AT1MTA AP Talo-1st MT angle, LT1MTA Lateral Talo-1st MT angle, FDL flexor digitorum longus, MDCO medial displacement calcaneal osteotomy, LCL Lateral column lengthening

[a]Preferred over calcaneo-cuboid lateral column lengthening, fusion procedures if inadequate correction

Fig. 6.7 Intraoperative image demonstrating location of medial displacement calcaneal osteotomy

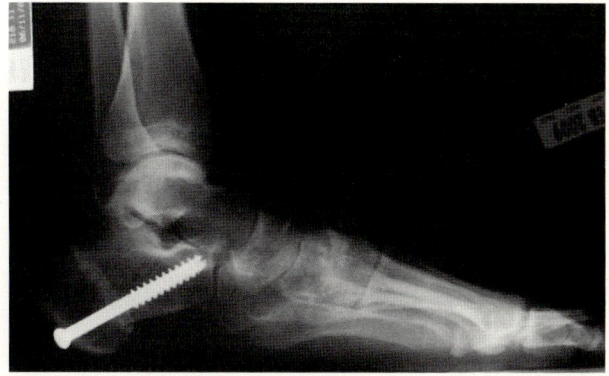

Post-operatively, we splint the extremity in approximately 20° of plantar flexion if FDL transfer was performed. Weight-bearing is not permitted for 6 weeks to allow for consolidation of osteotomies and incorporation of the tendon transfer. After the initial postoperative dressing is removed and sutures are removed, a cam-boot is applied, also in 20° of plantar flexion for an additional 4 weeks. However, we allow active dorsiflexion/plantar flexion as well as inversion with range-of-motion exercises against gravity, but not against resistance. The patient is cautioned to avoid dorsiflexion beyond 20° from neutral and eversion is avoided. The ankle is brought to neutral at the 6-week follow-up visit and we begin progressive weight-bearing at that time. Overall, however, each patient is counseled that 3 months are required for 75% of maximal healing, 6 months are required for 90% of healing, and that often 1 year is required for maximal rehabilitation.

Medial Displacement Calcaneal Osteotomy (MDCO)

Through an oblique calcaneal osteotomy performed proximal to the Achilles insertion (Fig. 6.7), our goals are to realign the axis of the hindfoot, provide inversion power through medial shift of the Achilles insertion, and restore the medial longitudinal arch. We obtain 1 cm of medial translation, and perform a "crush-plasty" of the prominent lateral cortex to optimize bony apposition and restore the contour of the calcaneus.[26] Fixation is achieved with one or two 6.5-mm or 7.3-mm cannulated partially threaded cancellous screws, with all threads passed beyond the osteotomy site.

FDL Transfer

The FDL transfer remains the optimal choice for supplementation or replacement of posterior tibialis function. Anatomic proximity and ease of transfer have led to reliably successful outcomes, although the flexor hallucis longus and peroneus brevis are also viable options.[27,28] We rarely perform the tendon transfer in isolation, as correction of alignment ensures maximal benefit and longevity of the repair.

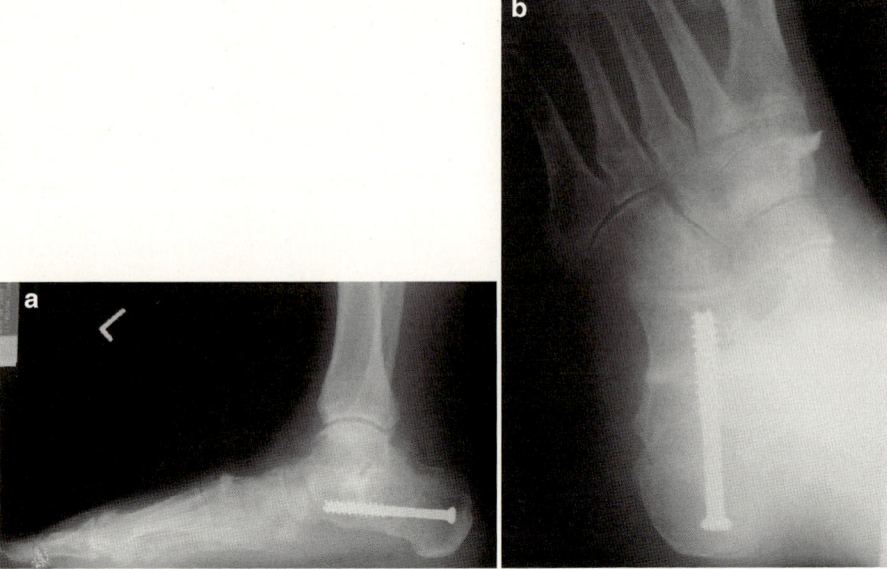

Fig. 6.8 Radiographic appearance of incorporated graft following Hintermann modification of Evans' lateral column lengthening procedure. The osteotomy is performed just anterior to the posterior facet of the calcaneus, and a femoral head allograft soaked in platelet-rich plasma is utilized to maintain lengthening. (**a**) Lateral view, (**b**) anteroposterior view

A whipstitch is placed in the FDL tendon after harvest and an interference screw is used to fix the FDL in the bone tunnel within the naviculum under appropriate tension. The tendon is additionally secured to the posterior tibialis insertion and joint capsule to further reinforce fixation. We do not routinely excise the posterior tibialis tendon; we have obtained good resolution of pain and restoration of strength with adequate debridement of degenerative tendon, correction of malalignment, and structural reinforcement with FDL transfer. Use of an interference screw allows for a less extensive FDL dissection and more proximal harvest; if the surgeon intends to suture the tendon onto itself, the FDL should be harvested at or distal to the knot of Henry in the midfoot. The transfer is tensioned prior to fixation to obtain approximately 15° of plantar flexion and 15° of inversion.

Lateral Column Lengthening

Due to the associated morbidity of these procedures, including lateral column overload and restriction of subtalar range of motion,[29] we tend to reserve these procedures for severe cases, with uncoverage of 40–50%. If performed, we utilize Hintermann's modification of the Evans procedure, with our osteotomy placed just anterior to the posterior facet (Fig. 6.8).[30] Clinically, when compared to more distal osteotomy between the middle and anterior facets,[31] we have found better graft incorporation, less restriction of subtalar motion, and less incidence of calcaneo-cuboid sublux-ation. Regardless of which technique is used, care is taken to preserve the sural nerve which can be encountered during the surgical approach. In our practice, lateral col-umn lengthening is only performed if the medial displacement calcaneal osteotomy does not provide adequate correction intraoperatively. Our preference is to perform the double calcaneal osteotomy as opposed to isolated lateral column procedures. In general, femoral neck allograft soaked in bone marrow–derived PRP is used for both structural and biologic benefits. It should be noted that severe midfoot abduction (>50% talonavicular uncoverage) may require fusion procedures as lateral column lengthening may be insufficient to correct this magnitude of deformity.

Cotton Osteotomy

If residual supination of the forefoot remains after tendon transfer and calcaneal osteotomy, our preference is to perform a dorsal opening wedge osteotomy of the medial cuneiform (Fig. 6.9). A dorsomedial incision is made overlying the medial cuneiform, carefully avoiding the medial branch of the dorsal cutaneous nerve. The extensor hallucis longus (EHL) is retracted laterally, and dorsal capsule and a small portion of tibialis anterior insertion is lifted in a sub-periosteal fashion to expose the osteotomy site. An approximately 7-mm wedge-shaped graft is prepared from a femoral head allograft after the osteotomy is made. Typically, we do not use internal fixation for the graft, as the graft is quite stable after insertion of the graft within the osteotomy.

Arthroereisis

As shown in a biomechanical study, the addition of arthroereisis to medial displace-ment calcaneal osteotomy (MDCO) and FDL transfer provided additional correc-tion in a severe flatfoot model.[32] In our practice, it is performed for patients with more significant deformity, obesity, or certain comorbidities such as diabetes or steroid use. We utilize the ProStop® (Arthrex, Naples, FL) arthroereisis implant which was designed by the senior author (LS). Its benefits include a conical design, availability of multiple diameters and lengths, and ease of insertion. Since we began using the implant, our incidence of removal due to implant pain has been reduced from 40% to less than 15% (unpublished data). Results from subtalar arthroereisis have been promising, with high levels of patient satisfaction, although implant removal for pain issues has been reported as a common complication.[33,34]

The implant is inserted via a 1.5-cm lateral incision overlying the sinus tarsi. Under c-arm visualization, the guide-wire is placed through the interval between the posterior and middle facets of the talus. The appropriate cannulated trial is inserted beneath the lateral one-half of the talar neck and subtalar range of motion is exam-ined. Care is taken to avoid excessive limitation of subtalar motion; the implant is intended to block eversion and medial and plantar rotation of the talus, typically

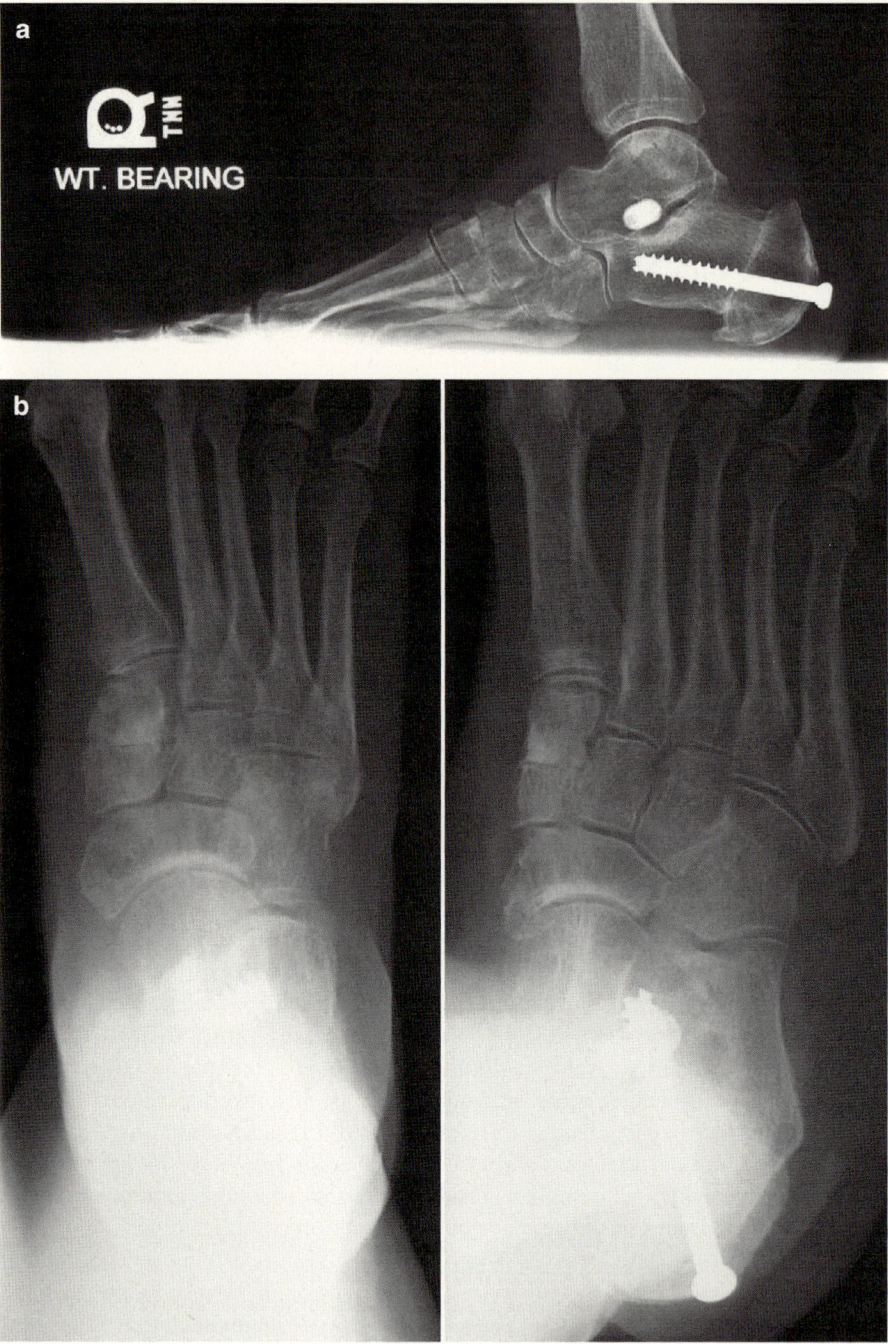

Fig. 6.9 Cotton osteotomy-dorsal opening wedge osteotomy of the medial cuneiform to correct residual forefoot supination after AAFD correction. (**a**) Lateral radiograph with femoral head allograft wedge in place. (**b**) AP and oblique radiographs

Fig. 6.10 Subtalar arthroereisis. Lateral radiographic image demonstrating arthroereisis with implant placed in sinus tarsi between the posterior and middle facets

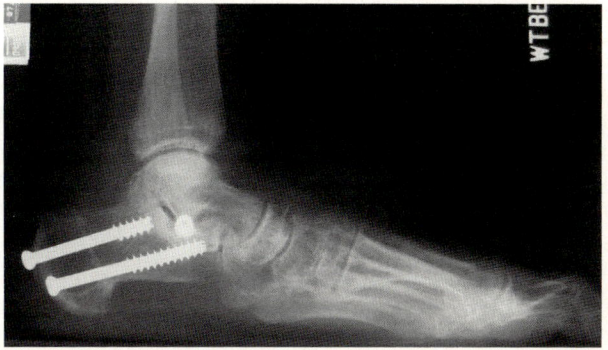

with 5–10° of residual hindfoot valgus. Our goal with this procedure is to allow for eversion that is symmetric to the unaffected, contralateral extremity. The final implant is inserted, the guide-wire is removed, and optimal position is again confirmed with c-arm (Fig. 6.10).

To date, there are no published prospective randomized studies regarding operative treatment for AAFD. Much of the literature is retrospective in nature, but does demonstrate good clinical results with a combination of bony and soft tissue reconstructive procedures. For example, for FDL transfer and medial displacement calcaneal osteotomy, the senior author (LS) demonstrated a 97% rate of pain relief, and 94% improvement in function in 129 patients.[35] Other authors have demonstrated similar outcomes from this combination of procedures.[36-38] There are no large outcome studies for more complex reconstruction protocols, and in our practice, individualized treatment is performed on a patient-specific basis according to our described treatment protocol.

6.5.3 Stage III

If a rigid deformity of the hindfoot exists, joint salvage procedures and tendon transfers are not indicated. For these cases, a triple arthrodesis is performed. It should be noted that proper alignment must be achieved with articular cartilage debridement and occasionally, osteotomies prior to fixation. As the positioning from a hindfoot fusion is permanent, alignment must be carefully considered. For example, in a female patient with a wide-pelvis gait and contralateral valgus heel, the hindfoot should be fused in appropriate valgus alignment to avoid excessive functional supination of the foot and lateral column overload during gait. This overload occurs due to the cyclical central to lateral shift in center of gravity which occurs during gait. As this shift can no longer be dissipated by subtalar range of motion, compensatory aberrant motion occurs between the foot–ground interface leading to functional supination. This phenomenon is manifested by excessive lateral heel breakdown in their footwear. Therefore, for these patients, the hindfoot should be positioned in comparable valgus alignment as the contralateral limb, with care taken to avoid subfibular impingement.

It is our practice to perform a calcaneo-cuboid sparing modified triple arthrodesis for these patients. Unless there is preexisting arthrosis at this joint, the minimal motion which remains may spare the lateral column and can protect against progressive degeneration of the four to five metatarso-cuboid articulations. With modern internal fixation techniques, nonunion is less of a concern, and we have noted good clinical results, without compromise of our fusion rates.

6.5.4 Stage IV and V

These patients represent a difficult population with complex deformities. As stated previously, proximal ankle deformity must be addressed with osteotomy, arthroplasty, or arthrodesis, and the hindfoot deformity frequently requires arthrodesis for optimal surgical outcomes for these patients. Preoperative discussion regarding the guarded nature of the outcomes from surgery and progressive degeneration of adjacent joints is crucial. Published data regarding the outcomes from operative treatment of these patients is sparse, and long-term follow-up on large cohorts is unavailable.

Adult acquired flatfoot deformity is a complex disorder with a broad spectrum of associated pathology and clinical presentation. The importance of early diagnosis and institution of conservative and operative treatment enables us to minimize pain, deformity, and dysfunction. Optimal surgical treatment requires utilization of a protocol involving a combination of soft tissue and bony procedures, tailored to address specific elements of pathology. Whenever possible, the goal of surgery should be to preserve joint motion, restore mechanical alignment, repair ligament integrity, and reestablish tendon function.

References

1. Key JA. Partial rupture of the tendon of the posterior tibial muscle. J Bone Joint Surg Am. 1953;35-A(4):1006-8.
2. Pell RF, Myerson MS, Schon LC. Clinical outcome after primary triple arthrodesis. J Bone Joint Surg Am. 2000;82(1):47-57.
3. Coetzee JC, Hansen ST. Surgical management of severe deformity resulting from posterior tibial tendon dysfunction. Foot Ankle Int. 2001;22(12):944-9.
4. Saltzman CL, Fehrle MJ, Cooper RR, Spencer EC, Ponseti IV. Triple arthrodesis: twenty-five and forty-four-year average follow-up of the same patients. J Bone Joint Surg Am. 1999;81(10):1391-402.
5. Deland J, de Asla R, Sung I-H, Ernberg L, Potter H. Posterior tibial tendon insufficiency: which ligaments are involved? Foot Ankle Int. 2005;26(6):427-35.
6. Niki H, Ching RP, Kiser P, Sangeorzan BJ. The effect of posterior tibial tendon dysfunction on hindfoot kinematics. Foot Ankle Int. 2001;22(4):292-300.

7. Van Boerum D, Sangeorzan B. Biomechanics and pathophysiology of flat foot. Foot Ankle Clin. 2003;8(3):419-30.

8. Supple KM, Hanft JR, Murphy BJ, Janecki CJ, Kogler GF. Posterior tibial tendon dysfunction. Semin Arthritis Rheum. 1992;22(2):106-13.

9. Petersen W, Hohmann G. Collagenous fibril texture of the gliding zone of the human tibialis posterior tendon. Foot Ankle Int. 2001;22(2):126-32.

10. Petersen W, Hohmann G, Stein V, Tillmann B. The blood supply of the posterior tibial tendon. J Bone Joint Surg Br. 2002;84(1):141-4.

11. Han S, Lee J, Guyton G, Parks B, Courneya J-P, Schon L. J. Leonard Goldner Award 2008. Effect of extracorporeal shock wave therapy on cultured tenocytes. Foot Ankle Int. 2009;30(2):93-8.

12. Sullivan JA. Pediatric flatfoot: evaluation and management. J Am Acad Orthop Surg. 1999;7(1):44-53.

13. Myerson M, Solomon G, Shereff M. Posterior tibial tendon dysfunction: its association with seronegative inflammatory disease. Foot Ankle. 1989;9(5):219-25.

14. Holmes GB, Mann RA. Possible epidemiological factors associated with rupture of the posterior tibial tendon. Foot Ankle. 1992;13(2):70-9.

15. Beals TC, Pomeroy GC, Manoli A. Posterior tibial tendon insufficiency: diagnosis and treatment. J Am Acad Orthop Surg. 1999;7(2):112-8.

16. Pinney S, Lin S. Current concept review: acquired adult flatfoot deformity. Foot Ankle Int. 2006;27(1):66-75.

17. Johnson K, Strom D. Tibialis posterior tendon dysfunction. Clin Orthop Relat Res. 1989;239:196-206.

18. Deland J. Adult-acquired flatfoot deformity. J Am Acad Orthop Surg. 2008;16(7):399-406.

19. Bluman E, Title C, Myerson M. Posterior tibial tendon rupture: a refined classification system. Foot Ankle Clin. 2007;12(2):233-49, v.

20. Myerson M. Adult acquired flatfoot deformity. J Bone Joint Surg Am. 1996;78:780-90.

21. Chao W, Wapner K, Lee T, Adams J, Hecht P. Nonoperative management of posterior tibial tendon dysfunction. Foot Ankle Int. 1996;17(12):736-41.

22. Augustin J, Lin S, Berberian W, Johnson J. Nonoperative treatment of adult acquired flat foot with the Arizona brace. Foot Ankle Clin. 2003;8(3):491-502.

23. Alvarez R, Marini A, Schmitt C, Saltzman C. Stage I and II posterior tibial tendon dysfunction treated by a structured nonoperative management protocol: an orthosis and exercise program. Foot Ankle Int. 2006;27(1):2-8.

24. Lin J, Balbas J, Richardson EG. Results of non-surgical treatment of stage II posterior tibial tendon dysfunction: a 7–10-year followup. Foot Ankle Int. 2008;29(8):781-6.

25. Teasdall RD, Johnson KA. Surgical treatment of stage I posterior tibial tendon dysfunction. Foot Ankle Int. 1994;15(12):646-8.

26. Schon LC. Crush-plasty of the calcaneus. Tech Orthop. 1996;11(3):222-3.

27. Sammarco GJ, Hockenbury RT. Treatment of stage II posterior tibial tendon dysfunction with flexor hallucis longus transfer and medial displacement calcaneal osteotomy. Foot Ankle Int. 2001;22(4):305-12.

28. Song SJ, Deland JT. Outcome following addition of peroneus brevis tendon transfer to treatment of acquired posterior tibial tendon insufficiency. Foot Ankle Int. 2001;22(4):301-4.

29. Tien T, Parks B, Guyton G. Plantar pressures in the forefoot after lateral column lengthening: a cadaver study comparing the Evans osteotomy and calcaneocuboid fusion. Foot Ankle Int. 2005;26(7):520-5.

30. Hintermann B, Valderrabano V, Kundert HP. Lengthening of the lateral column and reconstruction of the medial soft tissue for treatment of acquired flatfoot deformity associated with insufficiency of the posterior tibial tendon. Foot Ankle Int. 1999;20(10):622-9.

31. Evans D. Calcaneo-valgus deformity. J Bone Joint Surg Br. 1975;57(3):270-8.

32. Vora A, Tien T, Parks B, Schon L. Correction of moderate and severe acquired flexible flatfoot with medializing calcaneal osteotomy and flexor digitorum longus transfer. J Bone Joint Surg Am. 2006;88(8):1726-34.

33. Viladot R, Pons M, Alvarez F, Omaa J. Subtalar arthroereisis for posterior tibial tendon dysfunction: a preliminary report. Foot Ankle Int. 2003;24(8):600-6.
34. Needleman R. A surgical approach for flexible flatfeet in adults including a subtalar arthroereisis with the MBA sinus tarsi implant. Foot Ankle Int. 2006;27(1):9-18.
35. Myerson M, Badekas A, Schon L. Treatment of stage II posterior tibial tendon deficiency with flexor digitorum longus tendon transfer and calcaneal osteotomy. Foot Ankle Int. 2004;25(7):445-50.
36. Brodsky J. Preliminary gait analysis results after posterior tibial tendon reconstruction: a prospective study. Foot Ankle Int. 2004;25(2):96-100.
37. Fayazi A, Nguyen H-V, Juliano P. Intermediate term follow-up of calcaneal osteotomy and flexor digitorum longus transfer for treatment of posterior tibial tendon dysfunction. Foot Ankle Int. 2002;23(12):1107-11.
38. Guyton GP, Jeng C, Krieger LE, Mann RA. Flexor digitorum longus transfer and medial displacement calcaneal osteotomy for posterior tibial tendon dysfunction: a middle-term clinical follow-up. Foot Ankle Int. 2001;22(8):627-32.

Chapter 7
Cavus Foot

Sig T. Hansen Jr.

Cavus foot is not a diagnosis, but simply a description. It is as generic as its essential opposite – planus foot (pes planus), commonly known as "flatfoot." Just as "flatfoot" can vary from a quite normal and totally asymptomatic low-arched foot with normal sagittal alignment relative to the ankle, a high-arched foot also can be well aligned and relatively asymptomatic although it is usually a bit stiffer than a low-arched foot. "Flatfoot" can be accompanied by varying degrees of heel valgus and forefoot abduction and eventually the malalignment overpowers the posterior tibial tendon and the medial ligaments, making the foot markedly symptomatic. In its later stages, dorsolateral peritalar subluxation defines the deformity in relation to the stable position of the talus. Similarly, a cavus foot can be accompanied by various degrees of varus. The peroneus brevis may be overpowered, and the lateral foot and ankle ligaments may be stretched or become incompetent. The position of the foot then can be called plantar-medial peritalar subluxation. This describes the local anatomic deformity which is much more commonly called a cavovarus foot.[1]

Cavus foot certainly can occur without varus, but this involves a different muscle imbalance. Again, in contrast to a collapsing arch in flatfoot, virtually always caused by an overpowering triceps surae (most often gastrocnemius equinus, which is as much increased tone as actual contracture), a cavus foot, either calcaneocavus (as in meningomyelocoel) or global cavus, is generally associated with a weak or paralyzed triceps surae muscle and often intact long toe flexors. Usually the toe extensors and even the anterior tibialis and peroneus tertius are intact. The cavovarus foot usually has an overpowering posterior tibial tendon and/or peroneus longus muscle.

S.T. Hansen Jr., B.A., M.D.
Department of Orthopaedics (and Sports Medicine),
Harborview Medical Center, STH Foot and Ankle Institute,
325 9th Ave., 98104 Seattle, WA, USA
e-mail: hansetmd@u.washington.edu

A. Saxena (ed.), *Special Procedures in Foot and Ankle Surgery*,
DOI 10.1007/978-1-4471-4103-7_7, © Springer-Verlag London 2013

Early in my training, I was told "you must never lengthen a heel cord in a cavus foot." Certainly, this applies to the calcaneocavus and global cavus foot but not necessarily to a cavovarus foot, particularly a subtle one that causes frequent sprains and in which we often see gastrocnemius equinus as a secondary aggravating or predisposing condition to the chronic instability. There are, in addition to the muscle balance problems described, intrinsic bony deformities in many of these feet. These deformities may have been caused by subtle or significant muscle imbalance during growth. In other cases, a degree of bony deformity may be intrinsic to the bone or the cause is not clear. Regardless of cause, bony deformity nearly always must be corrected by osteotomy or fusion during treatment of a symptomatic cavus foot.[1-4]

With that introduction, it is surely apparent that the key to treating cavus deformities is in doing a very complete and accurate muscle examination of all the muscles affecting or residing in the foot. Ligament integrity or contracture and the plantar fascia must be assessed and functional weight-bearing x-rays obtained to assess bony deformities. Computed tomography (CT) scans occasionally may be helpful if coalitions or subtalar arthrosis are suspected, but magnetic resonance imaging (MRI) is rarely helpful. As has been recommended for years, a thorough spine and neurologic examination also should be done to see if there is a neurologically driven muscle imbalance perhaps from a tethered cord or another neurologic problem.

7.1 Muscles to Be Examined, Grade 1–5

7.1.1 Gastrocsoleus (Triceps Surae)

Test for strength by doing a heel raise.

Test for contracture of the gastroc and soleus with Silverskjold test. In this instance, the foot is locked in exact neutral position and tested for passive dorsiflexion with the knee bent and the knee straight. All the patient's muscles must be relaxed. This muscle is the antagonist of the anterior tibialis, the peroneus tertius, and body weight.

7.1.2 Anterior Tibialis

Test for strength and range. It is both a dorsiflexor and an inverter as well as an antagonist of the triceps surae and the peroneus longus.

7.1.3 Peroneus Tertius

This muscle is a lateral dorsiflexor. Test for strength and presence, as about 10% may be missing this tendon and replaced by the extensor digitorum longus (EDL). The intrinsic flexors have to stabilize the toes when the EDL acts to help with ankle dorsiflexion.

7.1.4 Extensor Hallucis Longus

This is an extrinsic great toe extensor. Test for strength and range and note if it is recruited when the ankle dorsiflexors are tested. It may cause a cock-up great toe if it overpowers the intrinsics.

7.1.5 Extensor Digitorum Longus

This is the extrinsic lesser toe extensor and must be tested for strength and range. Note if it is recruited for ankle extension when the anterior tibialis is weak or the gastrocnemius is tight as this can cause extensor claw toes. If the intrinsic flexors are overpowered or denervated, as in diabetes, or locally destroyed, as in rheumatoid arthritis, severe extensor claw toes will be present.

7.1.6 Posterior Tibial Tendon

On the flexor side, this tendon is a crucial muscle in the foot and is often very powerful in cavovarus. It is an inverter and internal rotator of the foot on the ankle. Test for strength and range, including the ability to passively move the foot into abduction and external rotation. In other words, watch for contractures in cavovarus foot caused by deep posterior compartment syndrome. Its antagonists are the peroneus brevis, functionally the triceps surae, and body weight.

7.1.7 Flexor Hallucis Longus

Test for strength and range. Flexibility is very important. It is tested largely to make sure that it is a good potential muscle to transfer in cavovarus foot. It can replace or augment the triceps surae in calcaneocavus and can replace the peroneus brevis in cavovarus.

7.1.8 Flexor Digitorum Longus

Test for strength and range. Look for extrinsic contractures if it is recruited as a plantar flexor in calcaneocavus. It is a potential replacement for the posterior tibialis if the posterior tibialis has to be moved to become a dorsolateral extensor in partial paralytic cavovarus. It may be contracted in old deep posterior compartmental syndrome, which can present as cavovarus.

7.1.9   Peroneus Brevis

In the lateral compartment, the peroneus brevis should be tested for strength and presence. Isolate the testing to pure eversion or external rotation of the foot not allowing long peroneal function, which plantar flexes the first ray to augment it. The peroneus brevis is a critical test because absence of the peroneus brevis alone can cause cavovarus foot. This muscle is usually very weak in Charcot-Marie-Tooth disease.

7.1.10   Peroneus Longus

Test for strength and range. It is usually surprisingly strong in cavovarus and its plantar flexing force on the first ray (medial column) against its antagonist, the anterior tibial tendon, can produce a plantar-flexed first metatarsal, a secondary cause of hindfoot varus and a cavovarus foot. This is tested by having the patient independently flex the first metatarsal, pushing the first metatarsal head down strongly with the foot in the everted position. When it is overactive or overpowering, there may be a callus under the first metatarsal or, in sensory neuropathy, even an ulcer under the first metatarsal head.

7.2   Evaluation of Ligaments and Plantar Fascia

This generally is done by manipulating the foot with the patient totally relaxed and assessing contracture vs. instability in various ligaments. For example, in flatfoot, the medial column is often very supple and unstable and when loaded under the first metatarsal head, the plantar fascia can be tightened so that passive dorsiflexion of the great toe is impossible.

In a cavovarus foot, the medial column may be quite unyielding in its plantar-flexed or adducted position, indicating contracture of the intact plantar fascia, the anterior deltoid, the spring ligament, the long plantar ligament, the medial capsule of the talonavicular joint, etc. It may be unstable in the lateral collateral ligaments of the ankle.

7.3   Bony Evaluation

Weight-bearing x-rays must be taken with the knee straight. That is, the patient should allow the foot to settle into its normal standing position. Anteroposterior (AP) and oblique x-ray views of the foot may be taken in the same position, although we rarely use the oblique view. If deformities are severe, AP and mortise ankle views should also be taken with weight-bearing to see if early tilting and/or narrowing of the joint is present.

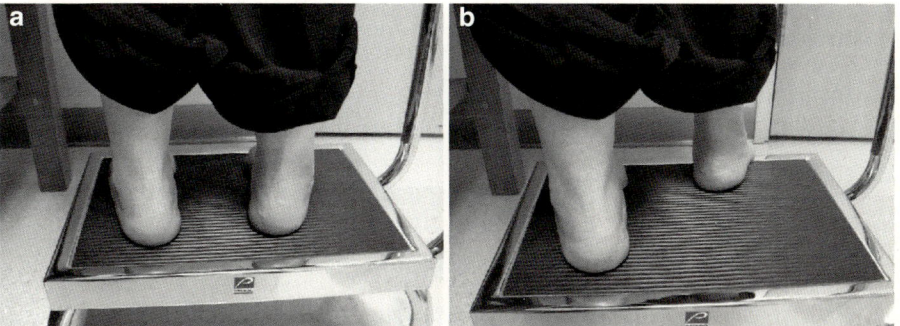

Fig. 7.1 (**a**) Coleman block test showing heel varus. (**b**) Coleman block test of right foot showing plantar-flexed first ray (forefoot driven heel varus) that allows eversion of the heel when forefoot is off-loaded (Photo courtesy of Amol Saxena, DPM)

Finally, a weight-bearing lateral view should be taken with the foot placed appropriately on a Coleman block. In other words, the patient stands on a one-half to three-quarter inch board under the heel and lateral foot and toes while the great toe and perhaps the second toe metatarsal heads drop down to the floor over the medial side of the block. This reveals the flexibility of the hindfoot and the degree of fixed plantar flexion in the medial column.[5,6]

In looking at the lateral view, the surgeon should look first at the amount of opening or closing in the sinus tarsi to see whether the hindfoot is in pronation or supination. A weight-bearing axial view of the heel both in natural stance and on a Coleman block is also helpful for giving a good measure of the amount of heel varus and hindfoot flexibility (Fig. 7.1). Sometimes the heel is quite curved into varus; at other times, it is just aligned in varus. The opening in the sinus tarsi seen on the lateral view indicates whether the varus is secondary to supination of the hindfoot.

After the initial physical evaluation, it is important to take a history of symptoms and disability. Of special interest is a family history of Charcot-Marie-Tooth disease, etc., any neurologic disease or infection such as polio or fracture, and diagnosis or classification of the deformity. From that, a treatment plan should be easily formulated.

7.4 Varieties of Cavus

There are many varieties of cavus, as we will see. Most are uncommon, but subtle cavovarus is very common. This is probably why it is often overlooked and sometimes even considered to be a "normal" foot. In fact, if initiated by an injury and/or abetted by gastrocnemius equinus, it can be the underlying cause of chronic ankle instability which is in my practice the single most common cause of end-stage ankle arthritis. Unfortunately, it is often just called osteoarthrosis and no etiologic factor for this is thought to be needed. However, the ankle is very resistant to arthrosis due

Fig. 7.2 Calcaneo-Cavus
(not the more severe variety
often seen in myelo-
Meningocoel patients)

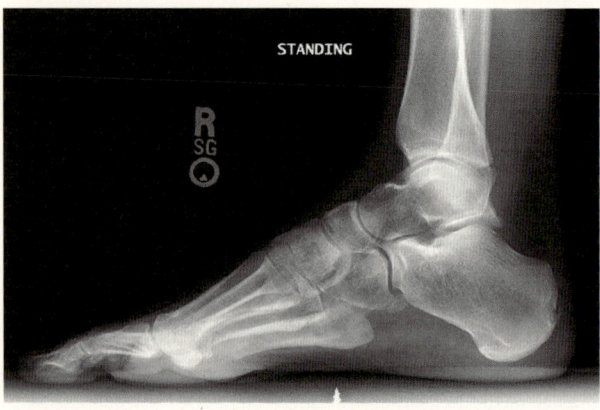

to overuse and no other cause. In my opinion, there is always a cause, be it a subtle injury to the bone itself or to the ligaments. Clearly, in subtle varus, the injury may be an ankle sprain that does not get well because of the increased stress on the lateral support structures in varus. This goes on to chronic instability and eventually over many years to severe degenerative arthritis. With this background, we will look at the varieties of cavus foot.

7.4.1 Calcaneocavus

This type of cavus is rare except in meningomyelocele clinic, where it is fairly common. It features a very high-arched foot usually in a good frontal plane alignment but this can be variable. The essential lesion is absence of muscle innervation below L-5 giving no power to the triceps surae. The lack of plantar flexion power in the ankle/hindfoot results in a very high calcaneal pitch angle and there is no pushoff by the forefoot.

Other muscles are variable, but the anterior tibialis and toe extensors are often present and occasionally the long toe flexors.

Treatment should include a calcaneal osteotomy at an obliquity that brings the heel proximal and back, lengthening its lever arm. Then a motor must be provided by some other active muscle. This often is done by transferring the anterior tibialis back through the interosseous membrane into the heel cord and using the toe extensors as ankle dorsiflexors. The long toe flexors, if present, are also put into the heel cord. If the long peroneal is present, it makes an excellent plantar flexor. If medial and lateral stability is needed, a fusion of the talonavicular joint or a midfoot or hindfoot fusion can be carried out as well (Fig. 7.2).

7.4.2 Global Cavus

This is possibly a subtle variant of calcaneocavus with no varus or valgus deformity but often with a high calcaneal pitch. More striking is a very high arch with the apex in the mid-tarsus, usually a tight plantar fascia. The long toe flexors are strong and the triceps surae is somewhat weak. The toe extensors are often strong and the anterior tib is a bit weak and extensor claw toes are present.

This is the cavus foot that is best treated by a mid-tarsal dorsal closing wedge osteotomy and balancing the muscle forces to increase triceps surae strength by inserting long toe flexors into the heel cord. The proximal plantar fascia is resected to help flatten out the foot and possibly the toe extensors are recessed to the midfoot level into the peroneus tertius and/or the anterior tibial tendons. Girdlestone-flexor to extensor transfers can be done, motored by the Quadratus plantae muscle, also called appropriately here the Flexor Accessorius Muscle.

The dorsal wedge osteotomy is a little tricky because the plantar apex of the wedge is low in the cuboid and the medial column has no low area. The cuts on the medial side do not actually converge completely if the osteotomy is done correctly and the foot is properly balanced and aligned in the two columns. The osteotomy can be stabilized by small plates placed medial and lateral and a couple of shear-resistant screws. It is quite stable in a cast for the 10 weeks of healing time (Fig. 7.3).

7.4.3   First Ray Cavus

This type of foot is quite common and the most likely to be symptomatic, particularly recurrent sprains. It often is seen with subtle varus either by itself or in association with a mild or even moderate intrinsic varus heel.

The first ray cavus can be either dynamic or fixed and may present either with or without intrinsic heel varus. The dynamic variety, by definition, has an overpowering or overactive long peroneal. When the muscle is relaxed, the metatarsal heads are fairly level although the first metatarsal head may have more callus. As the patient is asked to slowly plantar flex the forefoot, the first metatarsal drives down strongly and separately from the remainder of the forefoot. The problem may or may not be associated with findings or symptoms in the hindfoot. It is most serious in diabetic neuropathy, where it can cause a plantar ulcer under the metatarsal head. Fortunately, treatment is simple as the long peroneal can simply be divided as in an older diabetic or transferred to the peroneus brevis in a younger patient or when the overpull of the long peroneal was in compensation for a weak peroneus brevis.

The second variety, the fixed plantar-flexed first ray, is the more difficult problem. It is the deformity that is unmasked by the Coleman block test as the secondary hindfoot varus will straighten out when the first metatarsal is let down off the block. If the hindfoot goes all the way to slight valgus and the sinus tarsi closes down to the normal 7- or 8-mm opening with the hindfoot and midfoot now normal on the lateral x-ray view, the problem can be fixed by a dorsal closing wedge (extension) osteotomy at the base of the metatarsal. My preference is a dorsal closing wedge fusion through the first TMT Joint (Fig. 7.4). Any other muscle imbalance, e.g., gastroc equinus, extensor recruitment, intrinsic-minus toes, must be picked up on physical exam and should be treated at the same time.

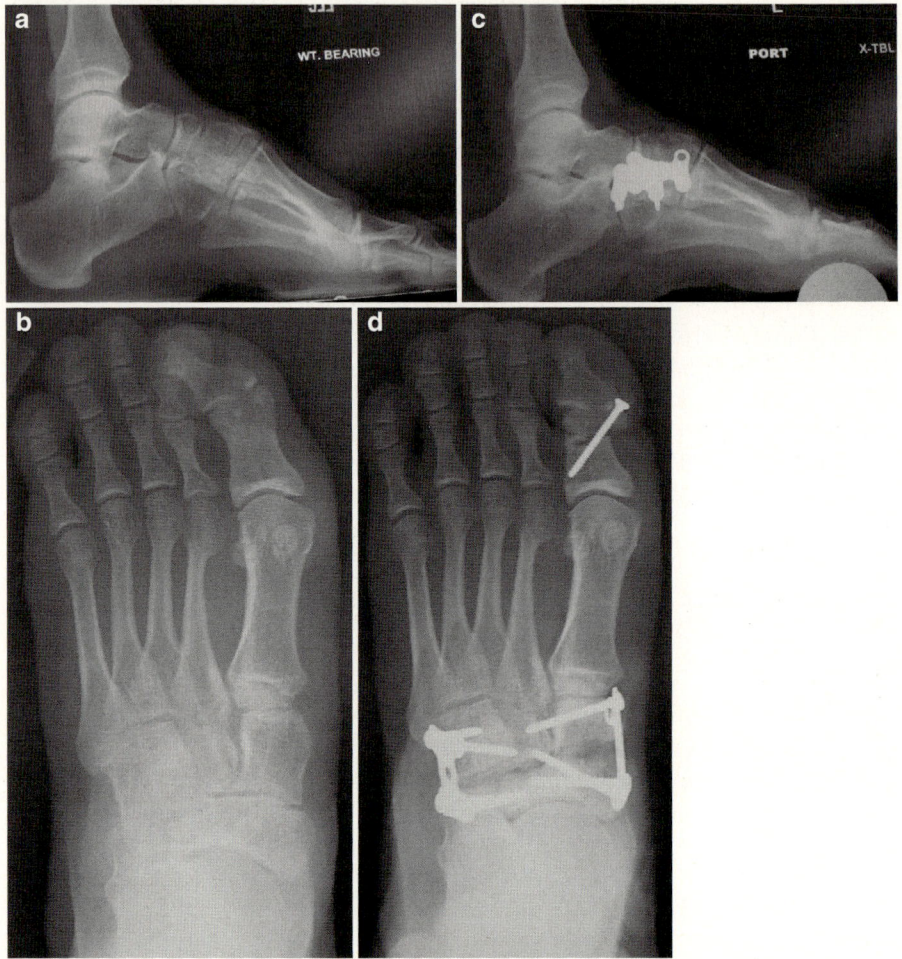

Fig. 7.3 Global cavus: (**a, b**) pre-op; (**c, d**) post-op

This kind of foot may be seen in old polio deformity with a weak anterior tibialis relative to the peroneus longus and also when the peroneus brevis has been damaged and the peroneus longus has attempted to compensate.

7.4.4 Cavovarus Foot

This term describes the foot most often seen in Charcot-Marie-Tooth disease, in which there is a plantar-flexed first metatarsal and occasionally a medial lesser metatarsal and a varus heel which may be intrinsic or secondary to posterior tibialis-induced supination.

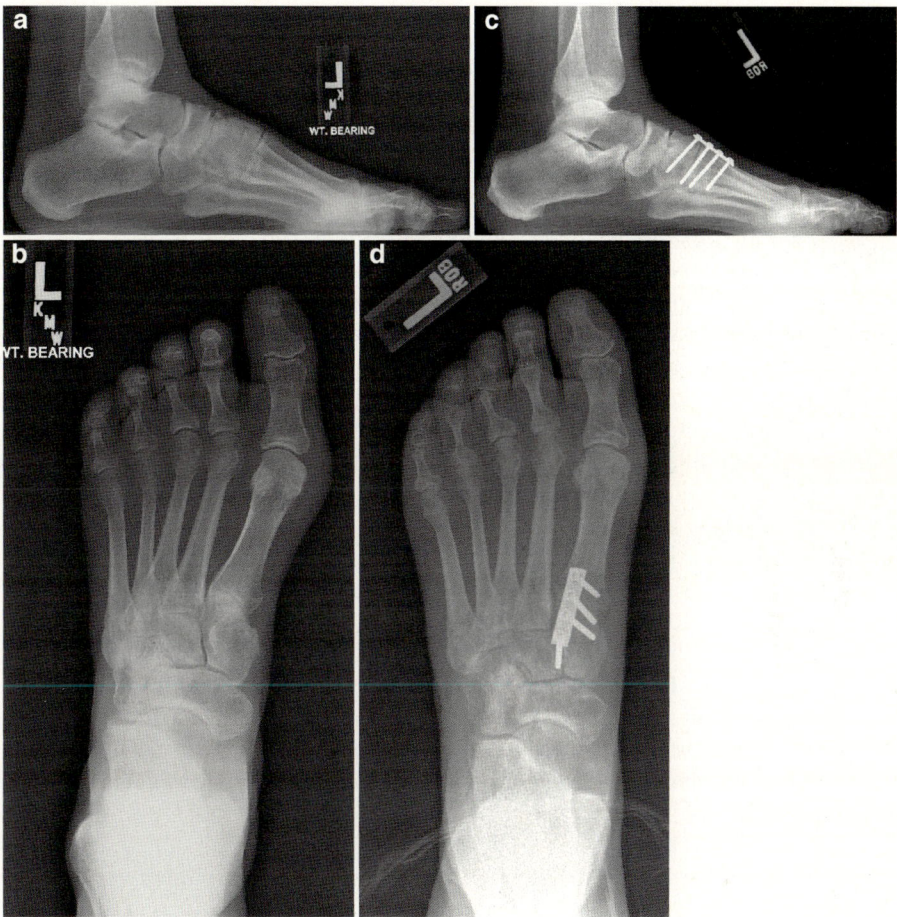

Fig. 7.4 First ray: (**a**, **b**) pre-op; (**c**, **d**) post-op

There are usually two muscle pairs out of balance: the long peroneal, which is stronger than the anterior tibialis, and the posterior tibialis, which overpowers the peroneus brevis. The two muscles that are typically weakened in Charcot-Marie-Tooth disease are the anterior tibialis and the peroneus brevis. This occurs primarily in males, as females in general have less deformity and more weakness. If the imbalance has persisted for a long period of time, particularly through growth and development, the deformity can be quite rigid. There will be deformity in the bone in addition to the marked contracture of the plantar-medial ligamentous structures. This foot deformity occurs under and around the talus and is called a plantar-medial peritalar subluxation. This is the opposite of the reversed failure of posterior tibial and medial ligament, which we call dorsolateral peritalar subluxation or posterior tibial tendon insufficiency.

Common sense and experience tells us from repair of muscle imbalance problems, the overpowering muscles must be weakened or transferred and the weak muscles must be augmented or replaced. Also, any fixed bony or joint deformity must be corrected by osteotomy or capsulotomy, respectively. There are numerous muscle transfers that can be done in keeping with the guidelines of using those with a similar phase and range. There are also a couple that break the rules but, in fact, work.

To begin a surgical correction, the most workable sequence is first to release the deforming structures to allow passive correction to the greatest degree possible if there is bony deformity. In the cavovarus foot, the primary deforming muscles are the posterior tibial tendon and the long peroneal tendon. These can be released to start, and then a proximal plantar fasciectomy can be done to allow the arch to lengthen and release some of the adduction. Next, the medial talonavicular capsule is excised. This may include the tibionavicular portion of the anterior deltoid, the calcaneonavicular spring ligament, and possibly a portion of the long plantar ligament. These structures are worked until the navicular can be brought dorsal and lateral into proper alignment with the talus. The medial capsule of the subtalar joint is also incised to let the anterior calcaneus rotate laterally under the talus following the navicular. If the gastrocnemius is tight, it can be released, as could the medial Achilles.

The long flexor of the toes is usually released distal near the Master Knot in preparation for transfer into the distal stump of the tibialis posterior. It will provide some adduction and internal rotation force, but much weaker than that of the posterior tibialis, which will have to be transferred. If needed, the flexor hallucis can be released distally and transferred around the back into the peroneus brevis to strengthen eversion.

Later, the posterior tibialis can be retracted up to 4 or 5 in. above the ankle and brought forward through the interosseous membrane through a very generous window. Traditionally, it has been freed medially as distally as possible and brought anterior all the way down to the second or third cuneiform or even the cuboid and attached there to bone. I did this for several years but found it overstretched the tibialis posterior and/or limited plantar flexion and/or pulled out or simply did not work well. I now leave the distal 1–2-cm of the posterior tibialis proximal to the navicular in which to attach the flexor digitorum longus to replace its function. The shorter posterior tibialis tendon is brought into the anterior compartment where I attach it into the tendon of the extensor digitorum longus and/or peroneus tertius (and into the anterior tib if the transfer was done for traumatic drop foot or anterior compartment syndrome rather than a varus foot). Then the distal extensor digitorum longus 3–4 tendons are attached by tenodesis into the lateral second or third cuneiform. This procedure is much simpler, allows better physiological tensioning, and has worked much better in my hands both for cavovarus and for anterior compartment syndrome.

The varus heel is addressed by lateral displacement calcaneal osteotomy. Realigning the medially displaced heel by moving the calcaneus laterally reduces the varus stress. A lateral incision is made in line with the proposed osteotomy (with the patient placed in the lateral position or supine with a bump under the ipsilateral hip), posterior to the Peroneal tendons, avoiding the sural nerve. The periosteum is dissected and an osteotomy is made taking care to avoid trauma to the medial neurovascular structures. The calcaneus is displaced laterally 6–10 mm; additional varus reduction can be achieved by removing a laterally based wedge. The osteotomy is fixated with two screws placed from posterior. Two transverse incisions are made to allow for placement of two 6.5-mm screws with 16-mm thread length, generally 55–70-mm long, coursing distally, avoiding the subtalar joint[6] (Fig. 7.5).

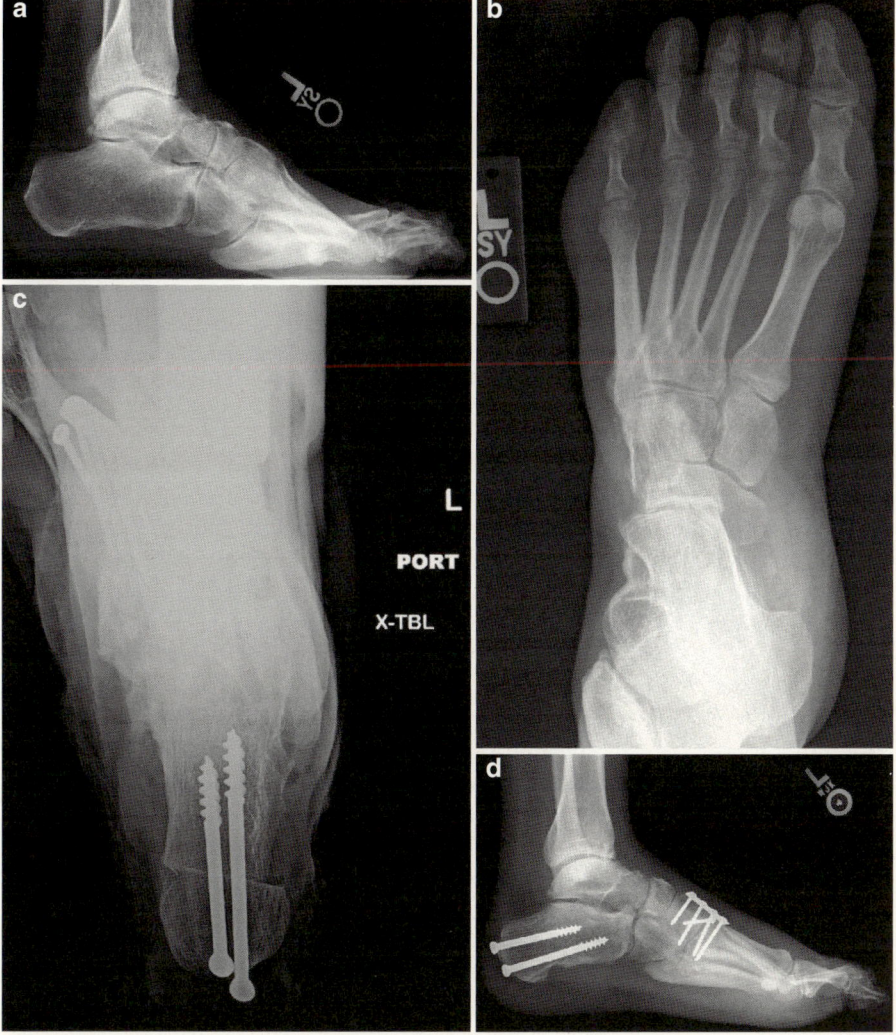

Fig. 7.5 Lateral-displacement calcaneal osteotomy: (**a, b**) pre-op; (**c**) intra-op; (**d, e**) post-op

Fig. 7.5 (continued)

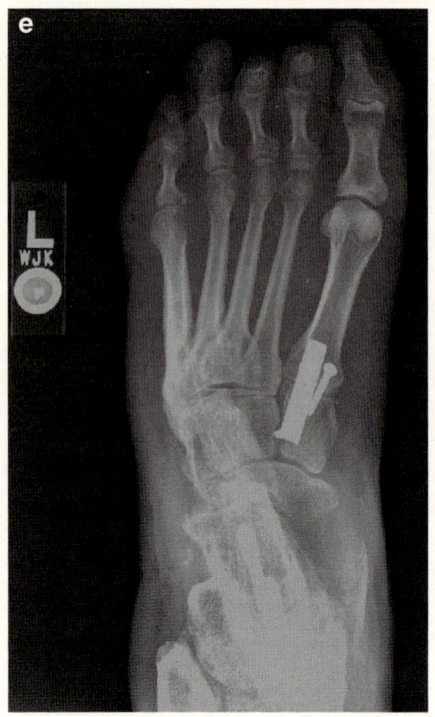

Another component of cavovarus deformity is supra-malleolar pathology. Varus malunion of ankle fractures can be responsible as well as neurological disorders. This may need to be addressed with supra-malleolar tibial and fibular osteotomies (Fig. 7.6). Reestablishing a stable ankle mortise is important, as some of these patients with longstanding deformity may require total ankle replacement (TAR), where alignment is critical. Varus positioning with TAR is poorly tolerated[7-10] (Fig. 7.7).

I have a word of caution about varus feet and residual function or, even worse, strong function of the tibialis anterior. The tibialis anterior can be a very strong inverter or source of varus working with the Achilles in the absence of normal evertors. In this case, either the talonavicular joint should be fused with appropriate medial column alignment to protect against inversion, or the anterior tibialis should be transferred laterally to the second or third cuneiform so that it cannot become an inversion force when it contracts. This is much more likely to happen if the foot had been in significant varus with marked medialization of the navicular on the head of the talus prior to surgery. Numerous authors have noted the same problem and solution when dealing with the same deformity in clubfoot.

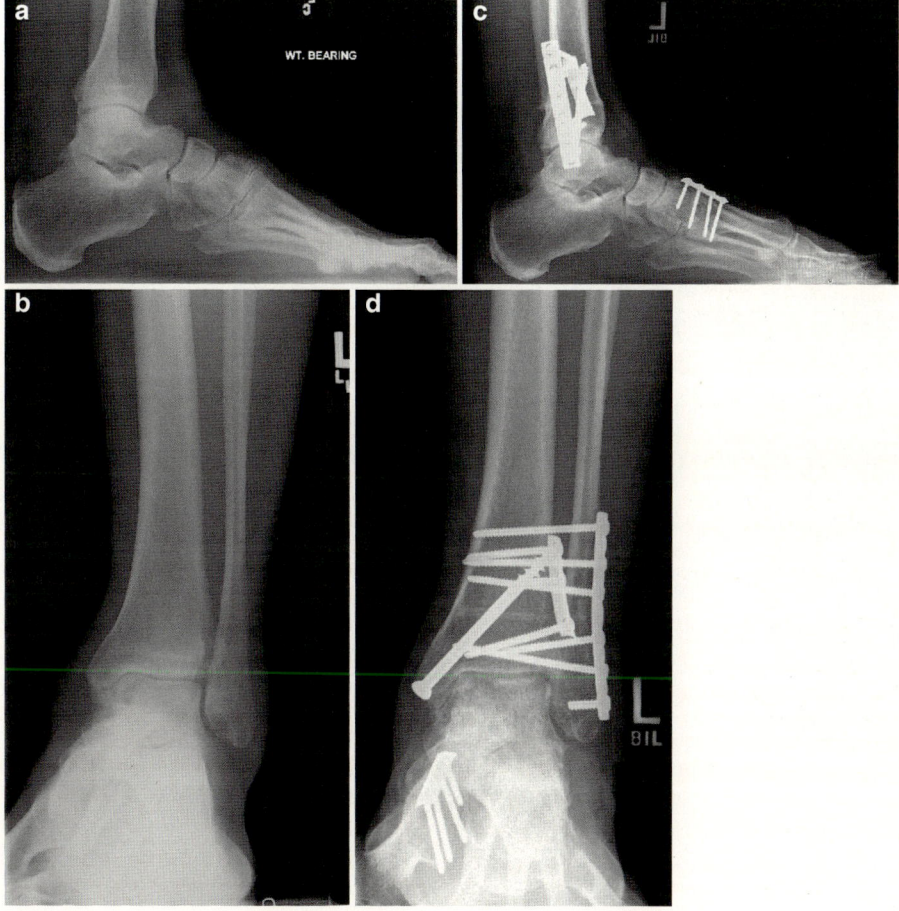

Fig. 7.6 Supra-malleolar osteotomies: (**a, b**) pre-op; (**c, d**) post-op

7.5 Take Home Messages

Treatment of complex but rare cavus feet is difficult and if it is not well understood, not much is lost. The subtle cavovarus foot, which leads to chronic ankle instability, is very common but fortunately very simple to deal with. A first tarsometatarsal dorsal fusion with or without lateralization of the calcaneal by osteotomy, possibly a gastrocnemius recession, and tenodesis of the extensor digitorum longus to the peroneus tertius is a simple and extremely effective group of procedures that would help a large number of people with minimal risk.

Acknowledgments   The author would like to thank Andrew L. Merritt, MD, for his assistance with this chapter.

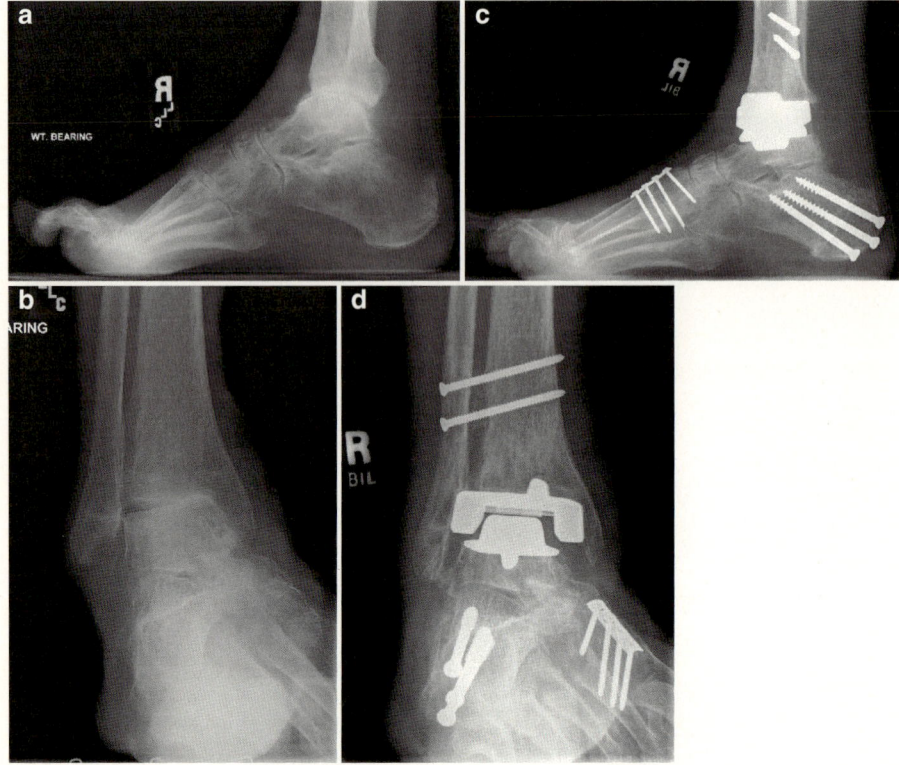

Fig. 7.7 Total ankle replacement in a patient with prior varus deformity: (**a, b**) pre-op; (**c, d**) post-op

References

1. Hansen S. The cavovarus foot (medial peritalar subluxation) in functional restoration of the foot and ankle. Philadelphia: Lippincott; 2000. p.209-13.
2. Fortin PT, Guettler J, Manoli A 2nd. Idiopathic cavovarus and lateral ankle instability: recognition and treatment implications relating to ankle arthritis. Foot Ankle Int. 2002;23(11):1031-7.
3. LaClair SM. Reconstruction of the varus ankle from soft-tissue procedures with osteotomy through arthrodesis. Foot Ankle Clin. 2007;12(1):153-76.
4. Younger AS, Hansen ST. Adult cavovarus foot. J Am Acad Orthop Surg. 2005;13(5):302-15.
5. Heckman DS, Reddy S, Pedowitz D, Wapner KL, Parekh SG. Operative treatment for peroneal tendon disorders. J Bone Joint Surg Am. 2008;90(2):404-18.
6. Hansen S. Calcaneal osteotomy for correction of heel varus. In functional restoration of the foot and ankle. Philadelphia: Lippincott; 2000. p.367-9.
7. Cornelis Doets H, van der Plaat LW, Klein JP. Medial malleolar osteotomy for the correction of varus deformity during total ankle arthroplasty: results in 15 ankles. Foot Ankle Int. 2008;29:171-7.
8. Coetzee JC. Management of varus or valgus ankle deformity with ankle replacement. Foot Ankle Clin. 2008;13:509, x.
9. Haskell A, Mann RA. Ankle arthroplasty with preoperative coronal plane deformity: short-term results. Clin Orthop Relat Res. 2004;424:98-103.
10. Saltzman CL, Tochigi Y, Rudert MJ, McIff TE, Brown TD. The effect of agility ankle prosthesis misalignment on the peri-ankle ligaments. Clin Orthop Relat Res. 2004;424:137-42.

Chapter 8
Endoscopic Gastrocnemius Recession

Lawrence A. DiDomenico, Thomas W. Groner, Jeffrey A. Szczepanski, and Amol Saxena

8.1 Introduction

Ankle joint equinus has been well known in the medical literature as a major deforming force connected with an assortment of foot and ankle pathologies. Ankle equinus is defined as a limitation of dorsiflexion at the ankle joint.[1,2] Limited ankle dorsiflexion has been defined as less than 3–15° with the knee extended. With the knee flexed, limited dorsiflexion has been described as less than 10–20°.[3] Traditionally, in the "normal" patient population, the accepted definition of range of motion continues to be the capability to dorsiflex the foot at the ankle joint a minimum of 10° with the knee extended.[1,2,4] For athletic patient populations, which will be discussed below, ankle dorsiflexion less than 10° may be considered "normal."[5]

There are numerous surgical approaches that have been well established for the correction of ankle joint equinus. Recently, endoscopic gastrocnemius recession (EGR) has gained worldwide recognition for the correction of ankle joint contracture,

L.A. DiDomenico, D.P.M., F.A.C.F.A.S. (✉)
Department of Surgery, Northside Medical Center,
500 Gypsy Lane, Youngstown, OH 44505, USA
e-mail: ld5353@aol.com

T.W. Groner, D.P.M., A.A.C.F.A.S.
Department of Surgery, Ankle and Foot Care Center,
Alliance, OH, USA

J.A. Szczepanski, D.P.M., PLLC
Munson Medical Center,
Traverse City, MI, USA

A. Saxena, D.P.M.
Department of Sports Medicine,
PAFMG-Palo Alto Division,
Palo Alto, CA, USA

A. Saxena (ed.), *Special Procedures in Foot and Ankle Surgery*,
DOI 10.1007/978-1-4471-4103-7_8, © Springer-Verlag London 2013

(specifically gastrocnemius equinus).[6-10] This is because of its relative ease, improved cosmesis, safety, ability to be performed supine and visualize neurovascular structures, along with a lower risk of complications.

8.2   Indications

Decreased ankle joint range of motion during the gait cycle becomes a deforming force that affects the function and position of the foot, leg, knee, hip, and spine.[11] Underlying ankle joint equinus is a contributing factor to many pathologic conditions. Surgical correction of equinus should be considered for conditions such as clubfoot, pediatric and adult flatfoot, Achilles tendinopathy, hypermobility of the first ray, Charcot arthropathy, and plantar forefoot ulcers.[12-15] Operative management of equinus may also be performed in conjunction with other procedures such as amputations, posterior tibial tendon reconstruction, triple arthrodesis, and total ankle arthroplasty.[11,16,17]

The gastrocnemius muscle in particular is the predominant deforming force in the foot and ankle leading to chronic pathological changes.[13] It has been well established that there is an association between isolated gastrocnemius tightness and patients who have chronic forefoot and midfoot symptoms such as plantar fasciitis, hallux valgus, symptomatic adult acquired flatfoot, metatarsalgia, synovitis of the metatarsalphalangeal (MTP) joints, and forefoot ulcerations.[12-15] Nonsurgical treatment such as stretching has been shown to be minimally effective.[18,19] Therefore, successful surgical management of these deformities should include assessment for ankle equinus as these patients are unlikely to experience full relief of symptoms unless this component is surgically addressed.

8.3   Anatomy and Etiology

The muscles of the superficial group of the lower leg are the gastrocnemius, soleus, and plantaris. The gastrocnemius and soleus form the triceps surae and share the Achilles tendon. The gastrocnemius muscle crosses the knee joint and is superficial and posterior to the deeper soleus muscle, which lies anterior. The plantaris is much smaller and arises lateral and directs medial to the gastrocnemius muscle but may have to be addressed during surgical correction of equinus deformities via tenotomy.[18]

The Achilles tendon is the strongest tendon in the human body. The gastrocnemius portion makes up the entire lateral aspect of the posterior surface and part of the lateral aspect of the anterior surface of the Achilles tendon. On the other hand, the soleus portion of the Achilles tendon usually comprises the medial two-thirds of the anterior surface and a small part of the medial posterior surface. Overall, the soleus and gastrocnemius contributions to the Achilles tendon are not easily separable.[18-21]

Ankle equinus may be classified according to different etiologies. Decreased ankle dorsiflexion may be due to muscular deformity, osseous deformity, or a combination of the two. In addition, muscular equinus is subclassified as either spastic, as in cerebral palsy, or the more common non-spastic. Gastrocnemius-soleus and isolated gastrocnemius are the two forms of muscular equinus.[2]

Osseous forms of equinus may be caused by exostoses that limit ankle range of motion with the knee either extended or flexed. Pseudo-equinus is the term often used for the false perception of true ankle equinus such as may be seen with pes cavus.[22] Although less frequent than muscular forms and osseous forms, pseudo-equinus must be ruled out before embarking upon surgical correction of equinus due to soft-tissue contracture.

8.4 Procedures

Various surgical procedures have been described for the correction of ankle equinus. Tendo-Achilles lengthening (TAL) may be performed in an open or percutaneous fashion. The Z-plasty technique was first performed through two transverse incisions 8–10 cm apart.[23] The open frontal plane Z-plasty became quite popular over the years due to its consistency in correction compared to other tenotomies.[2,23-25] Percutaneous TAL in a triple hemi-section fashion has been performed for 60 years.[25,26] The authors utilize this approach with two lateral and one medial incision in a valgus foot and with two medial and one lateral incision in a varus foot. Hansen describes a two-incision percutaneous technique.[10]

Gastrocnemius recession has been described as an open distal recession and was initially performed with variations of a transverse lengthening.[27,28]

Later modifications took the form of distally or proximally oriented tongue and groove lengthening of the gastrocnemius.[29,30] EGR has been reported as a viable alternative to open technique.[31-34] Studies have revealed average correction of equinus deformity after surgery to be about 18° using either open[35] or endoscopic[31] technique.

8.4.1 Clinical Examination and Procedure Selection

The preoperative physical examination is paramount to proper patient selection for EGR. It is necessary to distinguish between flexible and osseous equinus while ruling out any spastic component. Once it is established with a diagnosis of non-spastic muscular equinus, proper evaluation of ankle joint dorsiflexion can take place. There is much disparity in the literature to the exact measurement of ankle joint dorsiflexion when evaluating ankle equinus. The measurements range from 0° to 25°.[13] Note must be taken as to the position of the foot when measuring ankle joint dorsiflexion. In past studies, the foot position has not been consistent. When considering surgical correction, the Silfverskiold test should be performed to distinguish between muscular forms of ankle equinus.[36] The exam is performed with the patient in a supine or sitting position. The assessor extends the patient's knee and passively dorsiflexes the ankle with the subtalar joint in neutral position and the midtarsal joint adducted. It is very critical that the examining physician ensures that the patient's anterior tibial tendon is not actively functioning, performing a passive range of motion. The sagittal plane relationship of the bisection of the leg to the rearfoot is measured. Because the gastrocnemius muscle crosses the knee joint and the soleus does not, the gastrocnemius is shortened when the knee is flexed. Gastrocnemius equinus is present if there is less than 10° of dorsiflexion with the knee extended and an increase in ankle joint range of motion with the knee flexed.[31]

While the Silfverskiold test may help determine whether to perform an Achilles tendon lengthening or a gastrocnemius recession, other preoperative criteria must be considered. A percutaneous TAL may be selected for a patient who suffers from gastrocsoleus equinus and peripheral arterial disease,[3] e.g., patients who had undergone peripheral bypass surgery or amputations. On the other hand, a patient with gastrocnemius equinus can benefit from an open or endoscopic procedure.

Gastrocnemius recession in general may be preferable to a TAL in the athletic patient since the former maintains the propulsive strength of the soleus. One must note, however, equinus has been found in asymptomatic adolescent athletes, and since posterior lengthening has not been critically studied in this patient population, more study is needed.[5,8] Lengthening may be needed for posttraumatic contracture for an athletic patient.

Recurrent resection for anterior ankle exostoses is a good indication for consideration of a gastrocnemius recession. This is to reduce the deforming posterior contracture that may aid in the pathological development of anterior talo-tibial exostoses and is analogous to soft-tissue re-balancing in bunion deformity. Achilles tendon lengthening could produce weakness and is essentially a controlled rupture. Since gastrocnemius tears (also known as "tennis leg") allow for full functionality after adequate healing time, one could infer that gastrocnemius lengthening would be "safer" on athletic patients.

In addition, gastrocnemius recession allows for earlier weight-bearing as opposed to TAL and may be beneficial if the patient has a history of Achilles injury.[3,32,37] Furthermore, even in the non-athlete, patients with isolated gastrocnemius tightness who have had a TAL have been shown to lose plantarflexory strength and may develop calcaneal gait.[38] Overcorrection and loss of strength can be avoided when isolated gastrocnemius contracture is properly treated with a gastrocnemius recession.

Mistakenly, it has been understood by numerous clinicians that isolated gastrocnemius recession will not provide adequate correction when compared to TAL. In fact, 1-cm gapping of the gastrocnemius yields approximately 10–15° of increased ankle flexibility while diminishing instability from the midtarsal joint due to excessive sagittal plane rotation.[39]

Endoscopic gastrocnemius recession (EGR) may be preferred to open procedures for a number of reasons. It provides enhanced cosmesis and a lower likelihood

Fig. 8.1 A lateral and medial clinical view with marks demonstrating the leg broken into anterior, middle and posterior 1/3 of the leg

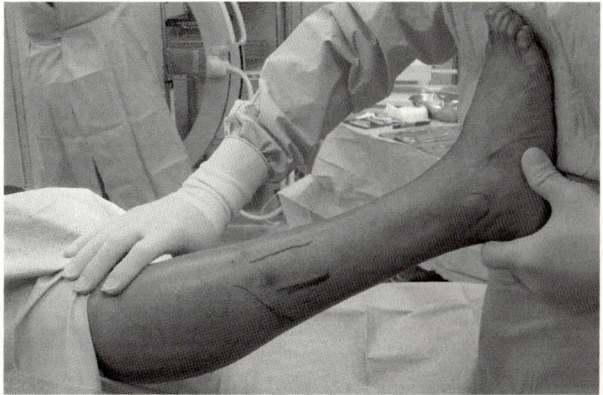

of hematoma formation due to its minimally invasive nature.[3,31,32] As a result, this decreases overall tissue trauma and allows for quicker healing postoperatively. An endoscopic procedure will necessitate only two small stab incisions (bi-portal) or a single (uni-portal) incision approach.[31,32] An open procedure may require the incision up to 10 cm in length.[8,33,40] Direct image through the endoscope allows for protection of vital structures such as the sural nerve and lesser saphenous vein. Also, EGR easily allows for supine or prone positioning of the patient and an associated decrease in operating room time.[12,31]

8.4.2 Technique

Following an appropriate time out and identification of the patient, the patient is placed in a supine position and anesthesia is induced. Typically, the patient is maintained in a supine position to allow ease of transition to additional procedures. A traditional prep and drape is performed to a level above the knee allowing the surgeon an entire view and function of the entire lower extremity. Normally, the endoscopic gastrocnemius recession is completed first and, in most cases, is performed in combination with other surgical procedures.

The incision landmarks are determined by the level of the inferior aspect of the muscle bellies of the medial and lateral head of gastrocnemius muscle. The gastrocnemius aponeurosis is typically identified at a level approximately 2–3 cm distal to the most inferior aspect of the medial head of the gastrocnemius muscle belly. (The medial head of the gastrocnemius muscle belly is more inferior than the lateral head of the gastrocnemius muscle belly.) The medial and lateral aspects of the lower leg (at the level of the gastrocnemius aponeurosis) are divided into thirds (Figs. 8.1 and 8.2). The small stab incisions are made longitudinally in line along the neurovascular structures in the posterior one-third of the lower leg at the gastrocnemius aponeurosis level. For a bi-portal technique, an incision is made at this level both medially and laterally. If utilizing a uni-portal technique, this incision is made medially at this

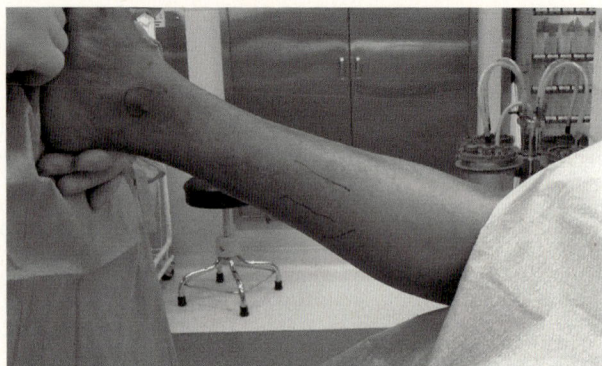

Fig. 8.2 The Endoscopic Gastrocnemius Recession Surgical Procedure incisions should be made at approximately the posterior 1/3 of the leg

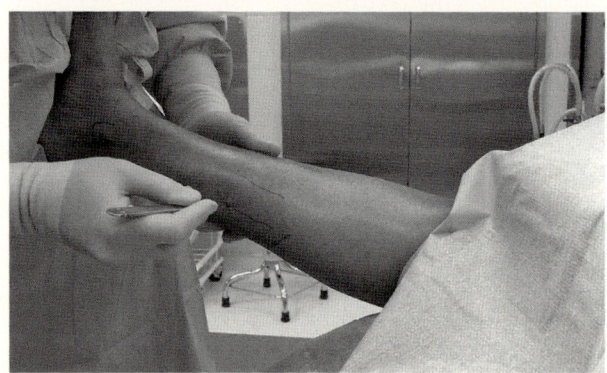

Fig. 8.3 A longitudinal stab incision is made in the posterior 1/3 compartment

level. The reason for the incisions being placed somewhat anteriorly is the gastrocnemius aponeurosis is shaped in a one-third tubular fashion. As the aponeurosis flares medially and laterally, it tends to advance anteriorly and by having the incisions placed in the posterior one-third of the lower leg, this allows for complete visualization of the gastrocnemius aponeurosis from medial to lateral.

The surgeon should then put the plantar aspect of the patient's foot against his or her chest (making sure the patient's knee is fully extended) and the surgeon should lean into the foot or have an assistant dorsiflex the ankle joint therefore applying tension to the posterior muscle group. A small stab incision is made medially, avoiding the greater saphenous vein and nerve (Fig. 8.3). The incision is deepened in the same plane to the deep fascia via blunt dissection. Any bleeders are identified and cauterized as necessary.

Attention is then carried down through the deep fascia to the gastrocnemius aponeurosis. A fascial elevator is slid along the posterior gastrocnemius aponeurosis from medial to lateral separating the deep fascia from the aponeurosis. Next, an obturator is inserted in the same plane and the obturator is inserted posterior to the gastrocnemius aponeurosis from medial to lateral (Fig. 8.4). For a bi-portal technique, the lateral skin is tented and a small stab incision is made laterally, parallel along the lines of the neurovascular structures (Fig. 8.5). Transillumination aids in

Fig. 8.4 The obturator is inserted from medial - lateral tenting the skin

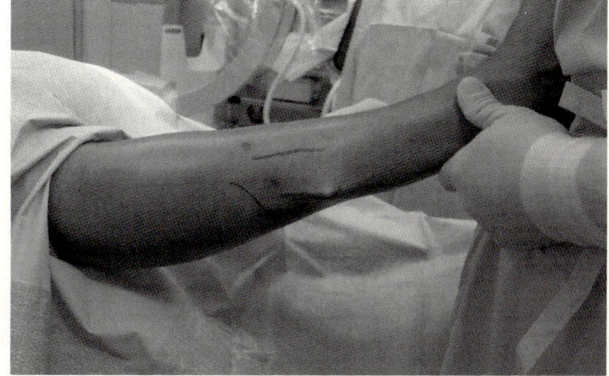

Fig. 8.5 A lateral view making a stab incision over the tented skin of the obturator

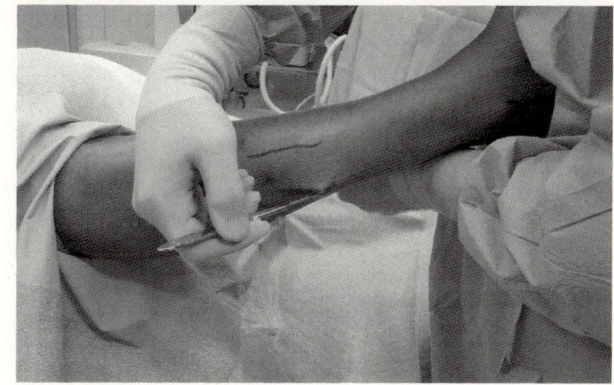

avoiding these structures. A cannula is then inserted over the obturator (Fig. 8.6). The cannula is inserted all the way across, thereby staying posterior to the gastrocnemius aponeurosis. The cannula is cleaned for good visualization with a cotton tip applicator, and the slotted aspect of the cannula should be facing anteriorly to allow for visualization of the gastrocnemius aponeurosis. Figure 8.7 with the open end of the cannula facing anteriorly against the gastrocnemius aponeurosis, a 4.0-mm 30° angled scope is inserted (Fig. 8.8). At this time, range of motion of the ankle joint is performed. This allows confirmation and visualization of the gastrocnemius aponeurosis only. If any other tissue is visualized, the equipment is exited and the blunt dissection separating the tissue planes is performed again in order to be posterior to the gastrocnemius aponeurosis and deep to the deep fascia and anteriorly to the sural nerve. Visualization of only the gastrocnemius aponeurosis fibers insures that the sural nerve and/or other neurovascular structures are not implicated. This also insures that the only tissue cut is the gastrocnemius aponeurosis. It is critical at this time that the gastrocnemius aponeurosis is the only anatomical structure visible in order to evade any possible neurovascular damage. The striations of the aponeurosis are very apparent and very distinct. It is also extremely important that the surgeon dorsiflexes and plantarflexes the ankle joint in order to allow for visibility

Fig. 8.6 The cannula fitted over the obturator going from lateral – medial

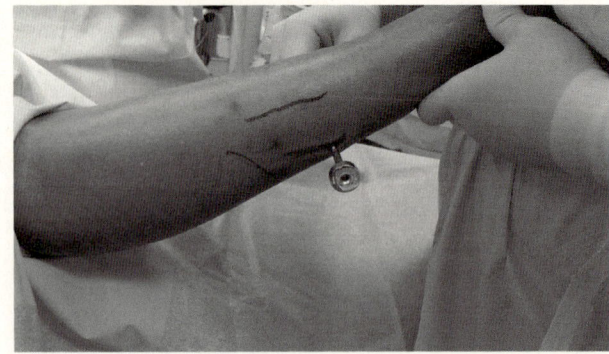

Fig. 8.7 A lateral view demonstrating the slotted cannula facing up (anteriorly) prior to insertion of the scope

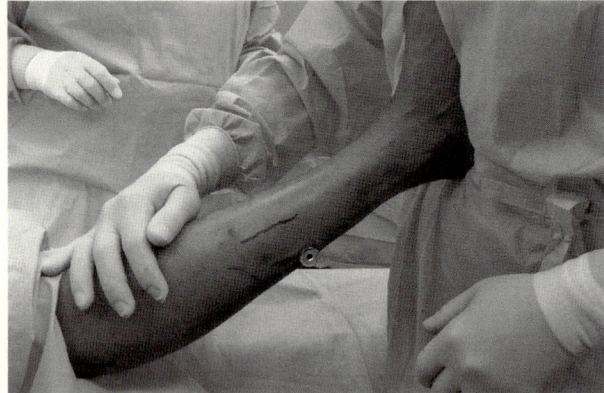

Fig. 8.8 Insertion of the endoscope from lateral to medial, please note that knee is extended and there is tension on gastrocnemius apenerosis by dorsiflexing the foot

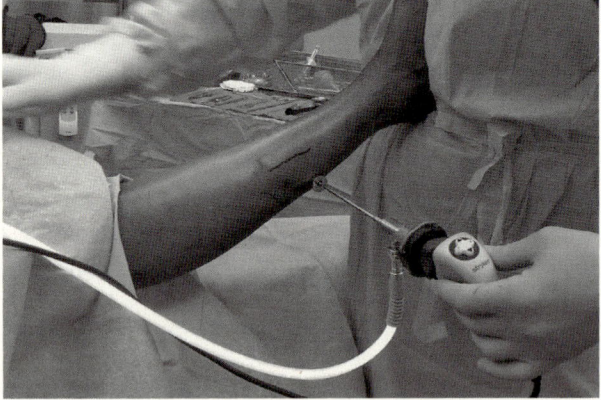

Fig. 8.9 Endoscopic insertion of a triangle blade from medial to incise the gastrocnemius aponeurosis (**a**) and endoscopic view (**b**)

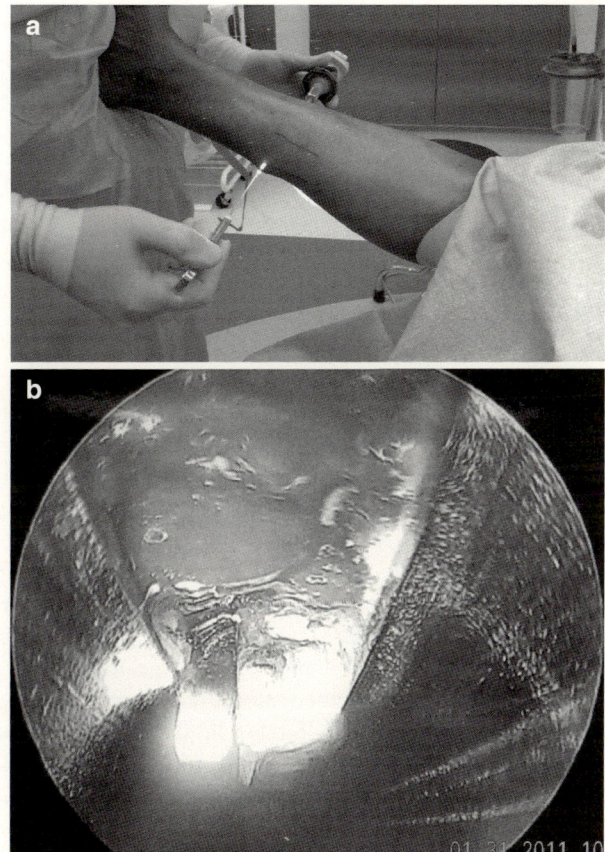

of these specific fibers of the aponeurosis moving proximal and distal to the anteriorly facing cannula. It should be noted that the surgeon performing EGR will often discover that the sural nerve may be located in the central posterior lower leg, and is not as laterally placed as many believe. It is possible in some patients to rotate the cannula posteriorly to view the sural nerve.

Once the cannula slot is facing anteriorly, a triangle blade, hook blade, or push blade can be used to incise along the gastrocnemius aponeurosis, performing a gastrocnemius recession (Fig. 8.9). This will allow a direct visualization of the soleus muscle belly and allow improved range of motion in the ankle joint. Many times there will be small portions of gastrocnemius aponeurosis septae in the soleus muscle belly. These fibers can be cut with the endoscope blade easily being careful not to cut the soleus muscle. The surgeon should be leaning into the foot prior to the release. As the cut is being performed and completed, the surgeon should "fall in" (feel the release) as the gastrocnemius aponeurosis is lengthened and increase in range of motion of the ankle joint is distinguished. With increased range of motion

Fig. 8.10 Demonstrating the small, cosmetically pleasing incision site following the procedure

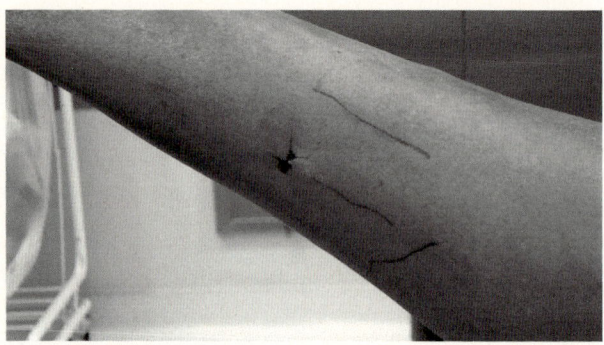

identified, the equipment is removed. Often times, the plantaris tendon will maintain its integrity and can be palpated following removal of the equipment. This small tendon can often times be very strong and prevent a complete increase in range of motion. In this scenario, a small blade is used to complete a plantaris tenotomy, yielding a complete release and increased range of motion of the ankle joint. Closure should consist of one simple skin closure per incision site (Fig. 8.10).

The surgeon must be well versed with gastrocnemius recession prior to embarking on the EGR procedure. It is mandatory that the surgeon knows how to convert an attempted EGR into a medial open gastrocnemius recession. This technique employs removing all of the endoscopic equipment and extending the medial "stab incision" approximately 3–7 cm. The incision is then carried down to the level of the deep fascia. The deep fascia is incised and retracted protecting the sural nerve. At this time, the gastrocnemius aponeurosis is recognized and the lengthening is performed with a pair of scissors or blade. Again, attention to detail is mandated to be certain to incise any isolated septae within the soleus muscle belly and the plantaris tendon. Once a complete release is obtained, the deep closure followed by skin closure is performed.

8.5 Contraindications and Complications

Contraindications to equinus correction ultimately only include associated medical issues that would negate any surgery or the use of anesthesia. Many complications, such as nerve damage or entrapment of the sural nerve, infection, wound dehiscence, hematoma, under-lengthening, over-lengthening, weakness, cutting into the soleus muscle, and painful scar formation, can be attributed to surgical technique. Recurrence of the contracture is usually associated with incomplete release, incorrect procedure selection, and is especially associated with spastic forms.[6] Overcorrection is more of an issue with TAL as opposed to gastrocnemius recession and can be avoided by properly examining the patient's range of motion preoperatively as well as intraoperatively. EGR demonstrates minimal risk of over-lengthening, thereby decreasing the chance of calcaneal gait which is fraught with further complications.[8,38]

Caution should be exercised when performing EGR in patients with an increased body mass index, specifically those with an obese lower leg and ankle region. These patients are typically the most difficult on whom to accurately perform an EGR as there is a very small area in which to appropriately place the incision. Proper placement of the incision cannot always be confirmed if gastrocnemius and soleus anatomy are not easily palpable. In such patients, the aponeurosis distal to the muscle junction can be especially challenging to accurately identify.

8.6 Conclusion

Despite the learning curve for this procedure (as compared to open techniques), the authors believe that the endoscopic approach could be superior to any of the open techniques available to the foot and ankle surgeon. Decreased likelihood for postoperative complications, the ability to position the patient either supine or prone, decreased surgical time, and a more cosmetically appealing incision are all advantages of the EGR over the established open approach.

Patient positioning is best done supine as opposed to many older techniques, which require that the patient be prone. Since most additional foot and ankle procedures require the patient be supine, placing the patient and rotating from the prone position greatly increases surgical time and anesthesia risks.

EGR may allow for improved recovery with earlier ambulation. In most cases, the procedures performed in conjunction with EGR will dictate the patient's postoperative recovery period and weight-bearing status. Total surgical time for this procedure is typically no more than 4–8 min, and requires minimal additional surgical equipment. When this technique is appropriately applied it may enhance surgical outcomes and is therefore advocated by the authors for the correction of gastrocnemius equinus.

References

1. Root ML, Orien WP, Weed JH. Normal and abnormal function of the foot. Los Angeles: Clinical Biomechanics Corporation; 1977.
2. Downey MS, Banks AS. Gastrocnemius recession in the treatment of nonspastic ankle equinus: a retrospective study. J Am Podiatr Med Assoc. 1989;79:159-74.
3. Schweinberger MH, Roukis TS. Surgical correction of soft tissue ankle equinus contracture. Clin Podiatr Med Surg. 2008;25(4):571-85.
4. Herzenberg JE, Lamm BM, Corwin C, et al. Isolated recession of the gastrocnemius muscle: the Baumann procedure. Foot Ankle Int. 2007;28(11):1154-9.
5. Saxena A, Kim W. Ankle dorsiflexion in adolescent athletes. J Am Podiatr Med Assoc. 2003;93(4):312-4.
6. Poul J, Tuma J, Bajerova J. Video-assisted tenotomy of the triceps muscle of the calf in cerebral palsy patients. Acta Chir Orthop Traumatol Cech. 2005;72(3):170-2.
7. Saxena A, Gollwitzer H, DiDomenico L, Widtfeldt A. Endoscopic Gastrocnemius Recession: a midterm report on 54 cases. Z Orthop Unfalllchir. 2007;145:1-6.
8. Saxena A, DiGiovanni C. Ankle equinus and the athlete. In: Maffulli N, Almekinders LC, editors. The achilles tendon. London: Springer; 2006.

9. Saxena A, DiGiovanni C. Endoscopic gastrocnemius recession. In: Scuderi G, Tria A, editors. Minimally invasive surgery in orthopedics. New York: Springer; 2009:365-70.

10. Hansen ST. Tendon transfers and muscle balancing techniques. Achilles tendon lengthening. In: Hansen S, ed. Functional reconstruction of the foot and ankle. Baltimore: Lippincott Williams & Wilkins; 2000:415-21.

11. Van Gils CC, Roeder B. The effect of ankle equinus upon the diabetic foot. Clin Podiatr Med Surg. 2002;19:391-409.

12. Meszaros A, Caudell G. The surgical management of equinus in the adult acquired flatfoot. Clin Podiatr Med Surg. 2007;24(4):667-85.

13. DiGiovanni CW, Kuo R, Tejwani N, et al. Isolated gastrocnemius tightness. J Bone Joint Surg Am. 2002;84(6):962-70.

14. Chang TJ. Surgical management of equinus. In: Master techniques in podiatric surgery: the foot and ankle. Philadelphia: Lippincott and Wilkins; 2005. p. 239-50.

15. Lavery LA, Armstrong DG, Boulton AJ. Ankle equinus deformity and its relationship to high plantar pressure in a large population with diabetes mellitus. J Am Podiatr Med Assoc. 2002;92:479-82.

16. Sammarco GJ, Bagwe MR, Sammaro VJ, et al. The effects of unilateral gastrocsoleus recession. Foot Ankle Int. 2006;27(7):508-11.

17. Shiha AE, Khalifa AR, Assaghir YM, et al. Medial transport of the fibula using the Ilizarov device for reconstruction of a massive defect of the tibia in two children. J Bone Joint Surg Br. 2008;90(12):1627-30.

18. Downey MS, Banks AS, Downey MS, Martin DE. Comprehensive textbook of foot surgery, vol. 1. 3rd ed. Philadelphia: Williams and Wilkins; 2001:715-60.

19. Grady J, Saxena A. Effect of stretching on the Gastrocnemius muscle. J Foot Ankle Surg. 1991;30(5):465-9.

20. Warwick R, Williams PL. Myology. In: Grays anatomy. Philadelphia: WB Saunders; 1973:574-5.

21. Cummins EJ, Anson BJ, Carr BW, et al. The structure of the Achilles tendon in relation to orthopaedic surgery. Surg Gynecol Obstet. 1946;83:107-16.

22. Groner TW, DiDomenico LA. Midfoot osteotomies for the cavus foot. Clin Podiatr Med Surg. 2005;22:247-64.

23. Sgarlatto TE, Morgan J, Shane HS, Frankenberg A. Tendo Achilles lengthening and its effect on foot disorders. J Am Podiatr Med Assoc. 1975;65:849-71.

24. Downey MS. Ankle equines. In: Mcglamry ED, editor. Comprehensive textbook of foot surgery. Baltimore: Williams and Wilkins; 1992:687-730.

25. Hatt RN, Lamphier TA. Triple hemisection: a simplified procedure for lengthening the Achilles tendon. N Engl J Med. 1947;236:166-9.

26. Haro AA, DiDomenico LA. Frontal plane guided percutaneous tendo achilles lengthening. J Foot Ankle Surg. 2007;46(1):55-61.

27. Vulpius O, Stoffel A. Orthopaedische operatioslehre. Stuttgart: Verlag von Ferdinand Enke; 1924.

28. Strayer LM. Recession of the gastrocnemius: an operation to relieve spastic contracture of the calf muscle. J Bone Joint Surg Am. 1950;32(3):671-6.

29. Baker LD. A rational approach to the surgical needs of the cerebral palsy patient. J Bone Joint Surg Am. 1956;56:313-23.

30. Fulp MJ, McGlamry ED. Gastrocnemius tendon recession: tongue in groove procedure to lengthen gastrocnemius tendon. J Am Podiatr Med Assoc. 1974;64:163-71.

31. DiDomenico LA, Adams HB, Garchar D. Endoscopic gastrocnemius recession for the treatment of gastrocnemius equinus. J Am Podiatr Med Assoc. 2005;95(4):410-3.

32. Saxena A, Widtfeldt A. Endoscopic gastrocnemius recession: preliminary report on 18 cases. J Foot Ankle Surg. 2004;43(5):302-6.

33. Tashjian RZ, Appel AJ, Banerjee R, et al. Anatomic study of the gastrocnemius-soleus junction and its relationship to the sural nerve. Foot Ankle Int. 2003;24(6):473-6.

34. Trevino S, Gibbs M, Panchbhavi V. Evaluation of results of endoscopic gastrocnemius recession. Foot Ankle Int. 2005;26(5):359-64.

35. Pinney SJ, Hansen ST, Sangeorzan BT. The effect of ankle dorsiflexion of gastrocnemius recession. Foot Ankle Int. 2002;23(1):26-9.
36. Silfverskiold N. Reduction of the uncrossed two-joint muscles of the leg to one-joint muscles in spastic conditions. Acta Chir Scand. 1924;56:315-30.
37. Panchbhavi VK, Trevino SG. Endoscopic gastrocnemius recession. Tech Foot Ankle Surg. 2004;3(3):149-52.
38. Delp SL, Statler K, Carroll NC. Preserving plantarflexion strength after surgical treatment for contracture of the triceps surae: a computer simulation study. J Orthop Res. 1995;13:96-104.
39. Sgarlato TE. Medial gastrocnemius tenotomy to assist body posture balancing. J Foot Ankle Surg. 1998;37:607-13.
40. Donley BG, Pinney ST, Holmes J. Gastrocnemius recession. Techn Foot Ankle Surg. 2003;2(1):35-9.

Chapter 9
Intramedullary Nail Fixation for Tibiotalocalcaneal Arthrodesis

Lawrence A. DiDomenico and Thomas W. Groner

9.1 Introduction

Tibiotalocalcaneal arthrodesis is used to treat severe arthrosis, deformity, and malalignment of the hindfoot and ankle. This may be accomplished by the utilization of crossed lag screws, plates, external fixation, or an intramedullary nail.[1] With a tibiotalocalcaneal arthrodesis, the goal is to create a solid fusion that corrects the deformity, maintains anatomic alignment, and allows the patient to function independently while relieving pain and providing a plantigrade foot and ankle that is shoeable or braceable.[2] Often the severity of the deformity affects not only the ankle but also the subtalar joint, thereby warranting fusion of both joints.

Intramedullary nail fixation, often termed IM nail, has been described in the literature for over 100 years. In 1906, Lexer described tibiotalocalcaneal arthrodesis in the form of an implanted cadaver bone "skewered" through the hind foot.[3,4] In 1915, Albee used a fibula as a makeshift IM nail.[5] The technique and hardware for this procedure have continued to be modified over the years.[6-19] Modern forms of the IM nail allow for a reproducible technique that provides stable fixation for tibiotalocalcaneal arthrodesis without extensive soft tissue damage.[20]

L.A. DiDomenico, D.P.M., F.A.C.F.A.S. (✉)
Department of Surgery, Northside Medical Center,
500 Gypsy Lane, Youngstown, OH 44505, USA
e-mail: ld5353@aol.com

T.W. Groner, D.P.M., A.A.C.F.A.S.
Department of Surgery, Ankle and Foot Care Center,
Alliance, OH, USA

A. Saxena (ed.), *Special Procedures in Foot and Ankle Surgery*,
DOI 10.1007/978-1-4471-4103-7_9, © Springer-Verlag London 2013

9.2   Indications and Contraindications

Appropriate utilization of an intramedullary nail in the hindfoot and ankle is limited to those patients who suffer from severe pathology of both the subtalar and ankle joint or those patients who have a nonviable talus. Tibiotalocalcaneal arthrodesis via an intramedullary nail is indicated in a number of situations. Indications include marked ankle and subtalar joint instability and severe deformities of rheumatoid, primary degenerative, and posttraumatic arthritis of both the ankle and subtalar joints. The procedure is also indicated for a talectomy and a tibial-calcaneal arthrodesis, for avascular necrosis of the talus, pseudoarthrosis, revision of failed ankle and subtalar joint arthrodesis, crush injuries, and severe deformity secondary to neuromuscular disease, cerebral vascular accidents, and residual or neglected clubfoot.[1,4,21] The use of an IM nail is also a powerful tool that can be very effective for the correction of severe Charcot deformities and after failed total ankle replacement.[2,22]

Charcot arthropathy is a very serious complication related with diabetic peripheral neuropathy (Fig. 9.1). The problem is most severe when the hindfoot and ankle are a major concern because of instability and progressive distortion which can lead to ulceration, infection, osteomyelitis, limb loss, and death. Indications for the surgical reconstruction of Charcot arthropathy of the ankle and hindfoot are the result of failure of conservative treatment to properly address the following: chronic recurrent ulcerations, osseous deformities, unstable joints, a non-braceable foot and ankle, acute displaced fractures, and malalignment.[2] Inadequate stabilization of the existing disease process may result in further breakdown and continued progression of the deformity. Oftentimes with multiple joint involvements at the ankle, subtalar joint, and midfoot, it is good appropriate medical care to initiate surgical stabilization and realignment as early as possible in an attempt to avoid the often inevitable severe deformity and skin breakdown. The surgical goal is to create a plantigrade weight-bearing surface free of ulceration and to restore stability and alignment so that shoe gear and bracing are possible (Fig. 9.2).

Salvage of a failed total ankle replacement may result in ankle and subtalar arthrodesis which can be associated with such sequelae as marked shortening of the limb. Other options consist of a below the knee amputation or a revisional ankle joint replacement which is technically difficult and potentially challenging for the patient.[23] The former may not be feasible if there is extensive bone loss or an active infection.[8,23,24] The latter is utilized only when limb salvage is considered impossible. Tibiotalocalcaneal fusion, especially in conjunction with an allograft if the talus is unsalvageable, provides an acceptable option after a failed total ankle procedure and decreases the amount of limb shortening.[23]

Contraindications to the use of intramedullary nailing for stabilization and realignment of severe hindfoot and ankle deformities are active infection and a dysvascular limb. Relative contraindications are acute phase Charcot disease, poor

Fig. 9.1 (**a, b**) A diabetic neuropathic patient with a neglected ankle fracture. A lateral (**a**) and Anterior-Posterior (**b**) radiograph demonstrating a neuropahtic ankle fracture with mal- alignment in the tibial - talar- fibula joint. This patient wound not benefit from an intramedullary nail as the subtalar joint is in good anatomical alignment and is well maintained

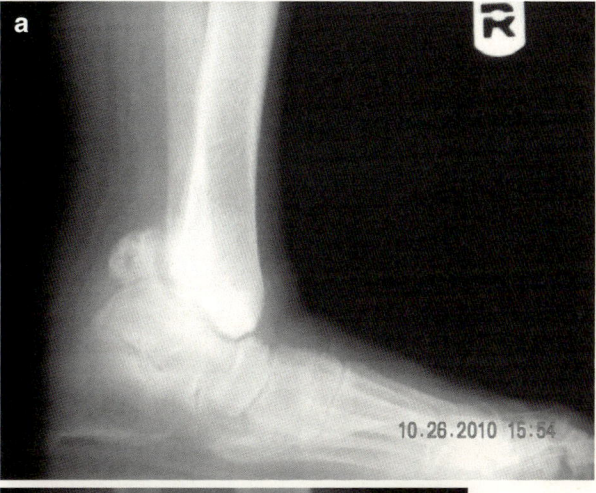

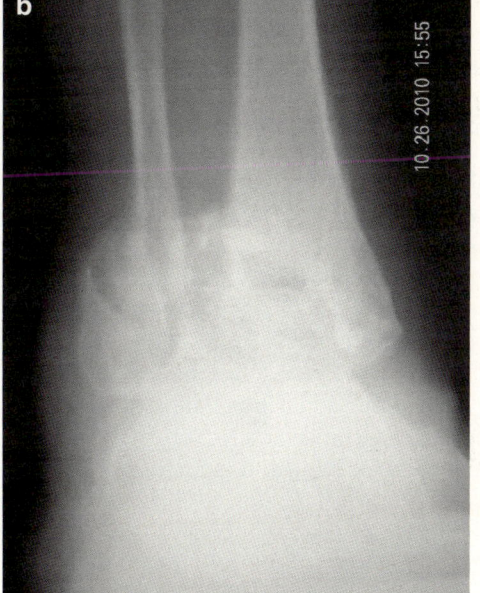

glycemic control, and nutritional status. Peripheral vascular disease; insufficient plantar fat pad; a significantly deformed calcaneus; previous infection involving the tibia, talus, and/or calcaneus; and severe comorbidities such as cardiac and renal disease are other relative contraindications.[2,25]

Fig. 9.2 A neuropathic patient with complete instability of the hindfoot and ankle. The radiograph demonstrates complete instability and dislocation of the tibial talar joint

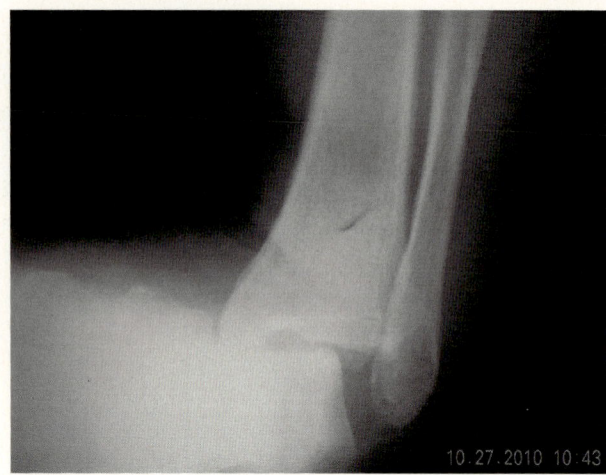

9.3 Advantages and Procedure

There are several advantages of IM nail fixation including maintaining length, alignment, and stability with relatively minimal soft tissue stripping.[4,20,22,25-27] Studies have concluded that the IM nail provides a significantly stiffer and more stable form of fixation for tibiotalocalcaneal arthrodesis when compared with lag screws.[28,29] IM nail fixation has proven successful as a salvage procedure in rheumatoid patients by providing an un-staged fusion while allowing for moderately early weight-bearing.[30] Kile reported good results when using an IM nail with autogenous bone graft.[11] Several other studies have deemed retrograde intramedullary nailing a useful alternative to other forms of tibiotalocalcaneal fusion.[13,22,31,32] While it has been cited as less appropriate in the neuropathic population,[13] other studies have determined IM nail fusion to be an excellent salvage procedure for patients with severe Charcot deformities.[2,22]

Several methods for IM nail fixation have been investigated.[17,19,20,22,33] Posterior-to-anterior distal screw orientation has become the norm since it provides increased rotational stability compared to a transversely placed lateral-to-medial distal screw (Fig. 9.3).[19,20] The authors have utilized multiple systems. Most current systems provide a lateral-to-medial screw as well as a posterior-to-anterior distal screw and have individual unique properties and modifications. More traditional systems offer a lateral-to-medial calcaneal screw. A number of the current systems have a dual stage compression mechanism with the ability to compress the ankle and subtalar joints independently. These systems normally utilize a special alignment arm to assist with proper positioning of the transfixation screws. A small number of the IM nails in the marketplace have a lateral bend to allow for better anatomical alignment and calcaneal screw purchase. Regardless of materials and configuration of each specific nail, the overall technique is not significantly different.

Fig. 9.3 Lateral projection demonstrating a posterior-to-anterior screw placement in the calcaneus

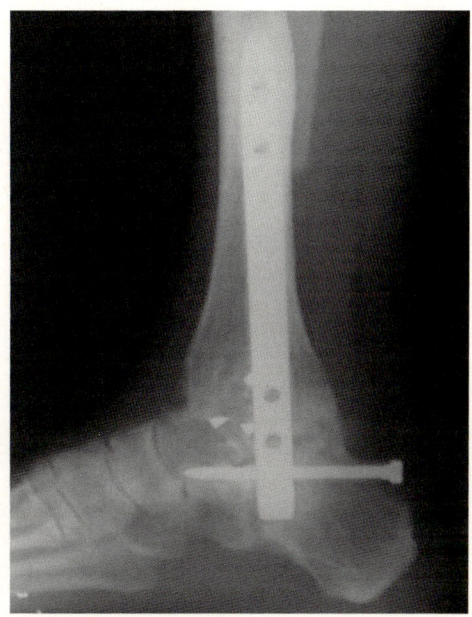

9.3.1 Technique

The patient is provided prophylactic antibiotic prior to surgery, and prophylactic deep vein thrombosis measures are also utilized. The patients wear support hose on the opposite leg as well as intermittent compression pumps during the course of the surgical procedure. Following the surgery, low weight molecular heparin is prescribed in effort to prevent a deep vein thrombosis.

Following proper identification of the patient and an appropriate time-out, the patient is placed in a lateral decubitus position for a lateral approach. If there is a significant soft tissue compromise to the lateral hind foot and ankle, then the patient is placed into a prone position and a posterior approach is utilized. A midthigh tourniquet is applied for hemostasis, and a typical prep and drape is performed. The prep and draping should be above the knee as this will provide excellent exposure to the entire lower extremity assisting the surgeon with alignment throughout the case.

In the presence of a severe hindfoot and ankle deformity, a gastrocnemius or gastroc-soleus equinus oftentimes will be present. Linked with these pathologies, a significant contracture will be present contributing as a major deforming force. The deformities can be addressed with a complete tenotomy, gastroc recession, or a tendo-Achilles lengthening based on the appropriate indication. This will reduce forefoot and midfoot pressures, aid in the realignment, and allow for restoration of the hindfoot beneath the leg (Fig. 9.4).[34]

Fig. 9.4 Intraoperative view demonstrating a performance of a percutaneous tendo-Achilles lengthening. This was needed in order to get the calcaneus in alignment with the lower leg

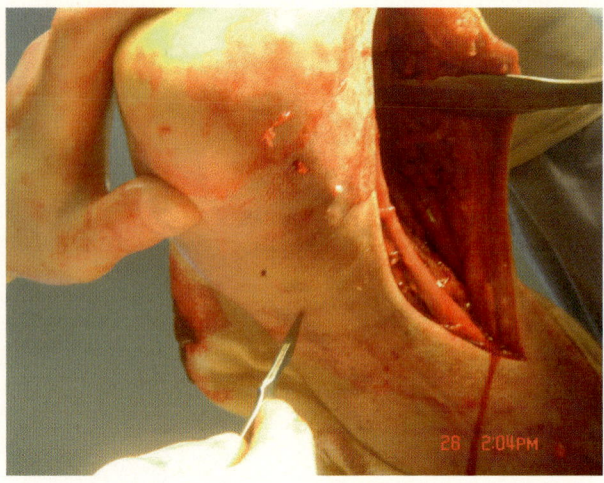

The lateral approach permits for outstanding exposure to the fibula, anterior and posterior ankle as well as the subtalar joint. The posterior approach provides an exceptional exposure to the posterior ankle, subtalar joint, syndesmosis as well as the medial and lateral malleoli.

9.3.1.1   Lateral Approach

The lateral incision is made over the distal one third of the fibula and carried out to the calcaneal cuboid joint. The lateral incision is carried deep to the level of the bony structures, avoiding all neurovascular structures. At this time, all soft tissues are retracted to allow for complete visualization of the bony anatomy (Fig. 9.5). An oblique fibular osteotomy is performed and retraction of the fibula from the distal tibia taking down the syndesmosis, in attempt to keep the calcaneal fibular ligaments intact providing excellent exposure to the ankle and subtalar joints.

9.3.1.2   Posterior Approach

In patients who have experienced soft tissue compromise laterally, a posterior approach should be considered. The posterior incision is made directly over the Achilles tendon onto the calcaneus. The Achilles can be completely excised and/or be retracted via a tenotomy. Next a breakdown of the remaining syndesmosis is performed allowing for separation of the distal fibula from the distal tibia and providing excellent exposure to the ankle and subtalar joint as well as the medial and lateral borders of the tibiotalocalcaneal joint. The medial aspect of the viable remaining fibula and the lateral aspect of the distal tibia are prepared for fusion via a rongeur, osteotome/mallet, and curettes. It is important that this site is prepared for a syndesmotic arthrodesis.

Fig. 9.5 Intraoperative view of a lateral approach of the hindfoot and ankle providing excellent exposure to the fibula; lateral, anterior, and posterior ankle; and subtalar joint

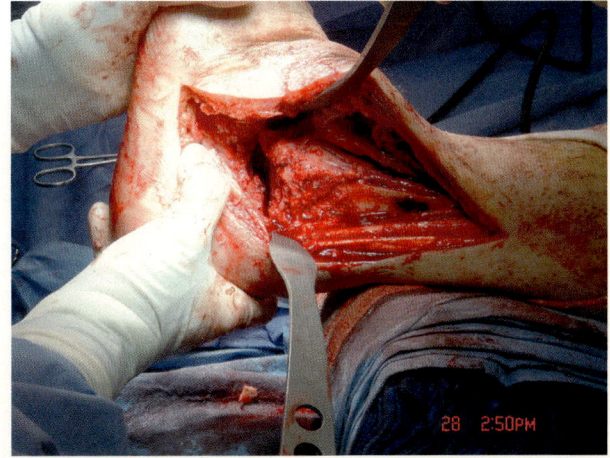

Following exposure either through a lateral or posterior approach, based on the degree of pathology present, a wide aggressive resection of all diseased bone, cartilage, fibrous tissue as well as any other unhealthy structures is obligatory. The involved joints need to be debrided to healthy viable bone. It is extremely important that the surgeon identifies the extent of bony disease involved. This is crucial as the surgeon must determine the amount of bone removal/resection necessary in order to obtain good anatomic alignment and to understand what bone is salvageable and nonsalvageable. Wide excision of the unhealthy bone is mandatory. It has been the author's understanding to leave as much healthy bone intact while being extremely aggressive in resecting the pathological-appearing bone. For example, when the nonpathological portion of the fibula can be salvaged, it is highly recommended that the fibula be used as an onlay graft or put into a bone mill to be utilized for autogenous bone graft. Another example is when a talectomy is being performed; it has been the authors' practice to leave the head and neck of the talus intact when there is no pathological process involved with the head and neck. This typically provides for a more stable construct which in turn has allowed for more favorable outcomes. In particular, with cases of osteomyelitis and Charcot joint resection, there will be areas of large resections that occur. It also has been the author's experience to leave the remaining viable bone intact as the resected areas can be backfilled with bone graft and the remaining viable bone areas provide a solid foundation for an arthrodesis (Fig. 9.6).

Following adequate joint preparation and certainty that all articular surfaces and nonviable bones are removed, clinical and radiographic assessment of anatomical alignment and temporary fixation is performed. Please note that in normal anatomy, the calcaneus falls lateral to the midline of the long axis of the tibia (Fig. 9.7). Based on the amount of bony destruction and involvement, the surgeon may be able to "medialize" the calcaneus directly under the long axis of the tibia.[6] In cases where the calcaneus cannot be "medialized," the surgeon may want to consider using an IM nail with a valgus design.

Fig. 9.6 Postoperative
anterior-posterior view
demonstrating the fibula used
as an onlay graft

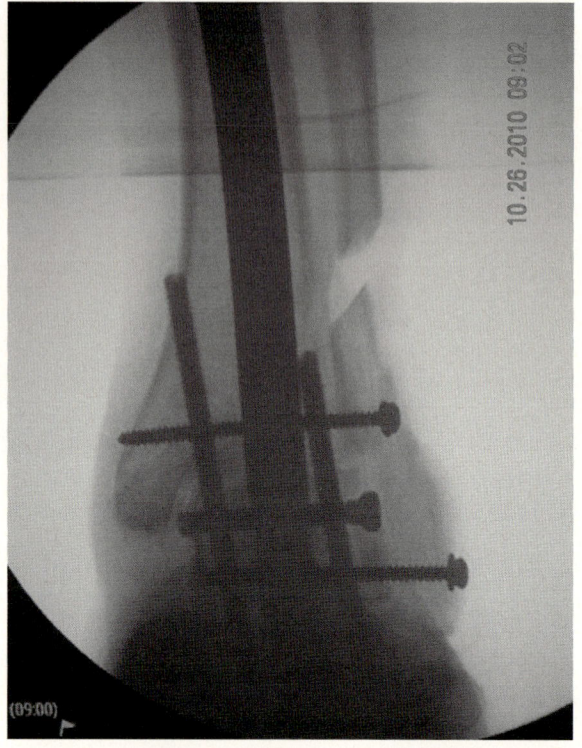

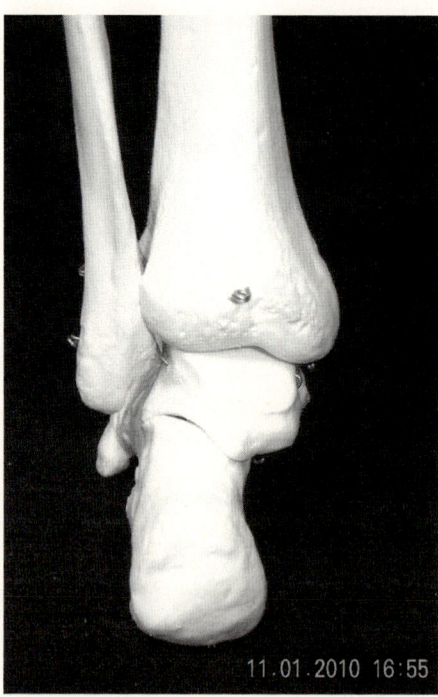

Fig. 9.7 The midline of the calcaneus is lateral
to the midline of the tibia in nonpathological
anatomy

Following adequate joint preparation, good anatomic alignment temporary fixation is inserted with large Steinman pins. Attention is directed to the plantar aspect of the calcaneus where a skin incision is made along the axial alignment of the distal tibia. This incision can be horizontal with the resting skin lines or it can be longitudinal.[2,6] Blunt dissection is carried down to the bone and care is taken to avoid neurovascular structures particularly the lateral plantar vessels.

After a satisfactory clinical and radiographic exam, a large guide wire is inserted through the plantar aspect of the heel up into the talus and into the tibial medullary canal. It is critical that the guide wire be placed into the central medial aspect of the calcaneus and centered in the medullary canal of the tibia. The body of the calcaneus is lateral relative to the alignment of the tibia in a nonpathological anatomy. In cases with significant pathology, it is usually necessary to medialize the calcaneus in order to get the calcaneus under the central portion of the tibia. Guide wire placement is evaluated using intraoperative fluoroscopy. It is very important at this time to evaluate the entire lower extremity for placement of the foot at 90° to the lower leg maintaining the heel in a neutral position with 10–15° of external rotation and/or maintain alignment that is consistent with the contralateral limb. With regards to the transverse plane, the second metatarsal should be aligned with the tibial tuberosity. It is critical that at this point – prior to insertion of the intramedullary nail – the most favorable alignment is obtained. Next a large drill is used to drill through the calcaneus and into the distal one third of the tibial canal. It is important to continuously check the alignment in all planes with fluoroscopy throughout the procedure in order to detect any shifting or malalignment that may occur. Next a flexible reamer is used to help determine the optimal diameter of the nail to be used. During the reaming process, the surgeon should experience "chatter." Chatter occurs when maximal diameter has been obtained and the reamer fits "tight" within the cortical walls. It is very important to reach this point in order to avoid the "wiper blade affect." The wiper blade affect occurs when too small of a diameter nail is inserted into the distal tibia allowing for toggle to occur with eventual loosening; therefore, it is desirable to obtain the largest diameter nail that will fit within the medullary canal for most favorable results. It is also important for the surgeon to be aware of "fatty emboli" which can occur during the reaming process. Once the nail size is determined, it is attached to the alignment jig and placed into the canal. The nail is driven into the tibia until the most inferior portion of the nail is slightly recessed into the plantar calcaneus. If a dynamic nail is desired, there are three techniques in order to obtain dynamic compression. One is by only using distal calcaneal transfixation and not utilizing proximal tibia transfixation. With this technique, the surgeon may apply a multi level external fixator and allow immediate weight-bearing. In this scenario, once a bony biological response is identified at the arthrodesis site, the external fixator may be loosened or "de-tensioned." The biology of healing with an external fixator is straightforward. Stiffness of the "construct" should be adjusted to match the biologic state of the bone. Some situations necessitate a very stiff construct while others require a flexible construct. In general, early phases of treatment start with stiff constructs, followed by progressive load transfer as the bone demonstrates a biologic response to healing (callus). Once a biologic response has been radiographically confirmed, the fixator can be adjusted to begin transferring load to the newly formed callus. This gradual load transfer is monitored closely by the surgeon and done by slowly "de-stiffening" of the fixator. This can be completed in

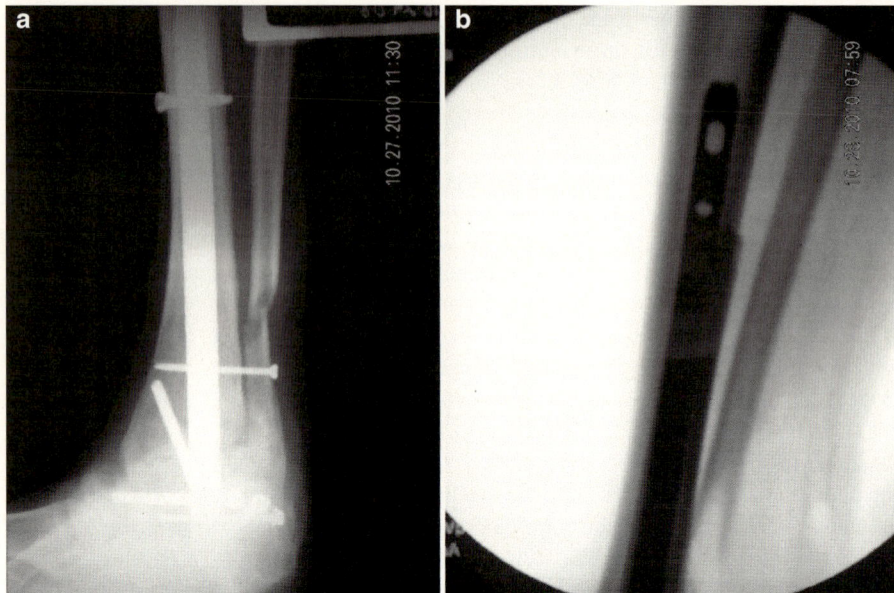

Fig. 9.8 (**a**) This radiograph demonstrates proximal and distal screw establishing a static nail. (**b**) This radiograph demonstrates how a dynamic compression construct can work. Note, once the patient is full weight-bearing and the proximal tibial transfixation screws are not utilized, this will create dynamic compression

many ways: removing bars, increasing the distance of bars from the load bearing axis (bone), removing fixation points (wires or pins), or using "dynamic" components that allow a predetermined spring stiffness. Once an appropriate amount of healing has taken place, the fixator can be completely "dynamized" by removing all connecting elements. The second technique is very similar to the external fixation described above with the difference being in utilizing a below-the-knee cast instead of an external fixator. Once the surgeon identifies an adequate biological response during the non-weight-bearing immobilization period, the patient is then transferred to a full weight-bearing walking boot. This will provide weight-bearing dynamization. The third technique is utilization of the more advanced systems. This technique involves the proximal screws being inserted first into the tibia. These systems have the ability to internally compress at the tibial–talar joint and/or the talar–calcaneal joint. Following the desired compression, the distal screws are inserted into the calcaneus to maintain compression. If a static nail is employed, an attempt to align the distal portion of the nail with the plantar calcaneus is made and the distal most transfixation screw (posterior to anterior or lateral to medial) is placed first. At this time, manual compression is applied from distal to proximal and the proximal tibial transfixation screws are inserted from medial to lateral in order to avoid the musculature lateral to the tibia (Fig. 9.8).

Regarding the calcaneal screw placement, the posterior-to-anterior screw offers more bone purchase. If a posterior-to-anterior calcaneal screw cannot be obtained, then a distal calcaneal transfixation lateral-to-medial screw is used, offering the least risk to the vital structures. Regarding the insertion of the proximal tibial screws,

Fig. 9.9 This intraoperative radiograph demonstrates the use of two temporary Steinman pin fixation while inserting the guide wire in the medullary canal of the tibia

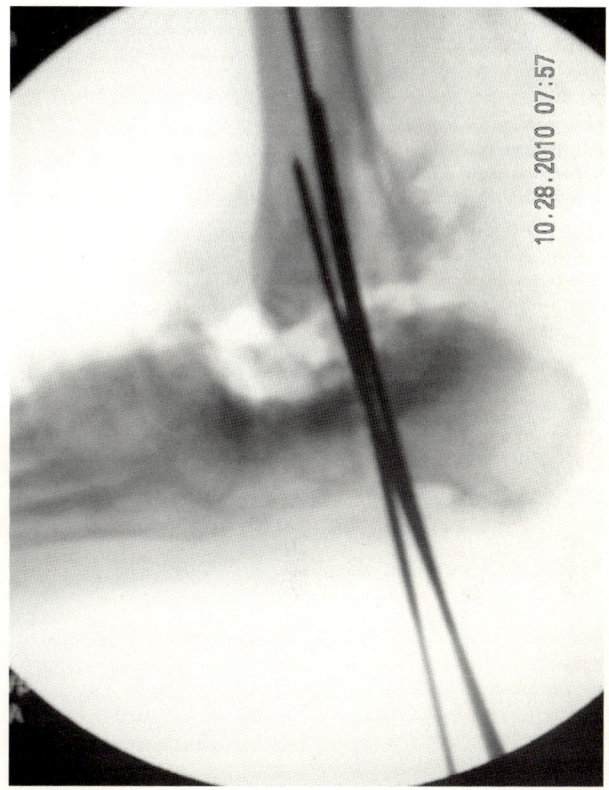

the screws should be inserted from medial to lateral, again avoiding vital structures. After evaluating the placement of the nail and fixation to the surgeon's satisfaction, the alignment jig is dismantled and an optional end-cap can be inserted at the most distal end of the nail to prevent fibrous ingrowth. This will offer an advantage should the nail need to be removed in the future (Figs. 9.9–9.11).

As stated earlier, it is the authors' recommendation to use tangential (peripheral) screws for additional stabilization. The authors have found that this provides a much more solid construct with the additional points of fixation (Fig. 9.12).

Following stabilization of the hindfoot and ankle, any osseous defects should be packed with some form of bone graft. The distal fibula is decorticated medially and the distal tibia and ankle are decorticated laterally allowing the fibula to be used as an onlay graft for added stability. The authors' experience has now recommended the use of additional fixation outside of the nail. The authors believe this obtains a more solid construct to have individual screw fixation inserted from plantar posterior calcaneus into the anterior distal tibia and or screw fixation inserted from the inferior midfoot into the posterior distal tibia. The surgical site is then flushed with irrigation solution. Care is taken not to wash away any bone graft. The tourniquet is deflated and hemostasis is obtained; typical deep tissue and skin closure is performed with the insertion of a closed suction drain.

Fig. 9.10 (a) A view of the plantar incision following insertion of the IM nail. (b) A calcaneal axial view postoperatively demonstrating the nail is in good position within the calcaneus

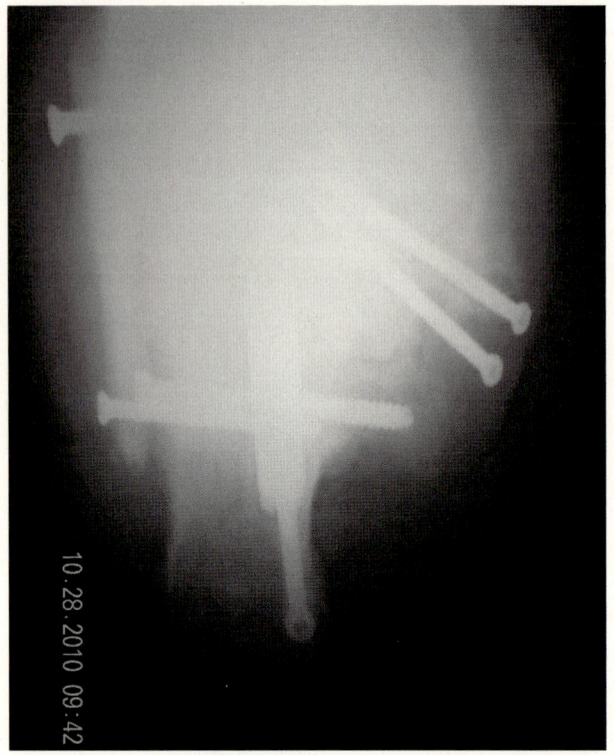

Fig. 9.11 An intraoperative view inserting the end-cap following insertion of the IM nail. Next, backfilling of bone graft is completed to allow for a solid bony union

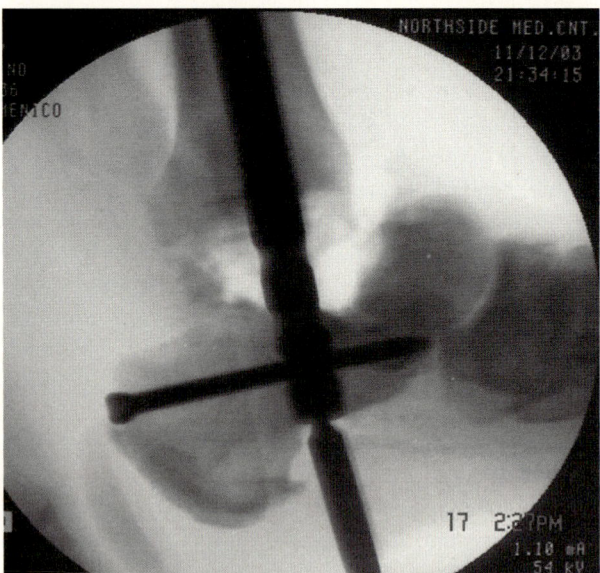

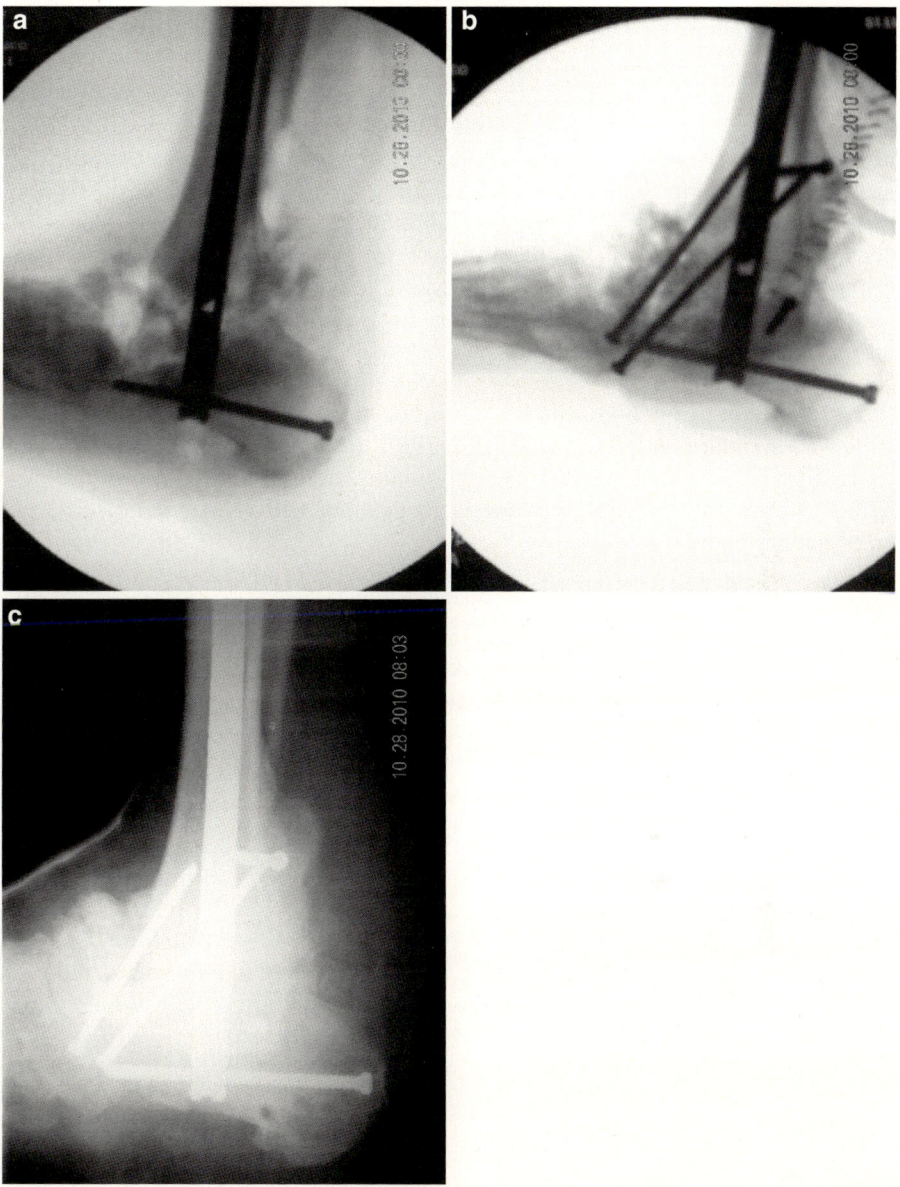

Fig. 9.12 (**a**) Lateral intraoperative view following complete insertion of the IM nail. (**b**) After the bone grafting is completed, the tangential screws are inserted providing additional stability. (**c**) Postoperative lateral radiograph demonstrating solid bony union with a stable hindfoot and ankle

9.4   Complications

General complications include infection, soft tissue complications, nerve injury, vascular injury, deep vein thrombosis, pulmonary emboli, fatty emboli, delayed union, nonunion, and malunion. A delay union and non union may result from inadequate resection of bone or hardware failure. Painful internal hardware may necessitate removal in rare instances. If a nonunion occurs with no gross evidence of hardware failure, the result may be uneventful as long as clinical stability and alignment is maintained. Nonunions, especially in patients who suffer from peripheral neuropathy, are generally not painful. Malunion (malposition), on the other hand, can be very difficult to manage and may require revisional surgery.

Fatigue fractures of the tibia have been observed at the proximal end of the nails with standard length (15 cm) following a successful tibio-calcaneal arthrodesis. Noonan et al. suggest the use of a long retrograde locked intramedullary nails for tibiotalocalcaneal arthrodesis in patients with systemic or localized osteopenia.[35]

Other complications include wound dehiscence, tibial or calcaneal fracture, and hardware failure. It is important to address any complication, such as ulceration, infection, or hardware failure, with extreme urgency and aggressive treatment since failure to do so may result in below-the-knee amputation (Figs. 9.13 and 9.14).

9.5   Conclusion

Intramedullary nails for tibiotalocalcaneal arthrodesis are used to treat severe arthrosis, deformity, and malalignment of the hindfoot and ankle. Often the severity of the deformity affects not only the ankle but may also affect the subtalar joint, thereby warranting fusion of both joints. The goal is to create a solid arthrodesis that corrects the deformity, maintains anatomic alignment, and provides a plantigrade foot that allows the patient to function independently while relieving pain. The objective is to have the patient be shoeable or braceable, thus maintaining the ability to ambulate unassisted.

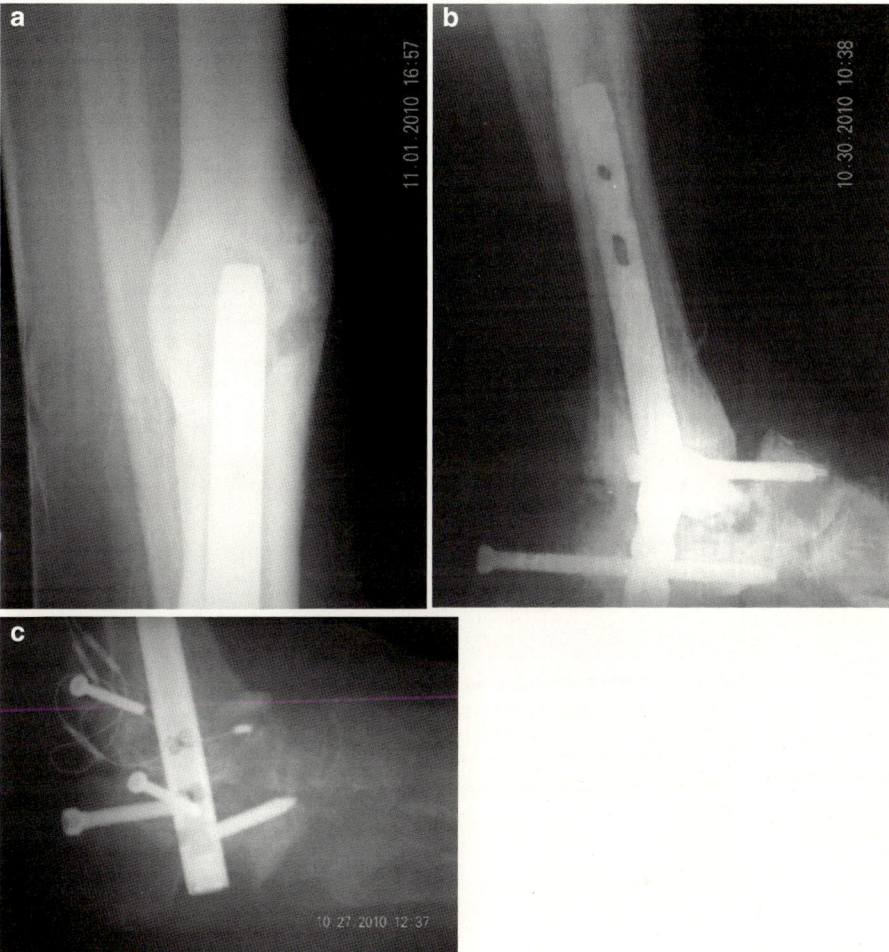

Fig. 9.13 (**a**) This view demonstrates a patient who had experienced a tibial fracture while inserting the nail. (**b**) This view demonstrates a nonunion and a fracture of the intramedullary nail. (**c**) This view demonstrates a fracture of the calcaneus with subsequent hardware failure, collapse of the calcaneus, and loosening with distal projection of the nail

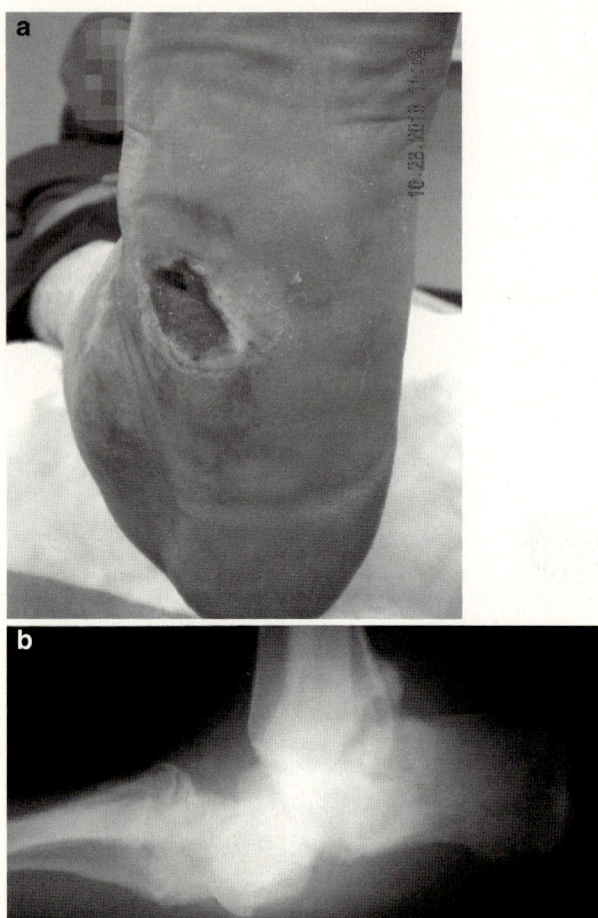

Fig. 9.14 (**a**) A non weight bearing view of a neuropathic patient with exposed bone secondary to an unstable charcot neuropathic deformity. (**b**) A lateral radiograph demonstrating malalignment of the midfoot, hindfoot, and ankle secondary to Charcot arthropathy. (**c**) A anterior-posterior radiograph demonstrating midfoot pathology and osteomyelitis secondary to the ulceration and Charcot arthropathy. (**d**) A lateral radiograph following insertion of an IM Nail. Not the hindfoot and ankle alignment and the use of the tangential screw from the posterior inferior calcaneus into the distal anterior tibia. (**e**) Anterior- posterior ankle view following the insertion of an IM Nail. Note the use of the fibula as an onlay bone graft. (**f**) Reconstruction utilizing a medial column fusion via a locking plate. (**g**) A post operative lateral radiographic view demonstrating a well healed and well aligned reconstructed mid foot, hindfoot and ankle

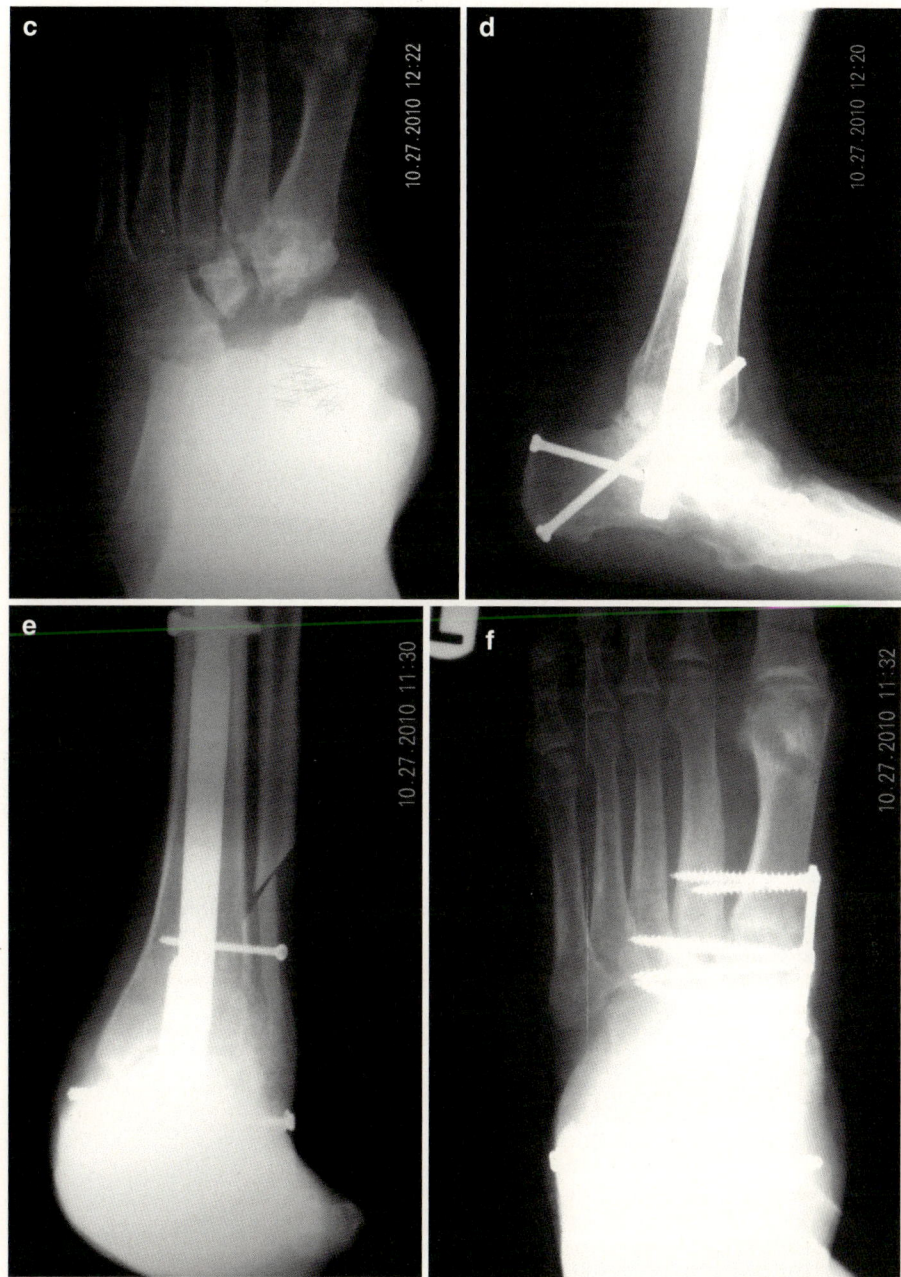

Fig. 9.14 (continued)

Fig. 9.14 (continued)

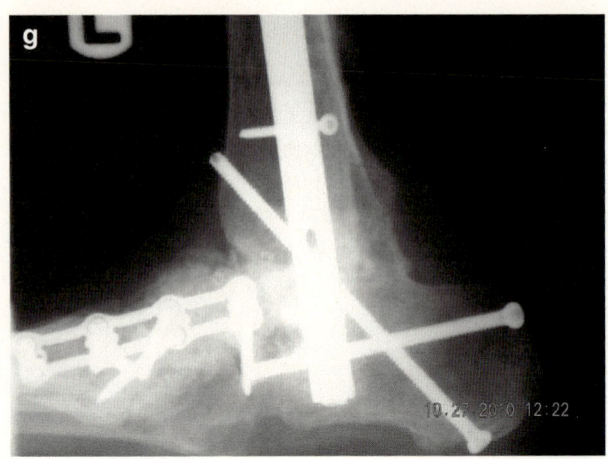

References

1. Myerson MS, Alvarez RG, Lam PW. Tibiocalcaneal arthrodesis for the management of severe ankle and hindfoot deformities. Foot Ankle Int. 2000;21:643-50.
2. DiDomenico LA, Adams HB. Intramedullary nailing for "Charcot" arthropathy of the hindfoot and ankle. In: Chang TJ, editor. Master techniques in podiatric surgery. Philadelphia: Lippincott Williams & Wilkins; 2005. p. 427-43.
3. Lexer E. Die verwedung der frein knockenplastik nebst versuchen uber gelenkversteifung und gelentransplanten. Langenbecks Arch Chir. 1906;86:938-42.
4. Mendencino RW, Catanzariti AR, Saltrick KR, et al. Tibiotalocalcaneal arthrodesis with retrograde intramedullary nailing. J Foot Ankle Surg. 2004;43(2):82-6.
5. Albee FH. Bone graft surgery. Philadelphia: Saunders; 1915. p. 335.
6. Roukis TS. Determining the insertion site for retrograde intramedullary nail fixation of tibiotalocalcaneal arthrodesis: a radiographic and intraoperative anatomical landmark analysis. J Foot Ankle Surg. 2006;45(4):227-34.
7. Bingold AC. Ankle and subtalar fusion by a transarticular graft. J Bone Joint Surg. 1956;38:862-70.
8. Adams JC. Arthrodesis of the ankle joint: experience with the transfibular approach. J Bone Joint Surg. 1948;30:506-11.
9. Carriar DA, Harris CM. Ankle arthrodesis with vertical Steinmann's pins in rheumatoid arthritis. Clin Orthop Relat Res. 1991;268:10-4.
10. Buratti RA, Johnson JD, Buratti D. Concurrent ankle and subtalar joint arthrodesis. J Foot Ankle Surg. 1994;33:278-82.
11. Kile TA, Donnelly RE, Gehrke JC, Werner ME, Johnson KA. Tibiotalocalcaneal arthrodesis with an intramedullary device. Foot Ankle Int. 1994;15:669-73.
12. Johnson KA. Tibiotalocalcaneal arthrodesis. In: Johnson KA, editor. Master techniques in orthopedic surgery: the foot and ankle. Philadelphia: Lippincott; 1994:483-96.
13. Quill GE. Tibiotalocalcaneal and pantalar arthrodesis. Foot Ankle Clin. 1996;1:199-209.
14. Quill GE. Tibiotalocalcaneal arthrodesis. Tech Orthop. 1996;11:269-73.
15. Quill GE. The use of a second generation intramedullary nail in the fixation of difficult ankle and hindfoot arthrodesis. Am J Orthop. 1999;1:23-31.
16. Quill GE. Tibiotalocalcaneal arthrodesis with medullary rod fixation. Tech Foot Ankle Surg. 2003;2:135-43.

17. Mader J, Penning D, Gausepohl T, Patsalis U. Calcaneotibial arthrodesis with a retrograde posterior to anterior locked nail as a salvage procedure for severe ankle pathology. J Bone Joint Surg. 2003;85:123-8.
18. Farber DC, DeOrio JK. Tibiotalocalcaneal fusion with a second generation intramedullary device. Presentation at: American Orthopedic Foot and Ankle Society Annual Summer Meeting; June 27, 2003; Hilton Head.
19. Mann MR, Parks BG, Pak SS, Miller SD. Tibiotalocalcaneal arthrodesis: a biomechanical analysis of the rotational stability of the Biomet ankle arthrodesis nail. Foot Ankle Int. 2001;22:731-3.
20. Means KR, Parks BG, Nguyen A, Schon LC. Intramedullary nail fixation with posterior to anterior compared to transverse distal screw placement for tibiotalocalcaneal arthrodesis: a biomechanical investigation. Foot Ankle Int. 2006;27(12):1137-42.
21. Niinimaki TT, Klemola TM, Leppilahti JI. Tibiotalocalcaneal arthrodesis with a compression retrograde intramedullary nail: a report of 34 consecutive patients. Foot Ankle Int. 2007;28(4):431-4.
22. Pinzur MS, Kelikian A. Charcot ankle fusion with a retrograde locked intramedullary nail. Foot Ankle Int. 1997;18:699-704.
23. Thomason K, Eyres KS. A technique of fusion for failed total replacement of the ankle: tibio-allograft-calcaneal fusion with a locked retrograde intramedullary nail. J Bone Joint Surg Br. 2008;90(7):885-8.
24. Bailey CC, Root HF. Neuropathic foot lesions in diabetes. N Engl J Med. 1947;236:397-401.
25. Fox IM, Shapero C, Kennedy A. Tibiotalocalcaneal arthrodesis with intramedullary interlocking nail fixation. Clin Podiatr Med Surg. 2000;17:19-31.
26. Muckley T, Eichhorn S, Hoffmeier K, et al. Biomechanical evaluation of primary stiffness of tibiotalocalcaneal fusion with intramedullary nails. Foot Ankle Int. 2007;28:224-31.
27. Moore TJ, Prince R, Pecatko D, Smith JW, Fleming S. Retrograde intramedullary nailing for ankle arthrodesis. Foot Ankle Int. 1995;16:433-6.
28. Mendencino RW, Catanzariti AR, Lamm BM, Statler TK. Realignment arthrodesis of the ankle. Posterpresented at: The American College of Foot and Ankle Surgeons National Meeting; February 7–11, 2001; New Orleans.
29. Berend ME, Glisson RR, Nunley JA. A biomechanical comparison of intramedullary nail and crossed lag screw fixation for tibiotalocalcaneal arthrodesis. Foot Ankle Int. 1997;18:639-64.
30. Stone KH, Helal B. A method of ankle stabilization. Clin Orthop Relat Res. 1991;268:102-6.
31. Pelton K, Hofer JK, Thordarson DB. Tibiotalocalcaneal arthrodesis using a dynamically locked retrograde intramedullary nail. Foot Ankle Int. 2006;27(10):759-63.
32. Santangelo JR, Glisson RR, Garras DN, Easly ME. Tibiotalocalcaneal arthrodesis: a biomechanical comparison of multiplanar external fixation with intramedullary fixation. Foot Ankle Int. 2008;29(9):936-41.
33. De Smet K, DeBrauwer V, Burssens P, et al. Tibiotalocalcaneal Marchetti-Vicenzi nailing in revision arthrodesis for posttraumatic pseudoarthrosis of the ankle. Acta Orthop Belg. 2003;69:42-8.
34. Armstrong DG, Stacpoole-Shea S, Nguyen H, Harkless LB. Lengthening of the Achilles tendon in diabetic patients who are at high risk for ulceration of the foot. J Bone Joint Surg. 1999;81:535-8.
35. Noonan T, Pinzur M, Paxinos O, Havey R, Patwardin A. Tibial calcaneal arthrodesis with a retrograde intramedullary nail: a biomechanical analysis of the effect on nail length. Foot Ankle Int. 2005;26(4):304-8.

Chapter 10
Pedal Amputations in Diabetes

Nicholas J. Bevilacqua, Lee C. Rogers, and David G. Armstrong

Diabetes is the leading cause of amputation worldwide. It has been said that "every 30 seconds a limb is lost as a consequence of diabetes."[1] In the United States, the annual incidence of lower extremity amputation in those with diabetes is 5–8 per 1,000.[2,3] The causes of amputation are well understood. Foot ulcer precedes amputations in 84% of the cases.[4] Up to 25% of those with diabetes will develop a foot ulcer over their lifetime.[5] More than half of those ulcers will become infected, and 1 in 5 will necessitate an amputation.[6] Approximately 60% of the limbs that are amputated are complicated by infection.[7] This prompted our group to conceptualize the "steps to an amputation" shown in Fig. 10.1. There are opportunities for intervention at each of these steps, which might prevent the progression of the patient toward the final step – amputation.

Amputation is not a benign treatment. The 5-year relative mortality rate is 48% after major limb loss, higher than many cancers (Fig. 10.2).[8] After a major limb loss, there is a 50% chance of developing a serious lesion on the contralateral limb within 2 years.[9] The more proximal the amputation level, the more energy is required for ambulation.[10] A patient with diabetes and comorbidities may not have cardiophysiologic reserves to ambulate effectively after proximal amputation, resulting in sedentariness and cardiovascular deconditioning.

N.J. Bevilacqua, D.P.M. (✉)
Associate, Foot and Ankle Surgery, North Jersey Orthopaedic Specialists,
Teaneck, NJ 07666, USA
e-mail: nicholas.bevilacqua@gmail.com

L.C. Rogers, D.P.M.
Amputation Prevention Center,
Valley Presbyterian Hospital, Van Nuys, CA, USA

D.G. Armstrong, D.P.M., M.D., Ph.D.
Southern Arizona Limb Salvage Alliance (SALSA),
Department of Surgery, University of Arizona,
Tucson, AZ, USA

A. Saxena (ed.), *Special Procedures in Foot and Ankle Surgery*,
DOI 10.1007/978-1-4471-4103-7_10, © Springer-Verlag London 2013

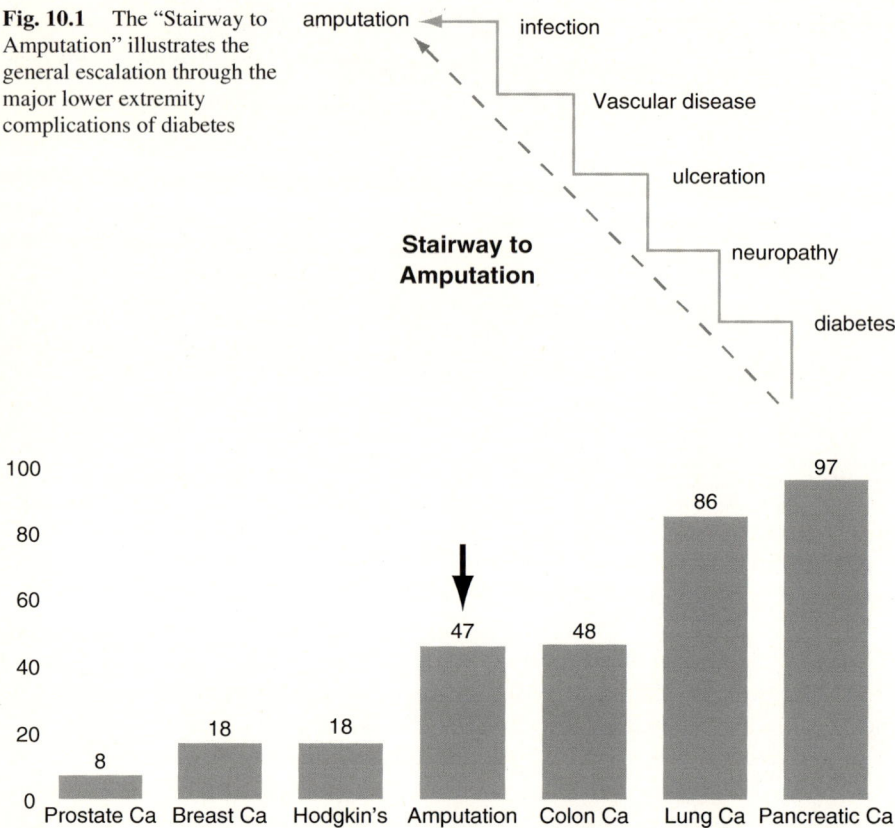

Fig. 10.1 The "Stairway to Amputation" illustrates the general escalation through the major lower extremity complications of diabetes

Fig. 10.2 The 5-year relative mortality rate of various cancers and major lower extremity amputation (*arrow*)

The average cost of a major amputation was estimated at approximately $70,000 per episode in 2007. Rogers et al. calculated that amputations in those with diabetes cost the US healthcare system $11.7 billion in 2007.[11]

Given these grave physical, psychological, and financial costs, every effort should be made to avoid a limb loss situation. Effective preventative care can help to avoid ulcers and infections, the common prequels to amputation. When the limb is at risk, specialized care involving a multidisciplinary team approach and organized care can reduce the rate of amputations.[12-14]

This chapter reviews the techniques and outcomes, when available in the literature, for the anatomic levels of lower extremity amputations.

10.1 Considerations in Pedal Amputation

The answer to the question "at which level to amputate" is not always obvious. In patients presenting with a limb-threatening infection, adequate debridement is paramount and the extent of infection will initially dictate the level of debridement. The goal is to perform the most distal, functional amputation. Certain lower-level amputations are generally better tolerated and result in a more functional outcome than higher-level amputations.

10.1.1 Infection

The immediate concern is to remove all infected and necrotic tissue, which will influence the final level of amputation, as debridement will always trump reconstruction. If there is an abscess, urgent incision and drainage can limit spread of infection and reduce the risk of a more proximal amputation. Appropriate empiric antibiotic therapy should take into account risk factors for methicillin-resistant *Staphylococcus aureus*. Proper cultures, including blood cultures when indicated, are paramount. Proper technique is essential for obtaining deep tissue cultures. It is important to obtain deep tissue cultures as opposed to a swap culture. The surgeon should remove outer gloves and use only sterile, unused instruments.

Due to immunopathy, less than half of all diabetic foot infections present with leukocytosis[15] and nearly 9 in 10 are afebrile.[16] In these cases of relative leukopenia, granulocyte colony-stimulating factor has been shown to reduce the rate of limb loss.[17] Once the infection is controlled, the surgeon must evaluate the vascular status to determine potential to heal and also the function of the resultant foot.

10.1.2 Vascular Status

It is important to determine the level of tissue perfusion and vascular outflow. A thorough history and physical exam is necessary to uncover any underlying vascular disease. Notation should be made of vascular comorbidities, such as coronary artery disease or cerebrovascular disease and precipitating factors like smoking, hypertension, and dyslipidemia. The patient should be questioned about intermittent claudication and rest pain. It is worth noting that the neuropathic patient may not have classic claudication and instead may present with lower extremity fatigue upon exertion that relieves after rest.

The physical exam should include observation of gangrene, dependent rubor, atrophic skin, and absent hair growth. Pedal pulses should be palpated, but if present do not always indicate adequate circulation.

Noninvasive vascular exams to assess macro- and micro-circulation assist the surgeon in determining the urgency of a vascular surgery consultation and appropriate level of amputation. Commonly employed noninvasive tests of macrovascular circulation include the ankle-brachial index, toe-brachial index, and pulse volume recording waveforms. Other noninvasive tests can estimate microvascular flow and function. TcPO2 may be useful in predicting the wound-healing capability at a specific level of pedal amputation. Values greater than 30 mmHg are associated with successful healing.[18,19] Skin perfusion pressure (SPP) is measured with a laser Doppler and may also aid in the determination of amputation healing. SPP measurements above 30 mmHg have 90% accuracy in predicting healing of the amputation site.[20] Hyperspectral imaging can measure tissue oxyhemoglobin and deoxyhemoglobin.[21] It is currently being investigated to predict diabetic wound healing and level of amputation healing.

10.1.3   Nutrition

Nutritional factors are important to consider for healing capability. Some preoperative parameters and factors predicting success include a serum albumin greater than or equal to 3.5 g/dL, prealbumin greater than 16 mg/dL, and total lymphocyte count greater 1,500.[22] Pinzur found a 92.2% healing rate after transmetatarsal amputation (TMA) with at least an ankle-brachial index (ABI) greater than 0.5, total lymphocyte count greater than 1,500, and serum albumin greater than 3.0 g/dL. In a review of 83 diabetic patients after a Syme amputation, Pinzur and coworkers reported 88% overall healing rate with serum albumin threshold of 2.5 g/dL.[23] Supplementation, when appropriate, should be given to those who are undernourished. In more severe cases, total parenteral nutrition is indicated.

10.1.4   Function

It is important to avoid nonfunctional amputations as this will lead to a biomechanically unsound foot. Even if limb salvage is successful, the patient may not truly benefit given the postoperative risks and potential morbidity following a nonfunctional amputation. Partial foot amputations often predispose diabetic patients to increased foot pressures and the development of foot deformities, which will further increase their risk for ulceration and amputation.[24] The resultant unstable foot frequently leads to the development of further neuropathic foot ulcerations leading to subsequent surgery, possibly resulting in a "high-level" or major amputation (Fig. 10.3). A disproportionate share of these adverse outcomes occur in high-level amputations and it has been shown that patients function better with a lower-level, more distal amputation.[10] Therefore, a prudent surgeon will preserve as much length to the foot as possible, but will also consider function and muscle imbalance and their associated risks for future ulcerations.

10.1.5   General Surgical Principles

Proper surgical technique is mandatory and the surgeon must adhere to basic principles to reduce the risk of complications. Procedures are generally performed without the use of a tourniquet. This will assist in determining the necessary extent of

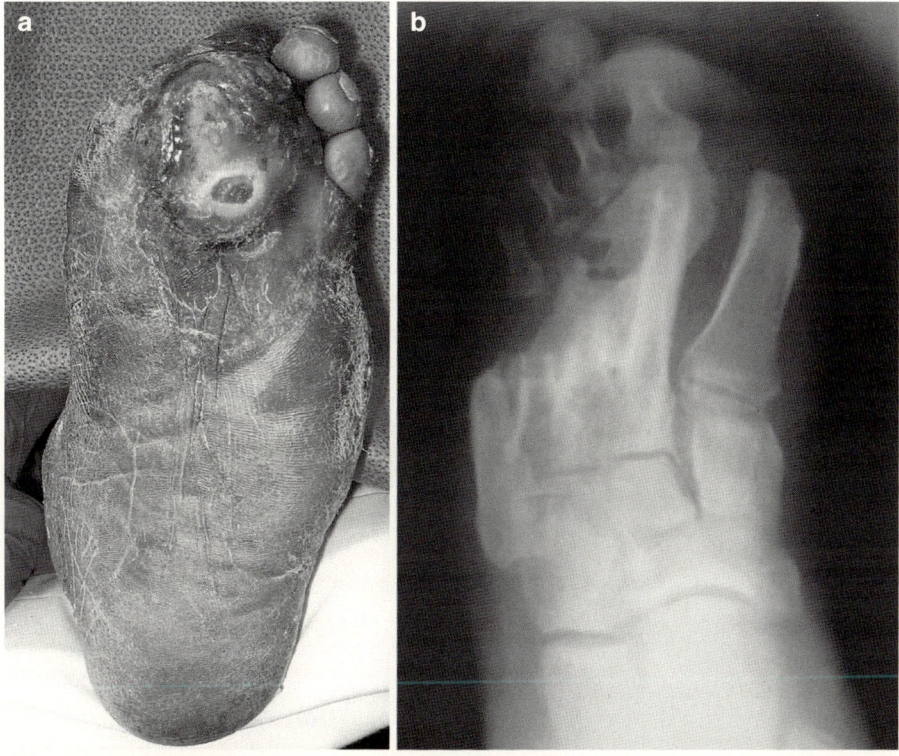

Fig. 10.3 (**a**) Clinical and (**b**) radiographic example of a biomechanically unsound foot resulting in increased foot pressures and skin breakdown and the need for subsequent amputation

debridement of the soft tissue and bone; bleeding is controlled on a local level. However, a tourniquet may be applied in case it is needed, and inflated if bleeding becomes extensive. A tourniquet is contraindicated in dysvascular patients and patients who have had recent revascularization. If a tourniquet is used, it is recommended that it be deflated before closure to ensure proper hemostasis is obtained.

Skin incisions should be made full-thickness with minimal undermining. Medial and lateral incisions should be performed at the glabrous juncture between the dorsal and plantar circulation. Dorsal and plantar incisions should be to bone, without undermining to preserve the metatarsal arteries in the flaps. Adequate removal of all infected and necrotic tissue is key to controlling infection. The goal is to excise the wound completely until only normal, soft, and well-vascularized tissue remains.[25] Bone and soft tissue are debrided layer by layer, until healthy bleeding tissue is reached. If you cut the tissue, and it does not bleed, it should be removed. Attinger et al.[26] recommends aggressively debriding infected bone until bleeding and normal appearing marrow is noted. Biomechanical considerations should not discourage the surgeon from debriding enough bone to ensure that all infection has been eliminated. Correction of the resultant biomechanical abnormality may be addressed after the wound has healed.[26] Any exposed unattached tendons are removed from the wound under traction.

Inspect, irrigate, and debulk the soft tissue to allow for adequate soft tissue coverage with minimal tension. If there is concern with residual infection, leave the wound open and return to the operating room for delayed primary closure once infection is controlled.

Recognition of potential muscle and tendon imbalances are essential for optimal long-term results. Tendon procedures, such as a tendo-Achilles lengthening, are often necessary, especially if it is determined that equinus is one of the etiologic factors that led to the original ulceration. The more proximal foot-sparing amputations will result in more pronounced muscle imbalance and deformity. Soft tissue balancing procedures and osseous reconstruction are sometimes needed.

Negative pressure wound therapy (NPWT) is a topical modality that can produce granulation tissue, speed closure, and reduce the rate of subsequent amputations. A multicenter, randomized, controlled trial compared NPWT (KCI Wound V.A.C.®) to standard moist wound care after partial diabetic foot amputation. The rate of wound healing and granulation tissue formation was faster in the NPWT group compared to the controls. Both groups had similar frequency and severity of adverse events. The NPWT group trended toward reduced risk for a subsequent amputation compared to the control.[27] NPWT is, in essence, a wound simplification device – transforming a deep, complicated wound to a more manageable, simple wound.

10.2 Anatomic Levels

10.2.1 Digital Amputations

Digital amputations are the most common amputations performed in the foot. This procedure is necessary when patients present with distal digital ulcerations with underlying osteomyelitis of the phalanges (Fig. 10.4a). The desired skin incision is placed proximal to open ulcerations. If the soft tissue and bone infection is limited to the distal aspect of the digit, a fish mouth-type incision is placed at the level of the proximal phalanx. The incision is planned with a plantar flap and the bone is resected leaving the base of the proximal phalanx to act as a buttress to prevent transverse migration of adjacent digits (Fig. 10.4b). If the infection extends more proximal, disarticulation at the metatarsophalangeal joint may be performed with a racket-type incision.

Postoperatively, patients may be placed in a surgical shoe or a removable cast walker. Sutures are removed when the incision appears healed and patients are transferred to extra-depth prescriptive shoes. Although no formal prosthesis is required, a plastizote insert provides dispersion of pressure areas. Complications include adjacent toe deformities with increased risk for ulceration and amputation.

Fig. 10.4   (**a**) Digital ulcer with underlying osteomyelitis of the distal phalanx. (**b**) Second digit amputation at the level of the proximal phalanx. The base of the proximal phalanx was preserved to act as a buttress to prevent transverse migration of adjacent digits

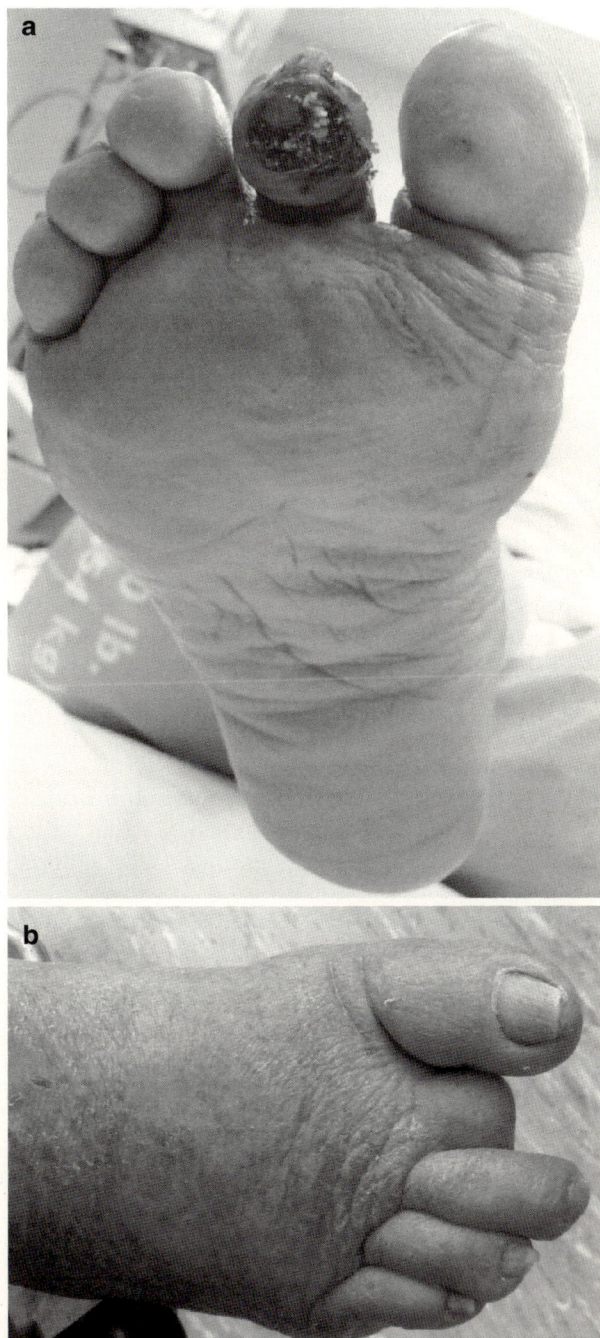

10.2.2   Hallux and First-Ray Amputation

Amputations of the hallux are most often indicated as a definitive procedure follow-ing surgical debridement of an infected distal hallux ulcer complicated by osteomy-elitis. Hallux ulcers are often the result of limited joint range of motion at the first metatarsal phalangeal joint (MTPJ). The limited joint range of motion leads to an increase in pressure at the distal hallux during ambulation resulting in ulceration. Once the wound and underlying bone become infected, surgery is often necessary.

If the ulceration is distal and the bone infection is confined to the distal phalanx, a fish-mouth incision is planned preserving a plantar flap. The incision is full-thickness and, if possible, incorporates the ulcer. The hallux is disarticulated at the interphalan-geal joint and the hallux is removed. The area is inspected, and all infected and necrotic tissue is excised. The proximal phalanx is debrided "slice by slice" until bleeding and normal appearing marrow is noted.[26] When possible, preservation of the base of the proximal phalanx preserves the flexor mechanism and markedly improves function (Fig. 10.5).[28] The resultant base of the phalanx will act as a buttress and prevent medial drift of the lesser digits as well (Fig. 10.6). However, if the infection extends proximal to the interphalangeal joint, the hallux is disarticulated from the metatarsal. Disruption of the joint capsule results in loss of vascularity to the cartilage; therefore, the cartilage is resected off the head of the metatarsal. The area is irrigated, deep tissue cultures are obtained, and if indicated, the wound is closed in layers.

The area is dressed and patients are placed in a surgical shoe or diabetic walker to eliminate the propulsive phase of gait. Patients ambulate postoperatively and are instructed to keep the surgical site clean and dry. Patients are followed weekly and sutures are removed when the incision is healed, often at 3 or 4 weeks after surgery. Patients are then placed in non-custom prescription footwear or, if neces-sary, are given a protective foot orthosis with a filler to prevent medial drift of the lesser digits.

If the infection spreads proximal to the MTPJ, a first-ray resection is indicated. We define a first-ray resection as an amputation of the phalanges and of at least part of the first metatarsal. A racket-type incision is made circumscribing the hallux and extended proximally at the medial glabrous juncture. A plantar flap is preserved and incisions are full-thickness with minimal undermining. The hallux is disarticulated at the MTPJ and removed. The wound is irrigated and inspected for any infected or nonviable tissue. The metatarsal is then debrided "slice by slice" until bleeding and normal appearing marrow is noted.[26] The metatarsal is ultimately angled from dor-sal-distal to plantar-proximal and proximal-medial to distal-lateral to avoid resul-tant bone prominences (Fig. 10.7).

The wound is irrigated and inspected. Extensor and flexor tendons are excised under traction and the soft tissue is debulked to allow for adequate soft tissue cover-age. The wound is closed being careful to avoid dead spaces. A closed suction drain may be used to prevent formation of hematoma post-op (Fig. 10.7b).

As mentioned earlier, the extent of infection and necrosis will dictate the level of debridement. Devitalized and nonviable bone and soft tissue impede healing and

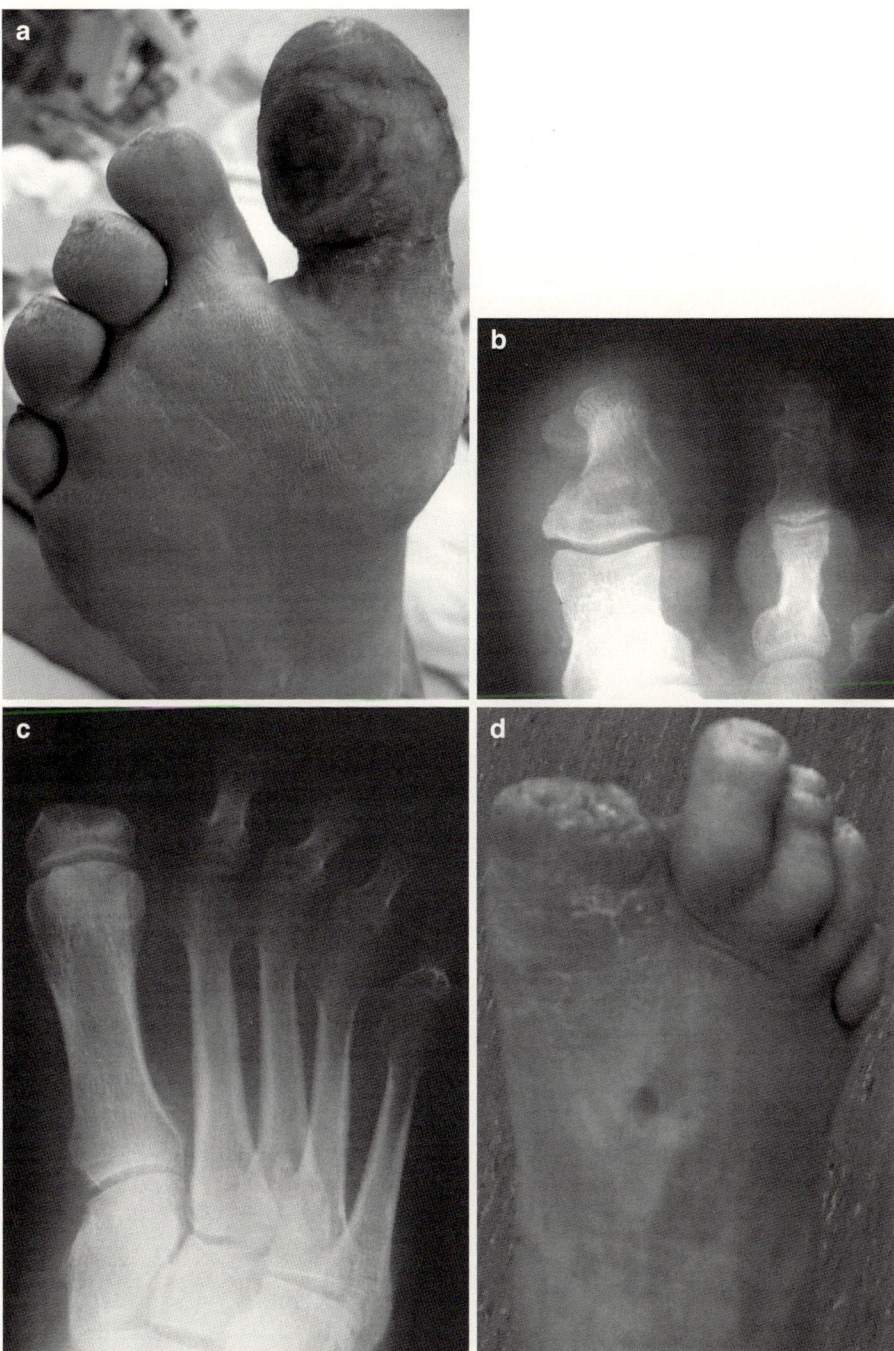

Fig. 10.5   (**a**) Plantar hallux ulceration with (**b**) underlying osteomyelitis. (**c**) Postoperative photo and (**d**) radiograph of a patient after a hallux amputation. The base of the proximal phalanx was preserved to improve function and act as a buttress and prevent medial drift of the lesser digits

Fig. 10.6 Medial drift of
the lesser digits after a hallux
amputation

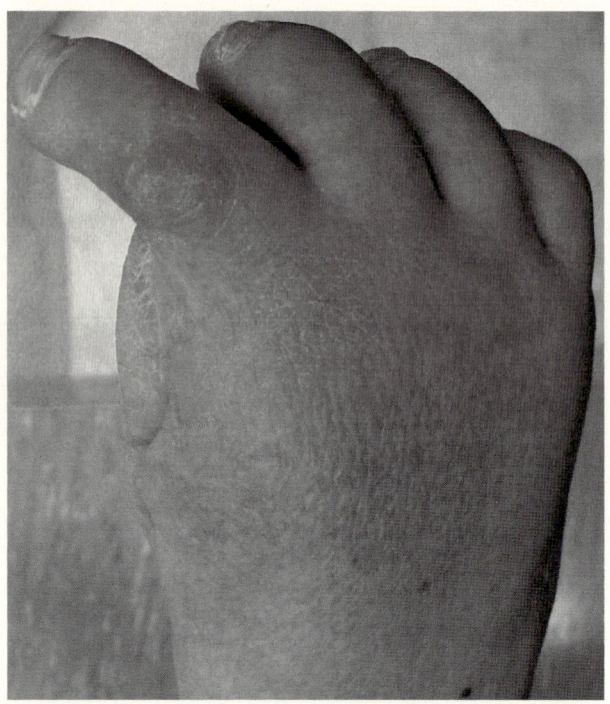

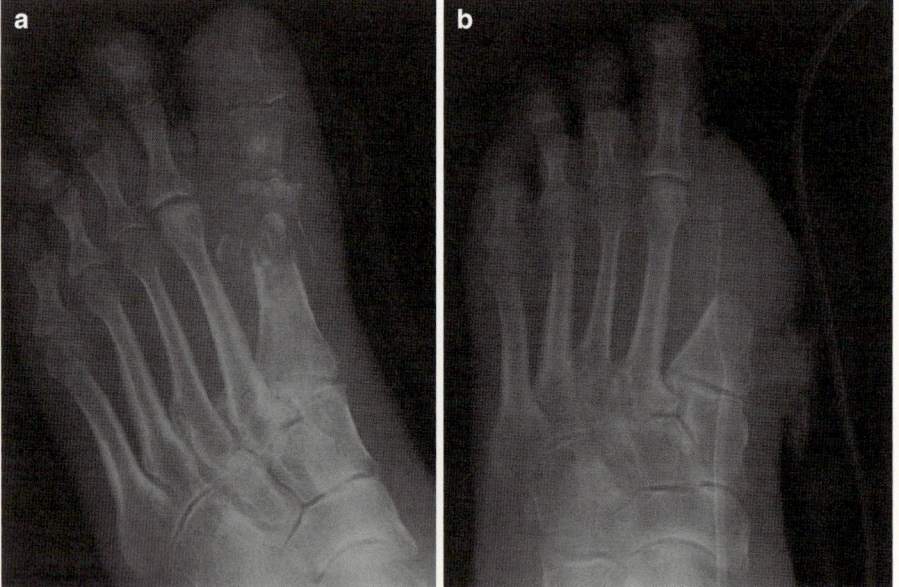

Fig. 10.7 (**a**) Osteomyelitis of the 1st MTPJ requiring a first-ray resection. (**b**) Postoperative
radiographs after a first-ray resection. The bone cut is angled from dorsal-distal to plantar-proximal and proximal-medial to distal-lateral to avoid resultant bone prominences

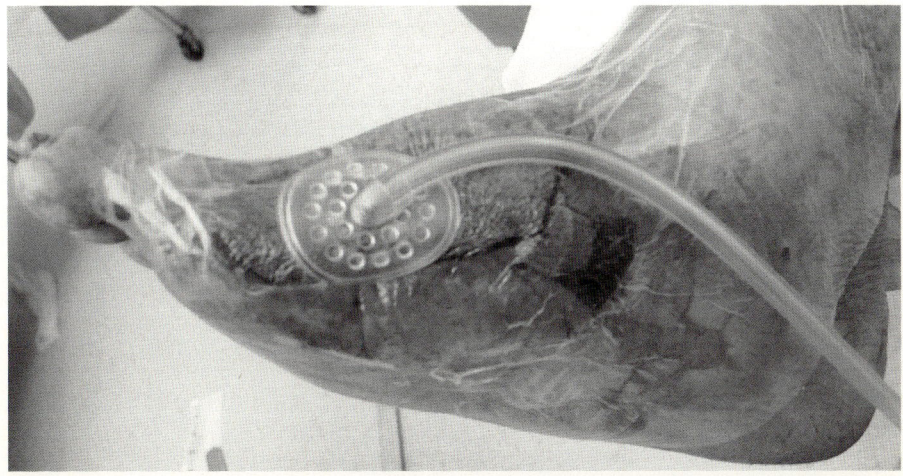

Fig. 10.8 First-ray resection with removal of all nonviable tissues resulting in a large wound. Application of NPWT, used to enhance granulation tissue and prepare wound bed for eventual skin graft

provide an ongoing nidus for infection and should be removed with adequate debridement. Optimal debridement may result in a large wound that is not amendable to primary closure. Here is a clear indication for NPWT (Fig. 10.8).

Postoperatively, patients are placed in a removable cast walker. Patients are followed weekly and eventually transitioned into prescriptive footwear. Plantar foot pressures transfer laterally after a hallux amputation; therefore, it is important to evaluate the residual foot and assess risk for further breakdown. The goals of postoperative management are to restore normal propulsion, reduce transfer of pressure, and provide a filler to stabilize the foot in the shoe. Extra-depth shoes with custom-molded inserts with a toe filler are indicated and a rocker sole shoe may be used to assist with ambulation.

First-ray amputations have an increased risk of undergoing a second amputation within 1 year.[29,30] The first MTPJ is an essential component of the normal gait cycle and removing this joint results in decreased stability and transfer of loads to adjacent rays. Oftentimes, this imbalance results in adjacent digital deformity leading to areas of increased pressure at risk for ulceration (Fig. 10.9).

Murdoch et al.[29] abstracted data from 90 diabetic patients who underwent great-toe and first-ray amputations over a 10-year period. The researchers found that 60% of the patients required a second amputation at a mean 10 months after surgery. Twenty-one patients went on to a third amputation, while 7% required a fourth. Seventeen percent of the patients had a subsequent below-knee amputation (BKA) and 11% had a transmetatarsal amputation (TMA) in the same extremity, whereas 3% had a BKA and 2% a TMA on the contralateral side. From the results of their study, the authors concluded that a large proportion of patients receiving an amputation at the level of the great-toe or first-ray receive higher-level amputations in the

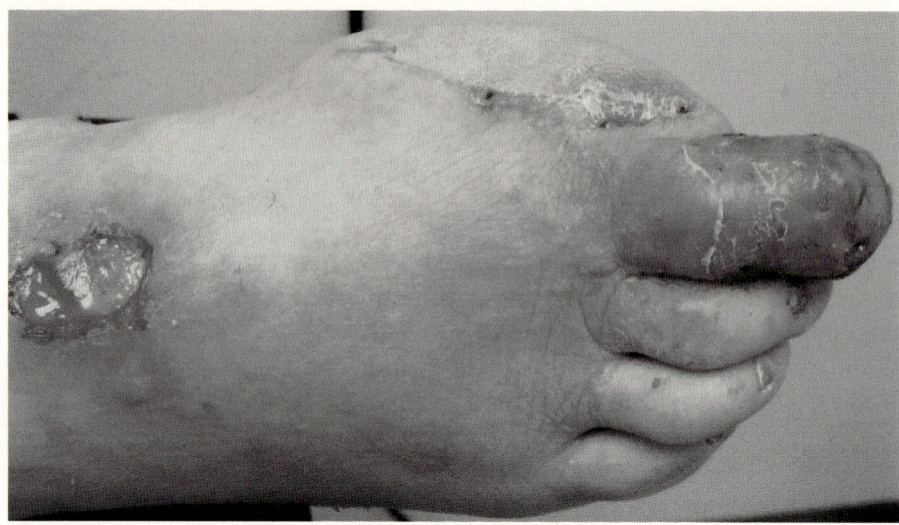

Fig. 10.9 First-ray resection causing a decrease in stability and transfer of loads to adjacent rays leading to a second digit ulceration with underlying osteomyelitis

first year following initial amputation. Understanding the risk for subsequent amputation, great efforts are needed to protect the affected and contralateral foot.

10.2.3   Central Ray Resection

Traditional management of plantar forefoot ulcers complicated with osteomyelitis consisted of partial or complete metatarsal resection resulting in a biomechanically unstable cleft foot often accompanied with a difficult-to-heal wound. The resultant deformity creates risk for further amputation. The forefoot narrowing technique is indicated following central ray resections and results in a stable plantigrade forefoot. This technique allows for primary closure of plantar incisions, foregoing prolonged wound care and lowering the risk for postoperative complications.[31] Strauss et al. first described the technique for the management of "problem" cleft wounds resulting from resection of a necrotic toe and adjacent metatarsal.[32] The authors preformed adjacent osteotomies, manually compressed the forefoot, and applied a large "cathedral-like configuration." The wounds were closed primarily, allowed to heal secondarily, or covered with a split-thickness skin graft. Oznur and Tokgozoglu described a similar technique as that of Strauss et al.[32] but instead used an Ilizarov external fixator consisting of half-rings.[33] Later, Zgonis used a similar construct as described by Oznur and Tokgozoglu,[33] but applied a split-thickness skin graft over the remaining soft tissue defect.[34] Bernstein and Guerin[35] and later, Bevilacqua et al.[31] presented the use of a lightweight, small, bone-lengthening external fixation device used to assist in wound closure flowing central ray resections.

Fig. 10.10   Full-thickness incisions are made with minimal undermining and the ulcer and digit are removed

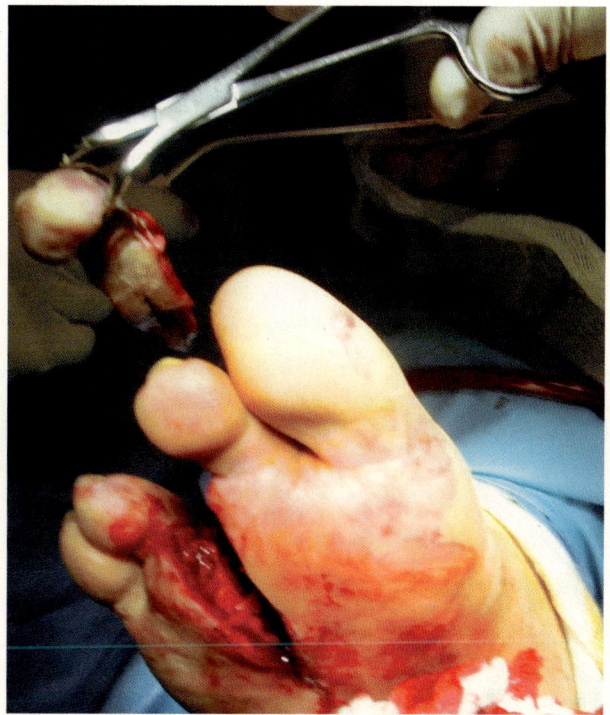

Full-thickness incisions are made along the margins of the digit extending proximal and converging dorsal and plantar on the metatarsal shaft and incorporates the ulcer. With minimal undermining, the ulcer and digit are removed (Fig. 10.10). The metatarsal is partially resected just distal to the base, the wound is inspected, and all necrotic and/or infected tissue is debrided.[36] Debridement of all infected and necrotic tissue is continued until viable tissue remains.[25] Adjacent osteotomies are not required with this technique.

An appropriate length DFS® MiniLengthener (Biomet, Parsippany, NJ) is chosen. The first and fifth metatarsals are identified. A 3.0-mm tapered threaded half-pin is percutaneously placed into the central aspect of the distal one third of the first metatarsal and a 2.0-mm threaded wire is placed into the central aspect of the distal shaft of the fifth metatarsal. All pins and wires are placed perpendicular to the metatarsal and purchase both the near and far cortex. Next, the fixator is loosely secured to serve as a guide and a second 3.0-mm tapered threaded half-pin and a 2.0-mm threaded wire are driven into the first and fifth metatarsals, respectively. After verifying the position of all half-pins and wires with fluoroscopy, the external fixator is firmly secured approximately 2 cm above the dorsum of the foot to allow for postoperative edema (Fig. 10.11).[35]

The forefoot is manually compressed until the plantar skin edges appose and the fixator is closed down to hold the position. The incision is either closed primarily,

Fig. 10.11 The DFS®
MiniLengthener is secured to
pins (first metatarsal) and
wires (fifth metatarsal). The
forefoot is manually
compressed and the external
fixator is closed down to hold
the position

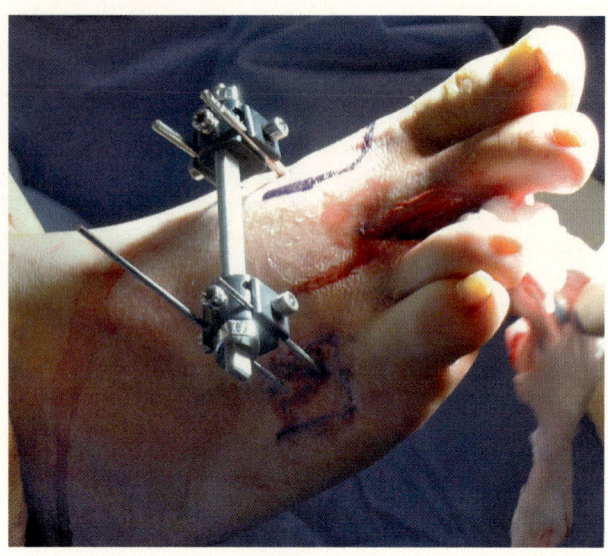

or if there is concern regarding residual soft tissue infection, the wound is left open and closed when deemed appropriate.

Patients are seen weekly in the clinic for assessment of incisions and pin sites. The mini-rail is small and lightweight allowing the use of a standard surgical shoe or a heel wedge shoe. Patients are kept non-weight-bearing for approximately 2 weeks, (longer if a tendo-Achilles lengthening is performed), then transitioned to partial weight-bearing. The external fixator is kept in place until complete healing of the incision and is easily removed in an office or clinic setting (Fig. 10.12). The patient is then placed in appropriate footwear usually consisting of custom-molded inserts in an extra-depth shoe.

10.2.4 Transmetatarsal Amputation

In 1855, Bernard and Heute first described the TMA for the treatment of trench foot. Later, McKittrick et al. described their series of diabetic patients in 1949. TMA is typically performed in patients with gangrene of the digits, chronic osteomyelitis involving the forefoot, or a non-healing ulceration with a previously resected first-ray. As mentioned earlier, a first-ray resection alters normal gait characteristics and patients are at heightened risk for developing transfer lesions putting them at risk for subsequent amputation. TMA is indicated in situations where the first-ray has been resected previously and the patient has a non-healing wound beneath an adjacent metatarsal.[37] Resection of multiple central rays results in a nonfunctional foot and a TMA is indicated to prevent multiple amputations. One should avoid putting multi-comorbid patients through multiple futile attempts at limb salvage (see Fig. 10.3).

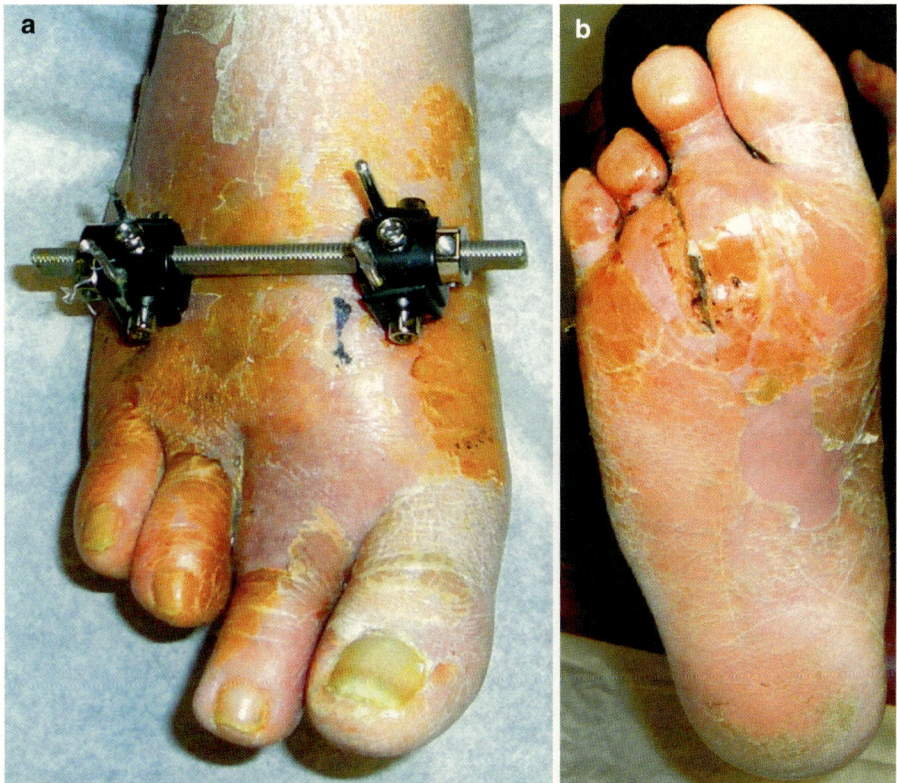

Fig. 10.12 (**a**) Dorsal and (**b**) plantar views of foot 4 weeks after a 3rd ray resection and forefoot narrowing technique with mini external fixator

The skin incision if placed proximal to all infectious and nonviable tissue. A fish-mouth incision with a plantar flap is created so that the final suture line lies on the dorsal aspect of the stump (Fig. 10.13a, b). All incisions are made full thickness with minimal undermining. The metatarsals are resected being careful to maintain the parabola. The metatarsal bone cuts are angled dorsal-distal to plantar-proximal, and the first and fifth metatarsals are beveled medially and laterally to reduce bony prominences. Leaving at least 20% of the metatarsal length will result in maximal function. The bases of the first and fifth metatarsals are left intact to preserve the attachments of tibialis anterior and peroneus brevis, respectively (Fig. 10.13c). The wound is closely inspected and all tendons within the flap are excised under traction. Adequate debridement is performed to remove all infected and necrotic tissues. The remaining soft tissue may be debulked to allow for primary closure with minimal tension (Fig. 10.13d, e). A closed suction drain may be used to reduce the risk of hematoma. If there is any concern with residual infection, the wound is left open until there are no signs and symptoms of infection before delayed primary closure.

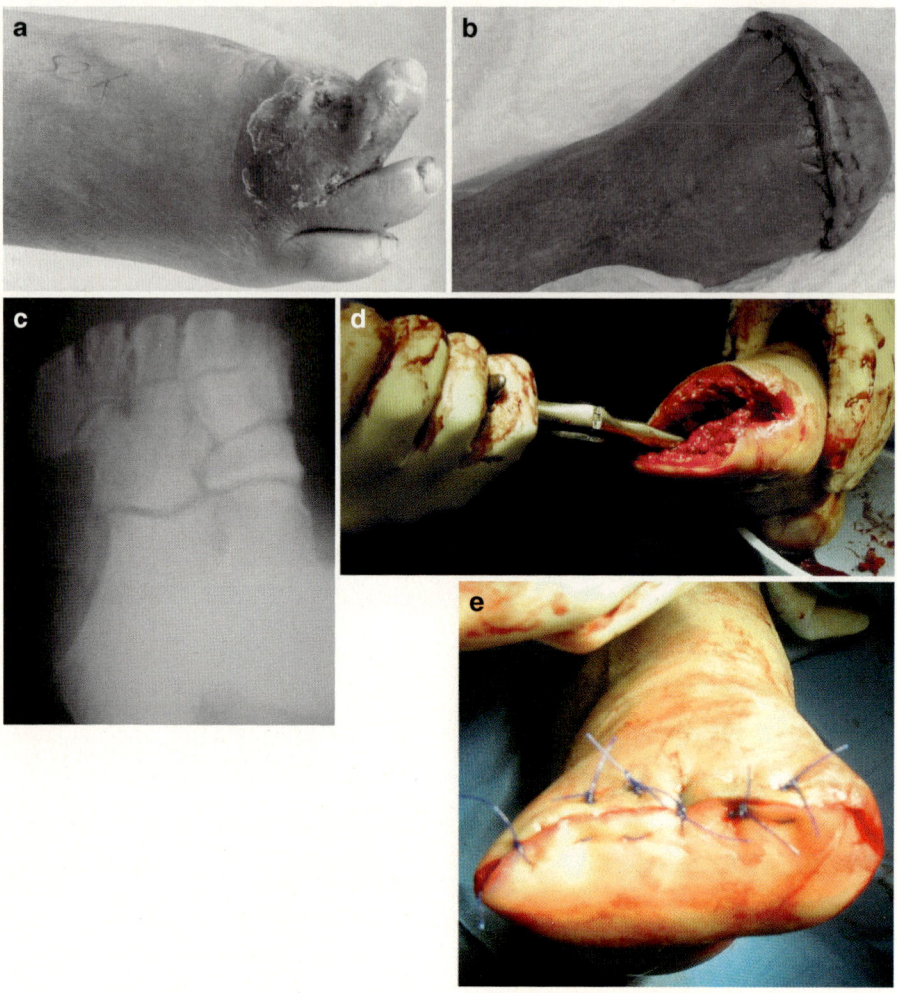

Fig. 10.13 (**a**) Previous failed 1st and 2nd ray resections with resultant wound. This is a clear indication for TMA. (**b**) A fish-mouth incision with a plantar flap is created so that the final suture line lies on the dorsal aspect of the stump. (**c**) Maintaining metatarsal parabola with bone cuts angled to reduce bone prominences. (**d**) All tendons are excised under traction and the remaining soft tissue is debulked to allow for primary closure with minimal tension. (**e**) Primary closure under minimal tension. Note the preservation of a plantar flap

The loss of some of the extensor tendons leads to muscle imbalance, and an equinovarus deformity is a commonly reported complication. The resultant excessive pressure and shearing forces result in ulceration of the plantar lateral aspect of the amputation stump (Fig. 10.14). An open or percutaneous tendo-Achilles lengthening or a gastrocnemius recession is performed to address the equinus component. Altered biomechanics may require tendon transfers to address the forefoot varus and at times, a split tibialis anterior tendon transfer or a peronius brevis tendon

Fig. 10.14 Equinovarus deformity after TMA leading to skin breakdown

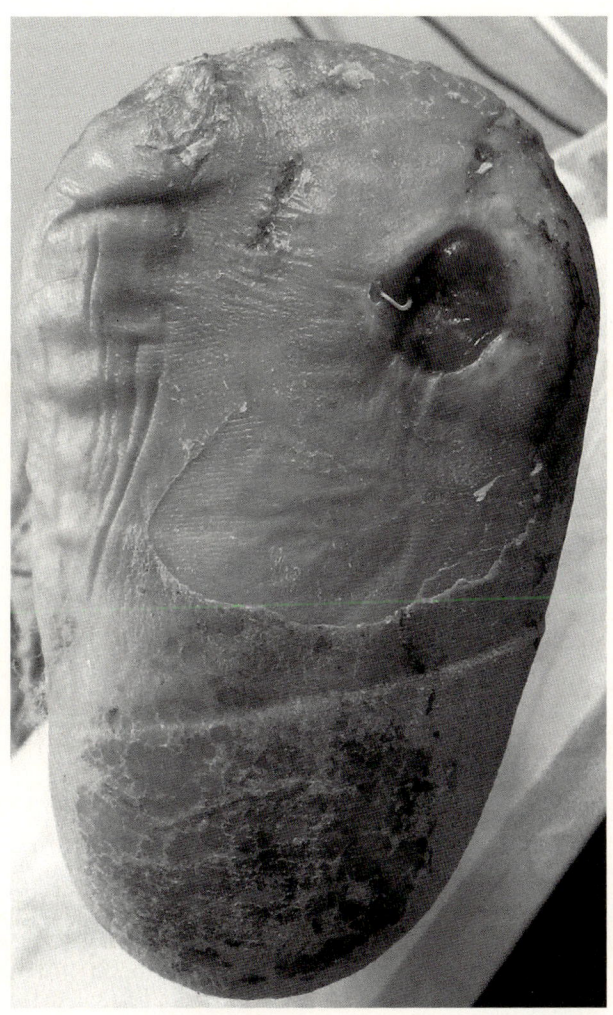

transfer may be used.[38] Recently, Roukis[39] described a flexor hallucis longus and extensor digitorum longus tendon transfer for balancing the foot following a TMA. Medially, the flexor hallucis longus tendon is transferred to the residual first metatarsal, and laterally, the extensor digitorum longus tendon is transferred to the residual fourth metatarsal. The tendons are passed through drill holes and secured with a suture anchor. Schweinberger and Roukis also employ intramedullary screw fixation across the medial and occasionally lateral column to stabilize and balance the TMA in the dysvascular patient. This technique avoids additional incisions that are required for tendon transfers.[40] The team led by Armstrong and coworkers has also described the potential use of spanning external fixation (SALSAstand) to (a) protect friable skin flaps/grafts in high-risk patients, (b) offload the posterior heel

during convalescence, and (c) hold soft tissue balancing procedures in a more corrected position (Fig. 10.15).[41]

Mueller et al.[42] reviewed the outcomes of 120 TMAs performed on 107 patients
over a 4-year period at a single institution. The researchers noted that 27% of
patients developed skin breakdown, and 28% required a higher-level amputation.
Most of the complications occurred within the first 3 months after the amputation.
These results highlight that the residual foot is at increased risk for skin breakdown

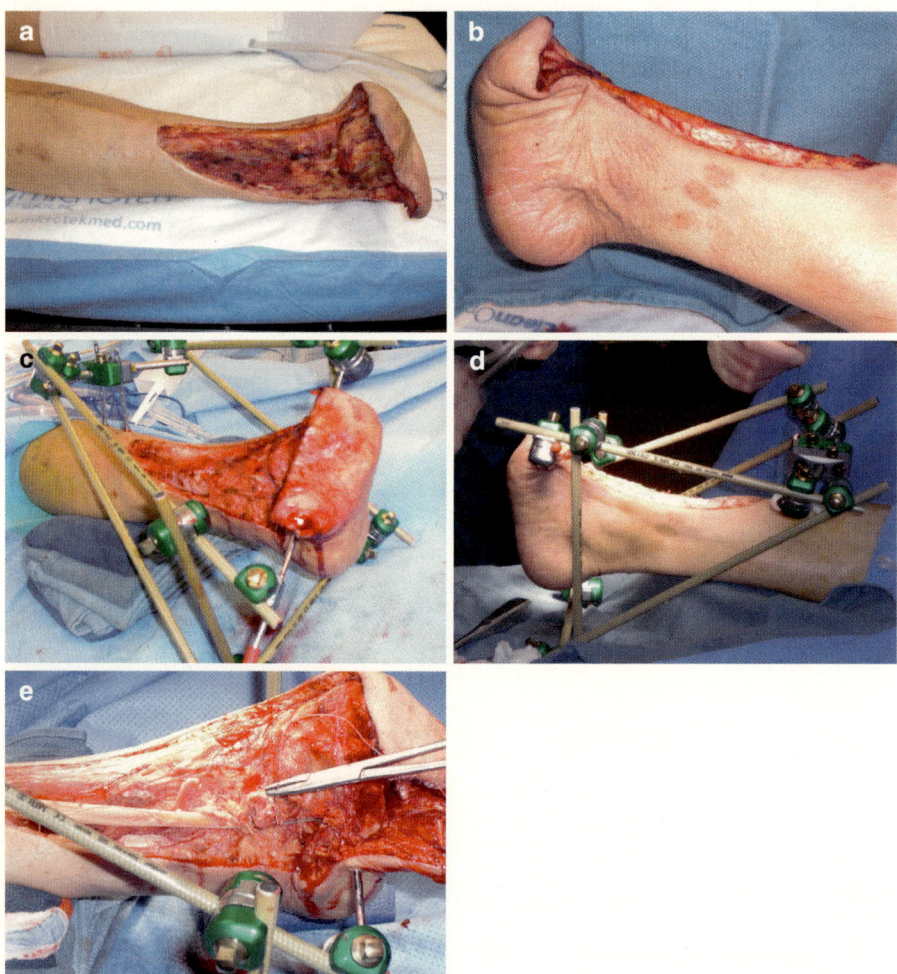

Fig. 10.15 (**a, b**) LisFranc's amputation with dorsal tissue loss and equinovarus deformity (**c, d**)
spanning external fixation used to stabilize and hold foot in corrected position (**e**) anterior tibial
tendon transfer (**f**) negative pressure wound therapy applied (**g**) free flap and split thickness skin
graft with foot held in corrected position during convalescence. Note this technique also offloads
the posterior heel

Fig. 10.15 (continued)

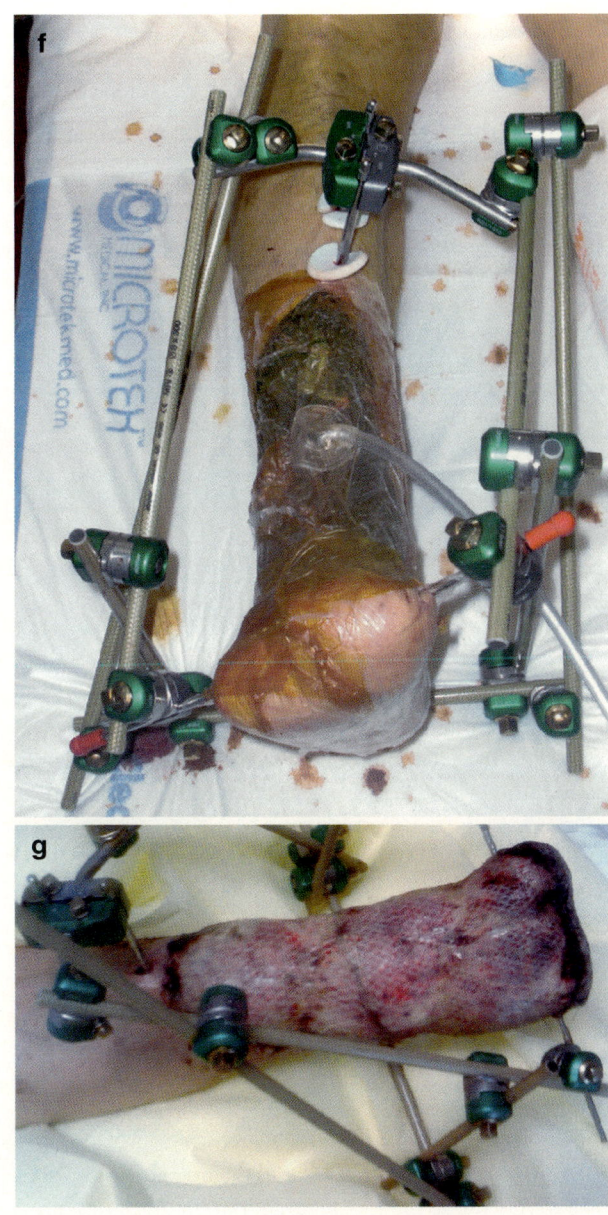

or higher amputation, especially during the first 3 months after surgery. The first 3 months after surgery is the time when patients begin to ambulate and may inadvertently injure their foot. The authors recommend and encourage a rehabilitation program emphasizing protection of the residual foot for at least 3 months to avoid complications.

Therefore, initial postoperative management consists of protecting the residual foot. Patients are placed in a compressive type dressing with a posterior splint and are non-weight-bearing with crutches, walker, or a wheelchair. Patients may be transitioned to a removable walker, and long-term management will depend on activity level, ambulatory status, and pain scores. Patients may be placed in a therapeutic shoe with a custom-molded accommodative insert with a forefoot filler. The shoe may also include a rigid rocker bottom sole to assist with ambulation. However, at times, patients may require the stability of an ankle foot orthosis (AFO) with a forefoot filler. The brace may be worn in extra-depth shoes.

10.2.5   Lisfranc Amputation

A TMA is preferred over a deformed, nonfunctional partial forefoot amputation. However, when the infection extends proximal, disarticulation at the tarsometatarsal joint (Lisfranc joint) is necessary. A Lisfranc disarticulation should be considered when there is inadequate soft tissue coverage for a TMA. Compared to a TMA, this more proximal amputation will result in a more pronounced muscle imbalance and deformity. Soft tissue balancing procedures are essential for long-term function. Laterally, the peroneal brevis tendon is transferred to the cuboid and the peroneous longus is sutured to peroneous brevis. Medially, the insertions of posterior tibialis and tibialis anterior are preserved and, if sacrificed, are reattached proximally. A tendo-Achilles lengthening or gastrocnemius recession is performed, and complete transection of the Achilles tendon may be performed. Postoperative management is similar to that described for the TMA and, initially, is concentrated on protecting the residual foot and later may require the stability of an AFO.

10.2.6   Chopart's Amputation

Chopart's amputation, as first described by the French surgeon, Francois Chopart, is a disarticulation through the midtarsal joint, leaving only the talus and calcaneus (Fig. 10.16). Historically, this amputation fell out of favor due to the equinovarus deformity that transpires. However, the combination of advanced surgical technique and effective, functional prosthetic care can result in a successful outcome.

Patients requiring a Chopart's amputation often present with infection extending proximal to the midfoot. The skin incision is placed proximal to all infected and necrotic tissues and a plantar flap is preserved. Proper surgical technique, as described above, is continued with disarticulation through the midtarsal joint. Special attention is directed to rebalancing the foot with appropriate tendon transfers. Tibialis anterior tendon is attached to the neck of the talus. The peroneal tendons are secured to the lateral wall of the calcaneus, and a tendo-Achilles lengthening or gastrocnemius recession is indicated. At times, a complete transection of the Achilles tendon may be necessary. If there is degeneration with resultant deformity of the hindfoot, a subtalar fusion or a tibiotalocalcaneal fusion may be performed.

Fig. 10.16 (**a**) Chopart's amputation with (**b**) preservation of a plantar flap

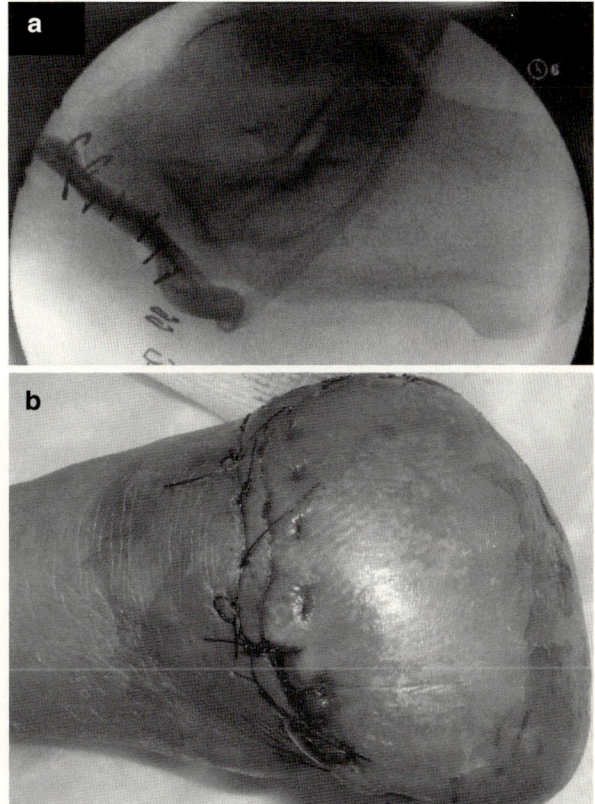

Initial postoperative care of the more proximal foot-sparing amputations focuses on protecting the residual foot. The surgical site is dressed accordingly and the limb is protected in a soft bandage and a posterior splint. Patients are non-weight-bearing with crutches, walker, or wheelchair. Generally, after allowing for soft tissue healing, patients are transitioned to a removable cast walker. Long-term management and choice of prosthetic will depend on the activity level of the patient. The choice of the prosthetic device depends upon the patient's ability to bear weight and ambulate. A common prosthetic used successfully is an AFO with a custom-molded insert and forefoot filler to be worn in an extra-depth shoe. If weight-bearing is painful, a Patella Bearing Orthosis (PTB) may be helpful in taking weight off the heel. For more control, patients may be fitted for a Charcot Restraint Orthotic Walker (CROW) or a clam-shell orthosis with a solid ankle.

10.2.7 Syme's Amputation

The Syme's amputation was originally described by Scottish surgeon, James Syme, in 1843 for definitive treatment for a non-salvageable foot infection with a viable heel pad.[43] This amputation preserves function of the knee with a long stump and independence by allowing patients to expend less energy walking than patients with higher-level amputations. Waters et al.[10] found that Syme amputees had greater gait velocity, cadence, and stride length and better function than below-knee and above-knee amputees.

The original technique included disarticulation of the foot at the ankle joint with resection of the malleolar projections. The procedure has been described as a 1-stage or 2-stage procedure. Wagner[44] popularized the 2-stage procedure for patients with diabetes with an active midfoot or rearfoot infection. The first stage involved disarticulation at the ankle, followed by resection of malleoli and revision of skin flap. Pinzur et al.[45] compared the 1-stage and 2-stage procedure and found similar results. The authors prefer the 1-stage procedure, as this avoids a return trip to the operating room.

The anterior incision essentially connects the tips of the medial and lateral malleoli, and the plantar incision connects the two malleolar points across the sole of the foot. Pinzur et al.[23] modified the technique as initially described by Wagner, in which the apices are located at a point 1–1.5 cm anterior and distal to the tips of the malleoli. The plantar heel pad is preserved, and an intact heel pad is key to successful outcomes. Careful dissection is carried down to the talus, and the talar collateral ligaments are transected. Care is taken to protect the posterior tibial artery, as this is the main supply to the plantar flap. The talus is disarticulated from the ankle, and the calcaneus is freed from the Achilles tendon and surrounding soft tissues. The malleoli are resected to the level of the tibial plafond maintaining a tibial flare. This tapered distal stump will assist with proper prosthetic fit postoperatively. All tendons are resected under traction and the plantar flap is prepared for closure. Soft tissue anchors or drill holes are placed in the distal anterior tibia to secure the heel pad. The wound is closed in layers with minimal tension and a drain may be placed to reduce the risk of formation of a hematoma post operatively.

The surgical site is dressed accordingly and patients are non-weight-bearing until the sutures are removed. Generally, patients are transitioned to a walking cast after 3 weeks and are fitted for a custom prosthetic when all wounds are healed and edema is controlled.

Pinzur et al.[23] performed a retrospective review of 97 patients and reported that 82 patients (84.5%) healed. Eighty of these 82 patients were able to walk with a prosthesis. Yu et al.[22] reported the results of Syme's amputation in 10 patients. Nine patients were able to ambulate in a prosthesis 4–6 months after surgery and 1 patient achieved ambulation 1.5 years postoperatively. Overall, 7 of the 10 patients reported improved quality of life and return to daily activities. Frykberg et al.[43] published their early experience with 26 cases in a high-risk population (majority of patients having diabetes and peripheral arterial disease). The authors reported that 50% healed at approximately 1-year follow-up with 46.2% (12/26) of the patients functioning well in a prosthesis.

10.2.8 Partial Calcanectomy

A partial calcanectomy is an alternative to below-knee amputation for calcaneal osteomyelitis with overlying tissue loss (Fig. 10.17a). Originally described by

Fig. 10.17 (**a**) Calcaneal osteomyelitis. (**b**) Vertical skin incision is deepened down to the level of the calcaneus, and the skin wedge and ulcer are excised. (**c**) The posterior body of the calcaneus is exposed, and a sagittal saw is used to make the bone cut. The bone cut is made transversely from immediately posterior to the posterior facet of the subtalar joint to proximal toward the calcaneocuboid joint. (**d**) Debridement of bone is continued "slice by slice" until bleeding and normal appearing marrow is noted

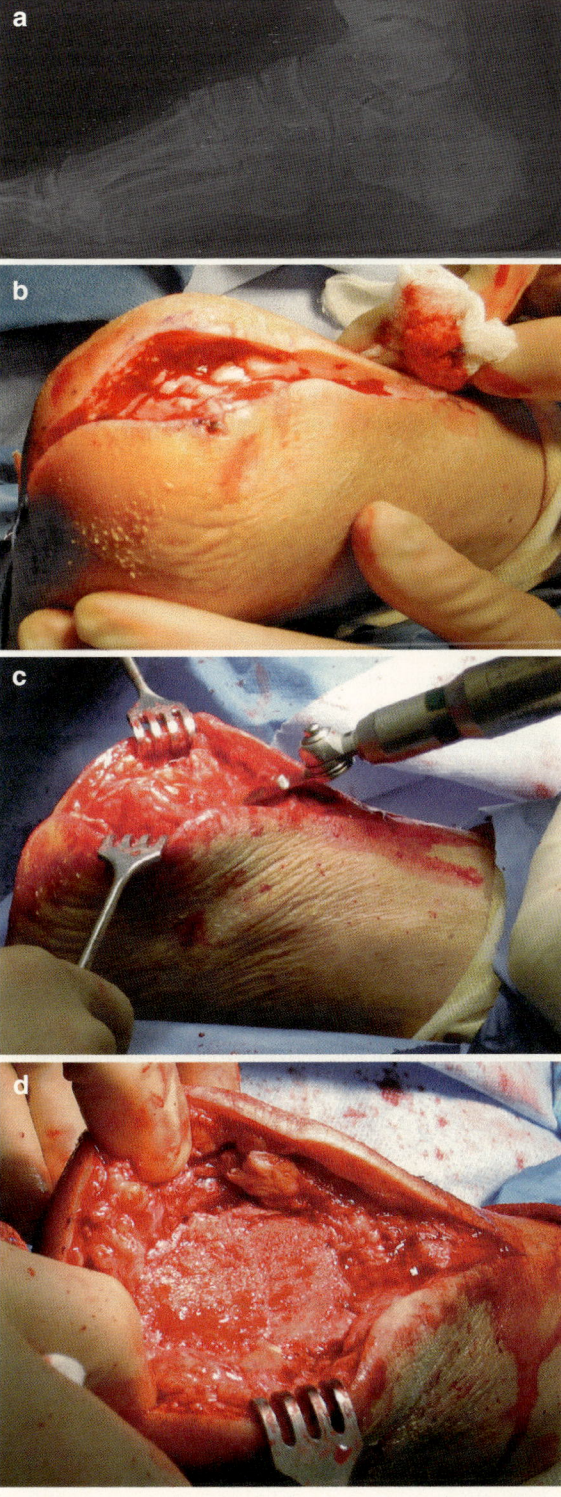

Gaenslen in 1931, this procedure is an excellent option for limb salvage with success rates approaching 70–80%.[46] Excellent results have been reported with strict adherence to preoperative criteria and thorough follow-up treatment with appropriate accommodative foot wear.[47] Once healed, most patients maintain ambulation and improved quality of life is achieved by preserving a functional limb.

The patient is placed in the prone or lateral decubitus position. Gaenslen originally described a split-heel incision, but a fish mouth-type incision may be used. The vertical incision has less of a chance of violating vascular structures and can be planned to incorporate a wound. The incision is deepened down to the level of the calcaneus, and the skin wedge and ulcer are excised (Fig. 10.17b). Dissection is continued to expose the posterior body of the calcaneus. Care is taken to protect the medial and lateral skin flaps, and a no-touch technique is employed. Medially, the neurovascular bundle is protected; laterally, the peroneal tendons are reflected; and posteriorly, the insertion of the Achilles tendon is identified and reflected.

The bone cut is made transversely from immediately posterior to the posterior facet of the subtalar joint to proximal toward the calcaneocubiod joint[47] (Fig. 10.17c). The integrity of the bone is inspected, and all necrotic and infected tissues are excised (Fig. 10.17d). Suture anchors or drill holes may be placed superior on the residual posterior body of the calcaneus for reinsertion of the Achilles tendon. Antibiotic-impregnated beads may be used in cases of osteomyelitis for local delivery of the antibiotic in high concentrations. The wound is closed in layers and a closed suction drain may be used to prevent formation of a hematoma postoperative. The surgical site is dressed accordingly and the foot is maintained in a slightly plantarflexed position. Patients are generally kept non-weight-bearing for a period of 6 weeks and then fitted for accommodative footwear. Depending on activity level and function, patients may be placed in an extra-depth shoe with accommodative inserts and a heel filler or an AFO to assist with ambulation.

Smith et al.[48] reported an 83% healing rate with partial calcanectomies used for the treatment of large heel ulcers and calcaneal osteomyelitis. Total calcanectomies have been described for the treatment of large heel ulcers with underlying osteomyelitis.[49] Additionally, Rogers et al. presented data on 21 partial calcanectomies and found that renal failure showed a trend toward a poor outcome, such as more proximal amputation or mortality.[50] Gait mechanics long term are an issue.

Maintaining as much of the distal limb is ideal for long-term gait. An alternative to partial calcanectomy is Boyd's amputation. Grady and Winters described their results of Boyd's modification of the Syme's amputation. In cases of forefoot and midfoot pathology necessitating amputation, the calcaneus is maintained after removing the talus, and fused to the distal tibia. This gives stability and maintains some length to the remaining limb, preserves the distal flap and plantar fat pad.[50]

10.3   Conclusion

The rapid increase in diabetes prevalence and subsequent improvements in medical care will result in more end-organ complications, such as limb-threatening conditions. The World Health Organization and the International Diabetes Federation have stated that 85% of lower extremity amputations in diabetes are preventable. Attention should be given to the patient's position on the "stairway to an amputation" (see Fig. 10.1) and interventions can be undertaken to prevent the escalation to the next step. In the unavoidable case, the most distal, functional amputation should be planned. Initially, removal of infected and necrotic material should be thorough. Functional reconstruction can then be completed. The care of the amputee continues long past the surgery. Post-amputation rehabilitation and prosthetic fitting is required to improve long-term prognosis. Frequent follow-up appointments to check for areas of skin breakdown and risk for reamputation or contralateral amputation are necessary. The principles presented in this chapter represent the most current strategies for best long-term outcomes in care of the amputee.

References

1. "Every thirty seconds, somewhere in the world, a limb is lost as a consequence of diabetes." Lancet. 2005;366:Cover.
2. Ollendorf DA, Kotsanos JG, Wishner WJ, Friedman M, Cooper T, Bittoni M. Potential economic benefits of lower extremity amputation prevention strategies in diabetes. Diabetes Care. 1998;21:1240-5.
3. Jeffcoate WJ. The incidence of amputation in diabetes. Acta Chir Belg. 2005;105(2):140-4.
4. Pecoraro RE, Reiber GE, Burgess EM. Pathways to diabetic limb amputation: basis for prevention. Diabetes Care. 1990;13:513-21.
5. Singh N, Armstrong DG, Lipsky BA. Preventing foot ulcers in patients with diabetes. JAMA. 2005;293(2):217-28.
6. Lavery LA, Wunderlich RP, Tredwell JL. Disease management for the diabetic foot: effectiveness of a diabetic foot prevention program to reduce amputations and hospitalizations. Diabetes Res Clin Pract. 2005;70(1):31-7.
7. Lipsky BA, Berendt AR, Embil J, De Lalla F. Diagnosing and treating diabetic foot infections. Diabetes Metab Res Rev. 2004;20(Suppl 1):S56-64.
8. Armstrong DG, Wrobel J, Robbins JM. Guest Editorial: are diabetes-related wounds and amputations worse than cancer? Int Wound J. 2007;4(4):286-7.
9. Goldner MG. The fate of the second leg in the diabetic amputee. Diabetes. 1960;9:100-3.
10. Waters RL, Perry J, Antonelle D, Hislop H. Energy cost of walking of amputees: the influence of level of amputation. J Bone Joint Surg Am. 1976;58:42-6.
11. Rogers LC, Lavery LA, Armstrong DG. The right to bear legs – an amendment to healthcare; how preventing amputations can save billions to the US health-care system. J Am Podiatr Med Assoc. 2008;98(2):166-8.
12. Canavan RJ, Unwin NC, Kelly WF, Connolly VM. Diabetes and non-diabetes related lower extremity amputation incidence before and after the introduction of better organized diabetes foot care continuous longitudinal monitoring using a standard method. Diabetes Care. 2007;31:459-63. Epub Dec 10, 2007.
13. Driver VR, Madsen J, Goodman RA. Reducing amputation rates in patients with diabetes at a military medical center: the limb preservation service model. Diabetes Care. 2005;28(2):248-53.
14. Rogers LC, Bevilacqua NJ. Organized programs reduce major amputations. J Am Podiatr Med Assoc. 2010;100(2):101-4.
15. Armstrong DG, Perales TA, Murff RT, Edelson GW, Welchon JG. Value of white blood cell count with differential in the acute diabetic foot infection. J Am Podiatr Med Assoc. 1996;86(5):224-7.
16. Lavery LA, Armstrong DG, Quebedeaux TL, Walker SC. Puncture wounds: the frequency of normal laboratory values in the face of severe foot infections of the foot in diabetic and non-diabetic adults. Am J Med. 1996;101:521-5.

17. Cruciani M, Lipsky BA, Mengoli C, de Lalla F. Are granulocyte colony-stimulating factors beneficial in treating diabetic foot infections?: a meta-analysis. Diabetes Care. 2005;28(2): 454-60.
18. Ballard JL, Eke CC, Bunt TJ, Killeen JD. A prospective evaluation of transcutaneous oxygen measurements in the management of diabetic foot problems. J Vasc Surg. 1995;22(4):485-90; discussion 490-2.
19. Bunt TJ, Holloway GA. TcPO2 as an accurate predictor of therapy in limb salvage. Ann Vasc Surg. 1996;10(3):224-7.
20. Adera HM, James K, Castronuovo JJ Jr, Byrne M, Deshmukh R, Lohr J. Prediction of amputation wound healing with skin perfusion pressure. J Vasc Surg. 1995;21(5):823-8; discussion 828-9.
21. Khaodhiar L, Dinh T, Schomacker KT, et al. The use of medical hyperspectral technology to evaluate microcirculatory changes in diabetic foot ulcers and to predict clinical outcomes. Diabetes Care. 2007;30(4):903-10.
22. Yu GV, Schinke TL, Meszaros A. Syme's amputation: a retrospective review of 10 cases. Clin Podiatr Med Surg. 2005;22(3):395-427.
23. Pinzur MS, Stuck RM, Sage R, Hunt N, Rabinovich Z. Syme ankle disarticulation in patients with diabetes. J Bone Joint Surg Am. 2003;85-A(9):1667-72.
24. Armstrong DG, Lavery LA, van Houtum WH, Harkless LB. Amputation and reamputation of the diabetic foot. J Am Podiatr Med Assoc. 1997;87(6):255-9.
25. Attinger CE, Bulan EJ. Debridement. The key initial first step in wound healing. Foot Ankle Clin. 2001;6(4):627-60.
26. Attinger CE, Bulan E, Blume PA. Surgical debridement: the key to successful wound healing and reconstruction. Clin Podiatr Med Surg. 2000;17(4):599-630.
27. Armstrong DG, Lavery LA. Negative pressure wound therapy after partial diabetic foot amputation: a multicentre, randomised controlled trial. Lancet. 2005;366(9498):1704-10.
28. Julien PH, Marcinko DE, Gordon S. Reconstruction of soft tissue defects about the great toe. J Foot Surg. 1988;27(2):116-20.
29. Murdoch DP, Armstrong DG, Dacus JB, Laughlin TJ, Morgan CB, Lavery LA. The natural history of great toe amputations. J Foot Ankle Surg. 1997;36(3):204-8.
30. Dalla Paola L, Faglia E, Caminiti M, Clerici G, Ninkovic S, Deanesi V. Ulcer recurrence following first ray amputation in diabetic patients: a cohort prospective study. Diabetes Care. 2003;26(6):1874-8.
31. Bevilacqua NJ, Rogers LC, DellaCorte MP, Armstrong DG. The narrowed forefoot at 1 year: an advanced approach for wound closure after central ray amputations. Clin Podiatr Med Surg. 2008;25(1):127-33.
32. Strauss MB, Bryant BJ, Hart JD. Forefoot narrowing with external fixation for problem cleft wounds. Foot Ankle Int. 2002;23(5):433-9.
33. Oznur A, Tokgozoglu M. Closure of central defects of the forefoot with external fixation: a case report. J Foot Ankle Surg. 2004;43(1):56-9.
34. Zgonis T, Oznur A, Roukis TS. A novel technique for closing difficult diabetic cleft foot wounds with skin grafting and a ring-type external fixation system. Oper Tech Orthop. 2006;2006(16):38-43.
35. Bernstein B, Guerin L. The use of mini external fixation in central forefoot amputations. J Foot Ankle Surg. 2005;44(4):307-10.
36. Attinger CE, Janis JE, Steinberg J, Schwartz J, Al-Attar A, Couch K. Clinical approach to wounds: debridement and wound bed preparation including the use of dressings and wound-healing adjuvants. Plast Reconstr Surg. 2006;117(7 Suppl):72S-109.
37. Wallace GF, Stapleton JJ. Transmetatarsal amputations. Clin Podiatr Med Surg. 2005;22(3): 365-84.
38. Schweinberger MH, Roukis TS. Soft-tissue and osseous techniques to balance forefoot and midfoot amputations. Clin Podiatr Med Surg. 2008;25(4):623-39. viii-ix.

39. Roukis TS. Flexor hallucis longus and extensor digitorum longus tendon transfers for balancing the foot following transmetatarsal amputation. J Foot Ankle Surg. 2009;48(3):398-401.
40. Schweinberger MH, Roukis TS. Intramedullary screw fixation for balancing of the dysvascular foot following transmetatarsal amputation. J Foot Ankle Surg. 2008;47(6):594-7.
41. Clark JC, Mills JL, Armstrong DG. A Method of external fixation to offload and protect the high-risk foot following reconstruction: the SALSAstand. Eplasty. 2009;9:e21.
42. Mueller MJ, Allen BT, Sinacore DR. Incidence of skin breakdown and higher amputation after transmetatarsal amputation: implications for rehabilitation. Arch Phys Med Rehabil. 1995;76(1):50-4.
43. Frykberg RG, Abraham S, Tierney E, Hall J. Syme amputation for limb salvage: early experience with 26 cases. J Foot Ankle Surg. 2007;46(2):93-100.
44. Wagner FW Jr. Amputations of the foot and ankle. Current status. Clin Orthop Relat Res. 1977;122:62-9.
45. Pinzur MS, Smith D, Osterman H. Syme ankle disarticulation in peripheral vascular disease and diabetic foot infection: the one-stage versus two-stage procedure. Foot Ankle Int. 1995;16(3):124-7.
46. Randall DB, Phillips J, Ianiro G. Partial calcanectomy for the treatment of recalcitrant heel ulcerations. J Am Podiatr Med Assoc. 2005;95(4):335-41.
47. Perez ML, Wagner SS, Yun J. Subtotal calcanectomy for chronic heel ulceration. J Foot Ankle Surg. 1994;33(6):572-9.
48. Smith DG, Stuck RM, Ketner L, Sage RM, Pinzur MS. Partial calcanectomy for the treatment of large ulcerations of the heel and calcaneal osteomyelitis. An amputation of the back of the foot. J Bone Joint Surg Am. 1992;74(4):571-6.
49. Baumhauer JF, Fraga CJ, Gould JS, Johnson JE. Total calcanectomy for the treatment of chronic calcaneal osteomyelitis. Foot Ankle Int. 1998;19(12):849-55.
50. Rogers LC, Bevilacqua NJ, Frykberg RG. Limb salvage with partial calcanectomy; a case series of 21 procedures. Paper presented at: American Podiatric Medical Association, August 2007; Philadelphia, PA.

Chapter 11
Charcot Foot and Ankle Disease

Ralph Springfeld

There are two sayings from India:
"If you talk, your talk must be better than your silence would have been!"
The other:
"The best knowledge is what you have when you need it!"

11.1 Introduction

Charcot disease of the foot and ankle is still a disease with unknown origin. The associated arthropathy is linked with diabetes mellitus (DM) and peripheral polyneuropathy (PNP). We know about the neuropathic and the vascular theory, called the French and the German theories, respectively. Repeated microtrauma and disturbance in the microvascular blood flow caused by the neuropathy of the autonomous nervous system change the integrity of bone and joints of the foot.[1-3] Newer findings suggest the possibility of changes of bone metabolism. Changes in the so-called RANK-L complex may interfere with the function of osteoclasts.[4,5]

One problem is that Charcot sometimes starts and ends without any therapy. We see patients with typical end-stage Charcot feet clinically (Fig. 11.1a) and radiographically (Fig. 11.1b, c) who never realized a problem and continued to wear normal shoes. Other patients get severe deformation, ulceration, infection, and life-threatening septic situations (Fig. 11.2).

R. Springfeld, M.D.
Head of Orthopedic Clinic, Klinik Dr. Guth
Juergensallee 46-48, Hamburg 22609, Germany
e-mail: dr.springfeld@drguth.de

A. Saxena (ed.), *Special Procedures in Foot and Ankle Surgery*,
DOI 10.1007/978-1-4471-4103-7_11, © Springer-Verlag London 2013

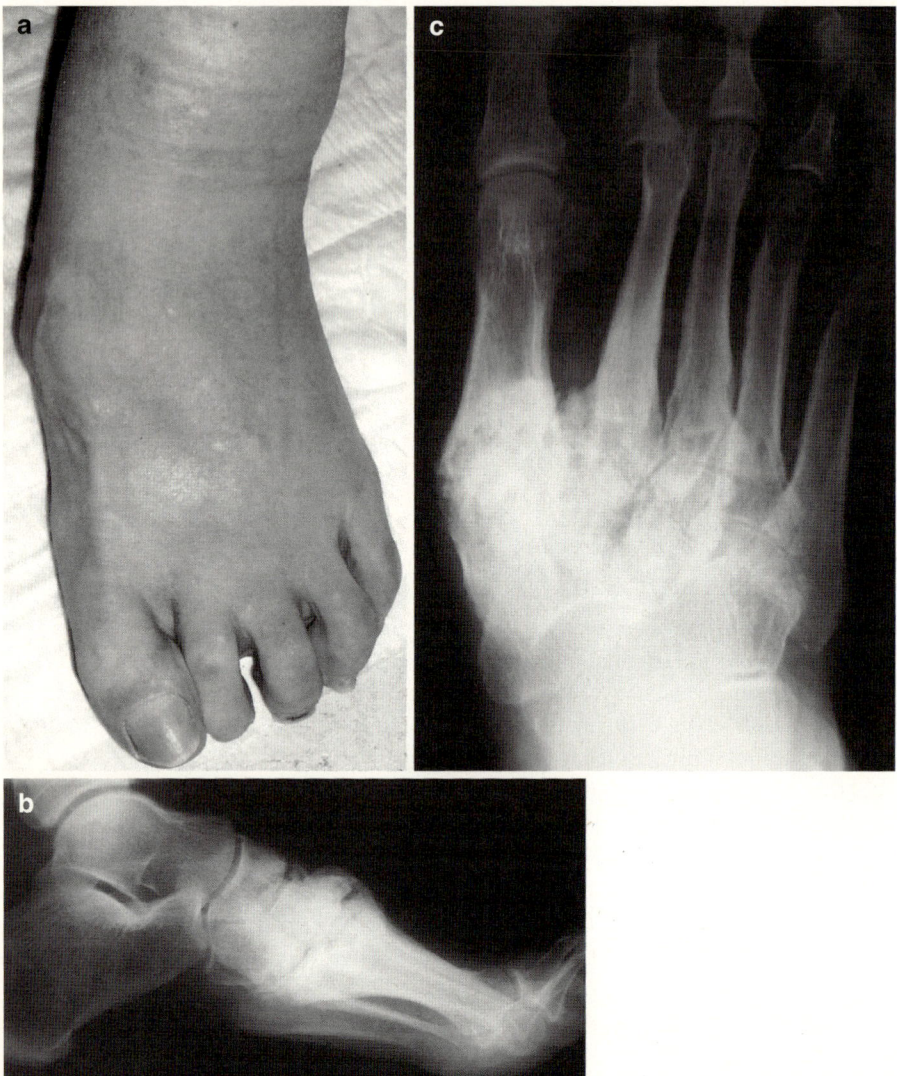

Fig. 11.1 Patient with D.M. type II for 12 years, PNP, dialysis, Charcot Type Sanders II, stage Eichenholtz III, without breakdown of the midfoot; (**a**) clinical appearence; (**b**) X-ray lateral view and (**c**) X-ray p-d view

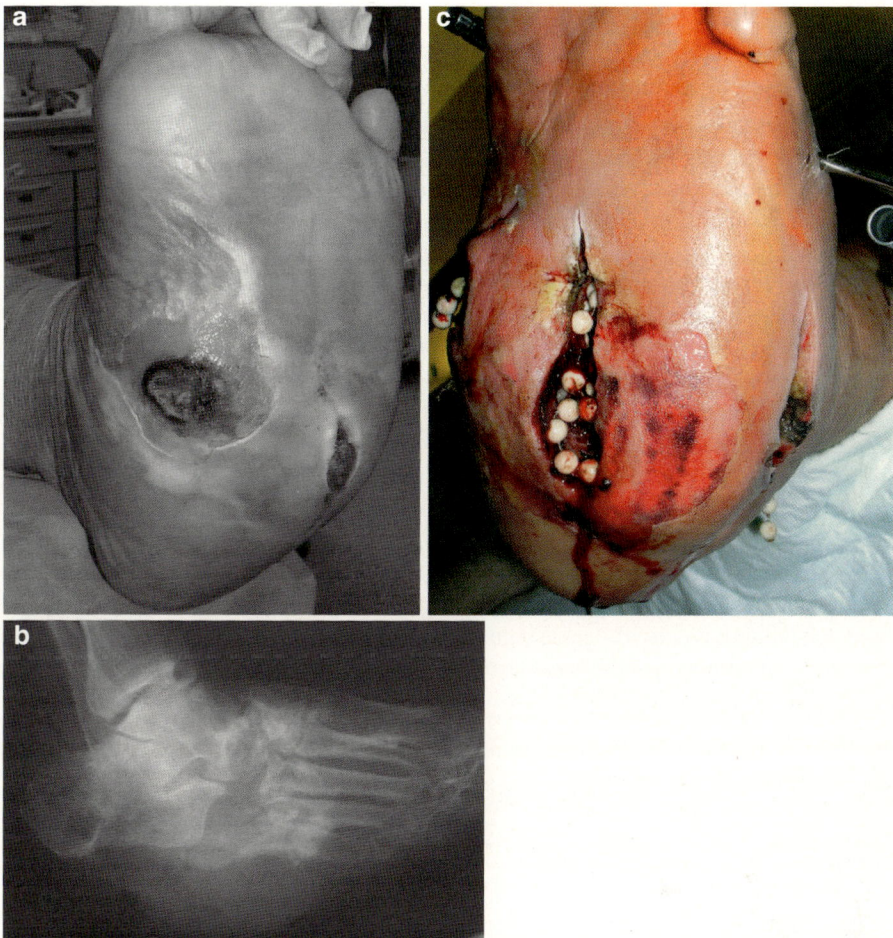

Fig. 11.2 (**a**) Staphylococcal sepsis in a 54-year-old male with D.M. II and Charcot type III and hemodilution therapy, temperature 39.6°C, leucocytes 20.6. (**b**) X-Ray with inclusion of gas in the soft tissue. (**c**) Incision, debridement, jet lavage, external fixateur, and antibiotic beads

11.2   Infected Charcot: Worst Case!

We know Charcot is not infection. As long as there is no ulceration of the skin or other injuries, there is no portal of entry. But this is not easy to decide. A red, hot swollen and mostly painless foot in an insensate patient with less inflammatory signs is rather an acute Charcot than an infection, or osteomyelitis. But if there is ulceration or other portals of entry, there is an opportunity of infection. Local situation and clinical signs are needed to decide acute infection and the need for immediate surgical intervention. X- Ray and MRI are helpful but often not confirmatory for infection or osteomyelitis. Most of the Charcot feet have a sufficient blood supply, but documentation of arterial inflow is a duty. Ultrasound detection is an easy and cheap method. If in doubt, further investigation is required. "Flow before toe" sounds simple and makes sense.

Acute infection needs to be treated like all infections – immediately! Surgical intervention to open all infected areas, joints, and tendon sheets, is essential. Incisions along the compartment lines and especially the tendon sheets of long flexors, Tibialis posterior and Peroneal tendons, if they are included, are important. Surgical debridement of all necrotic tissue and bone is performed. We remove all necrotic tissues from the wounds. Swabs from deep tissue and bone are a must. To clean the wound, we use the jet lavage with a disinfectant solution. Antibiotic beads with Gentamycin are available in Germany in different sizes and lengths. I use them for local antibiotic action and for drainage of the wounds. Repeated cleanings with lavage and a "second look" are needed until the infection is under control. Two other arms of treatment of infectious diseases are essential: antibiotic therapy according to the antibiotic testing and bed rest for the patient along with immobilization of the foot. External fixation that accomplishes both is a good option. The function control of all other organs is needed, coworking with the intensive care unit sometimes necessary.

After control of the septic situation, the reconstructive phase starts. The position of the foot can be controlled by the external fixation. Secondary bony procedures to enhance the position of the foot including lengthening of the Achilles tendon may be needed. The aim of all surgery in Charcot feet is a stabile, plantigrade, and shoe-able foot. Skin closure starts with dermatotraction. We use suture clips and vessel loops, suture clips around the wound parallel to each other and connected with the vessel loops. Because of the tension of the loops, the skin closes with the reduction of swelling and edema. The loops can easily be tightened with wound inspection (Fig. 11.3).

In spite of everything, we cannot protect every foot and leg. In severe infections or septic situations, we have to decide life before limb. That is a rule. We had great success (luck!); no amputation was needed for our Charcot foot patients over the past 3 years!

The combination and incidence of peripheral vascular disease and peripheral polyneuropathy, along with the predisposition for Charcot arthropathy for diabetic patients, is significant. The diabetic foot syndrome (DFS) is divided roughly into four groups: 25% peripheral vascular disease (PVD); 45% polyneuropathy (PNP);

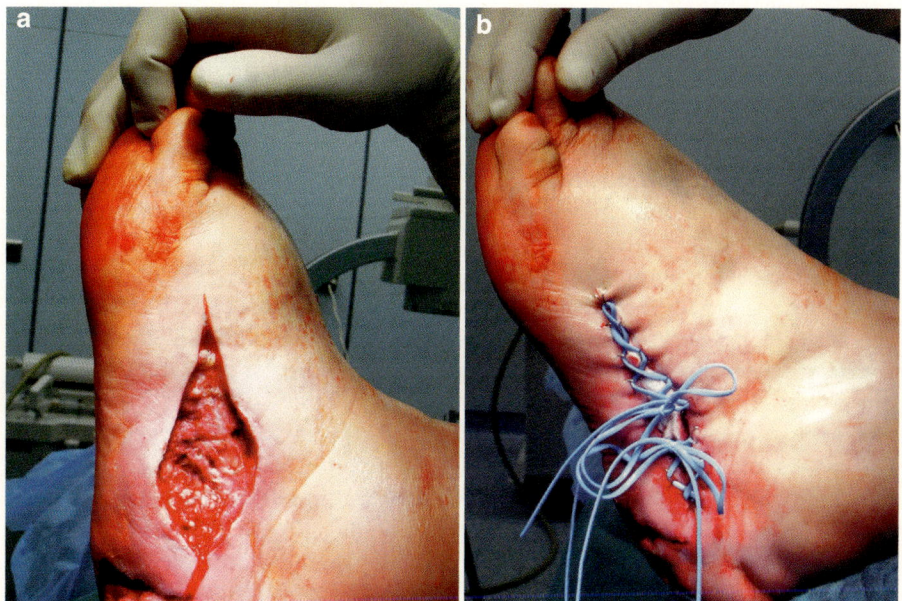

Fig. 11.3 (**a**) Charcot type Sanders V with a soft tissue infection of lateral aspect of the foot and heel; (**b**) debridement and closure with dermatotraction

25% PVD + PNP; and 5% Charcot. That means about 70% of the diabetic patients are at risk to get Charcot disease. The last estimation for Germany was 80,000 Charcot patients in 2008. A Charcot register is needed immediately in Germany.

It is not known who gets Charcot foot, or who does not get it. We know only a little about when, why, and which side Charcot joints will occur. The duration differs from patient to patient and a recurrence is possible every time. Trauma is an accepted cause to initiate a Charcot reaction. But the patients are insensate. They do not realize a trauma or they realize the breakdown of the foot as trauma but the Charcot exists still for weeks or month. On the other hand, traumas and fractures may cause a Charcot reaction.[6] The consequence is a different treatment and postoperative care in insensate patients. But there is much more to take into account; not all deformities in patients with DM, PNP, severe foot mal-alignment, and ulceration are Charcot feet.

11.3 Charcot: General Considerations

11.3.1 Classification

Two main scores are used to classify Charcot feet: first is the course of the disease. More or less useful is the staging according to Eichenholtz (1966): Stages: I–III. Stage I is the fragmentation, stage II is the coalescence, and stage III is the reconstruction. This staging was based on radiological findings.[7] Today we could add a Stage 0. The bone marrow edema marks the beginning of the disease, detected by MRI. There are different staging systems in debate[1,8]).

The second classification is the location of the destruction according to Sanders and Frykberg.[9] They stated five groups: Type I toe and distal metatarsals; Type II tarso- metatarsal joints: Lisfranc's joint line; Type III Chopart joints including Naviculo-Cuneiform joints; Type IV Ankle joint including subtalar joint, and Type V Calcaneus.

Often used and requested in Germany is the San Antonio classification according to Wagner and modified by the vascular and infectious status by Armstrong et al.[10] This is a useful system to classify wounds in diabetic patients and add the predicting outcome factors: blood flow and infection. But no information on status of bone and joints is made.

A very sophisticated system of Charcot staging was published by Sommerey.[8] This system classifies bony destruction, fracture type, luxation status, soft tissue defects, location of the destruction, and MRI findings (P1–3, F0–3; D0–2; S0-4; L1- 10; M0- 4). It covers all different problems but with the lot of subgroups and it is therefore not in clinical use. A reliable staging is still needed. A generally accepted and useful classification is needed based on research and scientific work.

I prefer to use a combination of the Eichenholtz stage, the location of the disease classified by Sanders and Frykberg, infectious status (with or without ulceration, with or without infection), and vascular status. Patient's general status is also taken into account.

Acute dislocation of Charcot feet is special problem. Classification systems should allow for this. Fusion is needed after reposition. But the reposition itself is also a problem. Primary fusion or secondary fusion after fixation in an External fixator depends still on the experience of the surgeon and patient's conditions.

Another main point of differentiation of Charcot feet is stability at later stages. Some become stable with bony fusion or fibrotic stability, others remain unstable. Beneath unstable joints we may find ulcerations. This is not easy to detect because in time of investigation we see a resting foot. The test of instability at the affected joints is mandatory. One good option in patients with stabile feet and plantar bony prominences is the "exostosectomy."[11] An approach is made at the medial or lateral margin of the foot to expose the bone. The bony cut creates a smooth surface parallel to the weight-bearing surface (Fig. 11.4).

The classification of Charcot depends on stage and location. But no information is given on the soft tissue condition with or without ulceration, with or without infection. Additionally the San Antonio classification can be used. According to the WHO Consensus Conference, the vascular status needs to be documented especially prior to surgical intervention.[12] Outcome studies for Charcot treatment are needed. To compare the different treatment attempts, an accepted staging system would be of great benefit.

Fig. 11.4 (**a**) Charcot type
Sanders II with dislocated
Cuneiforme bone with plantar
peak pressure; (**b**) medial
surgical approach with
exposition of the bone

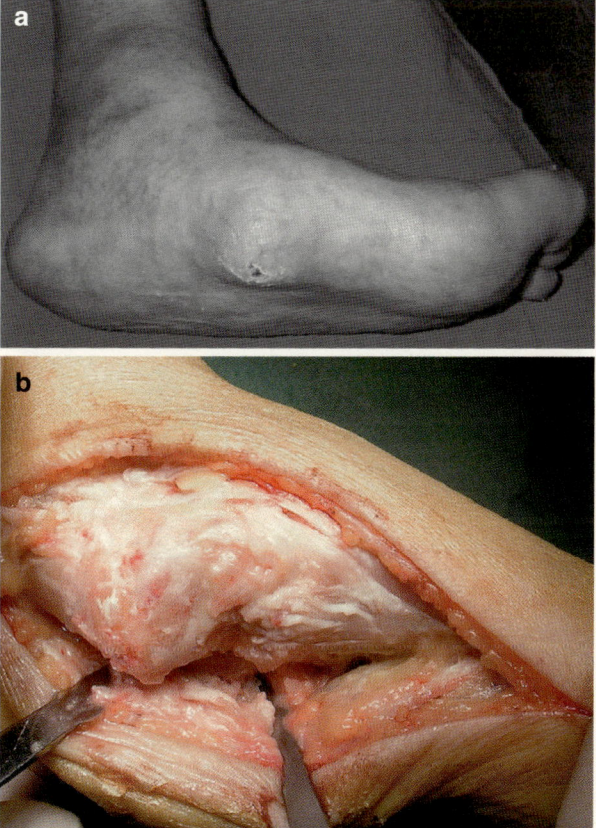

11.4   Charcot Treatment Principles

11.4.1   Treatment Principles According to Staging Eichenholtz (1966)

Eichenholtz 0 (bone marrow edema, MRI by Kessler,[1] and Eichenholtz 1 (fragmentation)[7] should be treated nonsurgically. Off-loading with a wheel chair and crutches is needed. For immobilization purposes and to reduce the rear foot rotation, a custom-made or over-the-counter walker should be used. The Total Contact Cast (TCC) provides the best off-loading and immobilization.[6,13-17] But we know about potential problems with the TCC. Over time we prefer to a system like a TCC but removable, manufactured by Lohmann/Rauscher Germany. It is applied by the orthopedic shoe technicians (Fig. 11.5).

Aim of immobilization and off-loading is to protect the bones and joints, and prevent the breakdown of the arch. Over a period of 3–6 months, the metabolism of bone

Fig. 11.5 (**a**) [15×] A 58-year-old patient with bilateral Charcot Sanders II, stage Eichenholtz I; TCC bilateral by Lohmann/Rauscher Germany applied by Trentmann/Gromotka Co. Hamburg, Germany; (**b**) [16×]: Patients with TCC do not feel as bad as we would expect

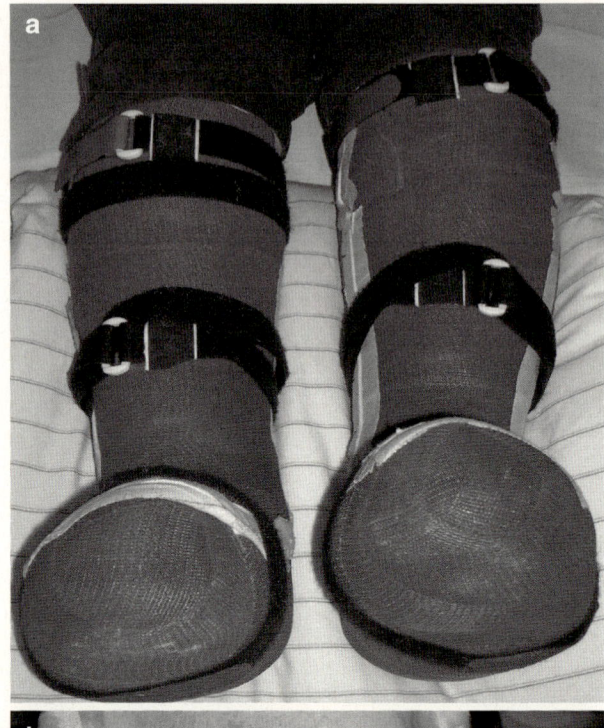

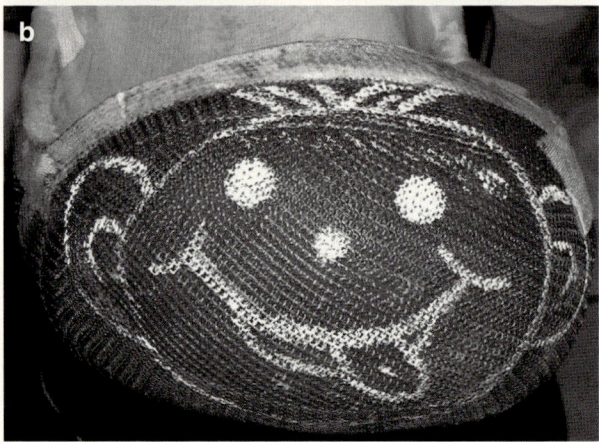

returns to almost normal. Today we have the option to visualize the change in bone marrow activity by MRI. This would be the optimal treatment of Charcot: Detect the onset in stage 0 and immobilize the foot as long as the marrow edema disappears. Potentially no change in the shape of the foot would happen. This condition is rare. Four out of 128 patients in the cohort collected by Sommerey[8] had stage 0. We had 3 patients with 4 ft directly treated with TCC. Our referrals are biased, however, since surgical departments get patients with complications and late stages of the disease.

Fig. 11.6 A 60-year-old patient, D.M. X 30 year, PNP 12 year, Charcot Sanders V since May 2009, note the cranial dislocation of the heel. (**a**) X-Ray and (**b**) MRI imagines

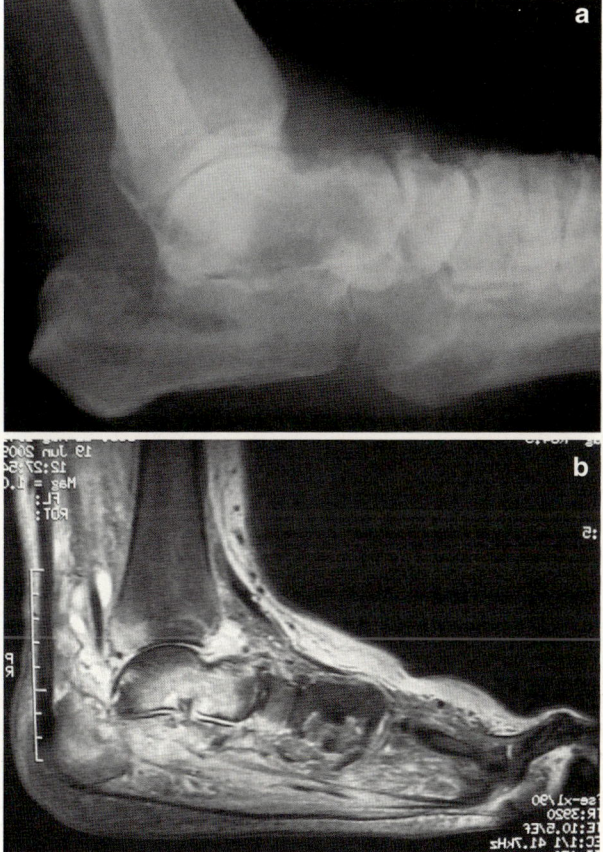

Eichenholtz Stage II and III (coalescence and reconstruction) are the typical well-known feet with slight-to-severe deformations. The x-ray shows the dislocation of joints and fractures with bony healing or pseudarthrosis and increasing deformation or stabile healing. Every Charcot seems to have its own clinical picture. The situation may be stabile or unstable. Bony prominences may occur. Soft tissue may be under pressure or tension. Keratoic disorders or subkeratotic hematomas may happen. Small ulcerations develop beneath this keratomas. This is the possible portal of infection.

The tension of Achilles tendon supports or causes the midfoot break. The power of the gastrocnemius complex triggers the collapse in Lisfranc or Chopart joint line. The typical late-stage rocker bottom foot starts to develop. In Charcot type V, the heel may fracture and heel bone or parts are pulled proximally (Fig. 11.6).

Stabile and plantigrade-orientated feet are best for custom-made shoes with soft two-layered insoles. The insoles cover the whole sole of the foot. This provides the best pressure distribution of the body weight on the sole of the foot. Pressure-measuring devices control the effect of reducing peak loadings. In Germany,

Fig. 11.7 A 47-year-old patient Charcot Sanders III, Eichenholtz III post Ex Fix and healing of ulceration and infection, custom-made rocker bottom boot with internal shoe and integrated insole worn in the boot

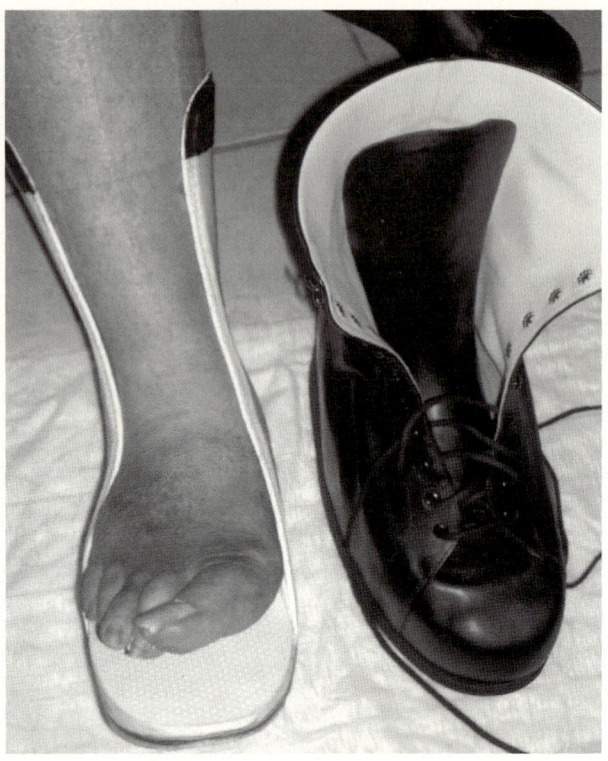

custom-made orthopedic boots are recommended and reimbursed by the insurance since January 2007 (Leitlinien DFS; 2007: www.leitlinien.de) for Charcot patients (Fig. 11.7).

First maxim of treatment irrespective of Eichenholtz stage: Consider conservative treatment. Off-loading and immobilization in an adequate orthotic is mandatory.[14] TCC is the best option, but today prefabricated, removable boots are more often used. The problem of patients' compliance is well known. David Armstrong's idea to make those devices irremovable by using additional fixation like cast or cables is a good option. He called this type of TCC "instant orthotic" (personal communication). Off-loading or how much weight is allowed to secure the healing and the duration of orthotic use is still in debate. MRI is expected to support the treatment decisions.[8]

11.4.2 Treatment According to Sanders and Frykberg Classification (1993)

Sanders I classifies the Charcot of toes and distal metatarsal heads. Our series showed Sanders type I Charcot feet in four postsurgical cases. Postoperative development was seen by other groups too.[12] One worse possible complication

Fig. 11.8 A 73-year-old
male, D.M. type II,
polyneuropathy, amputation
of the great toe and proximal
first metatarsal, note the
fracture and dislocation of the
metatarsal heads II and III

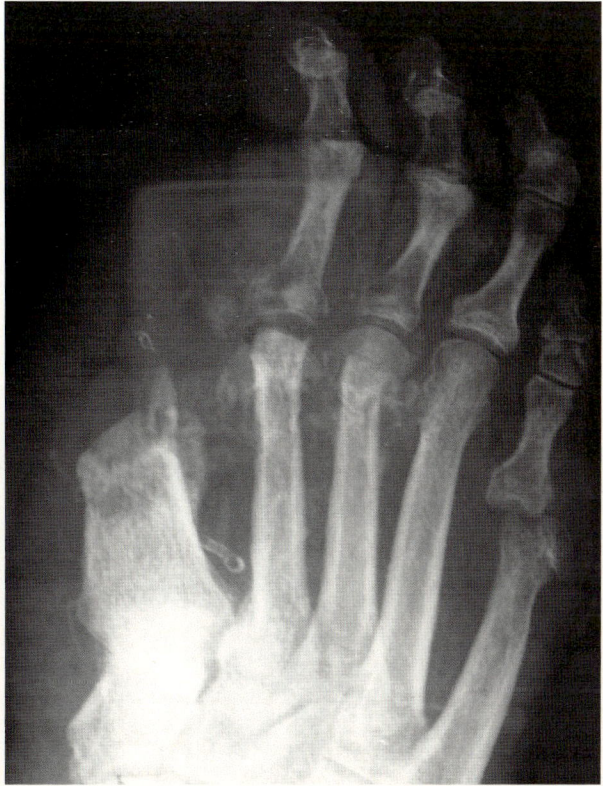

in patients with polyneuropathy is to trigger a Charcot reaction. Interestingly, this Charcot may not occur in the surgical region. We have seen patients after surgical intervention at the first ray with Charcot reaction of the lesser metatarsals (Fig. 11.8). In one case, we assume the surgery was indicated because of a misdiagnosed Charcot type I with osteolysis of the first metatarsal head to be an osteomyelitis (Fig. 11.9).

A lot of Charcot Sanders type I are not treated, because complications are not as often as with midfoot Charcot's. We treat Charcot Sanders type I conservatively (nonsurgically). Boots or orthotics are used. A stiff sole with rocker bottom is applied. Surgery is only needed in cases with ulceration or infection. Charcot Sanders type I does not exist in other classifications, e.g., Brodsky.[13] For treatment of plantar ulcerations, metatarsal heads are often resected. That may be the second reason for few reported Sanders type I patients.

Sanders type II attacks the Lisfranc joints. Untreated different dislocation and fracture types occur. Main problem is the break of the arch with bony prominences at plantar side of the foot, often described as an "exostosis." This is pathologically incorrect. The prominences are dislocated bones but no "exostosis" in sense of new bone formation (Fig. 11.10).

Fig. 11.9 A 38-year-old male, D.M. type I, polyneuropathy, head resection of the first metatarsal (probably misdiagnosed Charcot type I), note break and dislocation of the metatarsal heads II and III

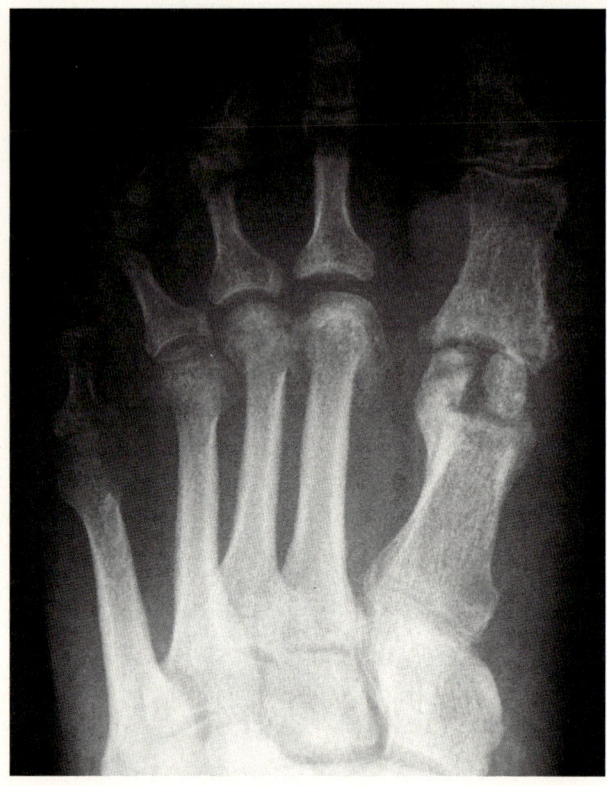

The different destruction patterns from Lisfranc to Chopart joint are covered by the Schon et al. classification.[18] The classification depends on the different involved joints including the articulation between the navicular and the cuneiforms. A more useful classification by Schon et al. is the foot shape: **A** normal arch; **B** flat foot, and **C** rocker bottom.[19] This is clinically very useful. Types A and B can be treated conservatively if the skeleton of the foot is stabile. Custom-made shoes are the solution; 2-layered insoles covering the whole sole in addition provide good protection. Type C will create ulcerations by so-called internal decubitus.

Charcot Sanders type II may cause a breakdown of the arch with a rocker bottom deformity of the foot. Ulcerations may be present, healed or impending. The foot may be mechanically unstable. These are situations that we consider for surgical intervention: osseous correction and stabilization.[1,15,19-21]

Surgical intervention is preferred for feet in Eichenholtz stages II and III. Stage I surgery should be avoided because of the high metabolic turnover in the involved bones. The bones are mechanically weak and fixation is tricky. But in dislocated types we could expect problems, or in extremely unstable situations surgery should be taken into account. Best surgical technique is still in debate. External fixation is a safe method but reposition and retention and infection control at the pin track areas are well-known problems.[15,22-24] Internal fixation has different problems: open

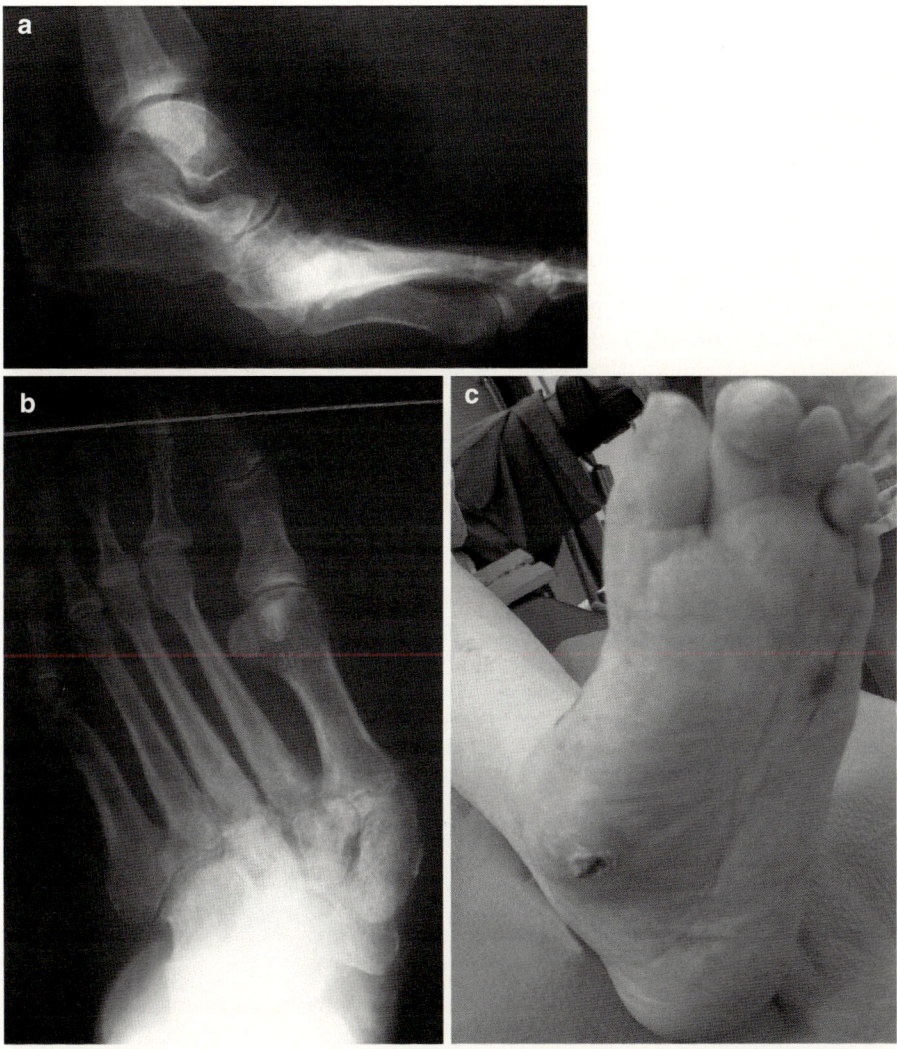

Fig. 11.10 A 68-year-old male, D.M. II. (**a**) Syme amputation right foot, Charcot Sanders II left foot, stage Eichenholtz III; (**b**) X-ray and (**c**) clinical appearance with mal perforans medially

surgery with danger of infection, all problems connected with hard ware, especially in long term with recurrence of Charcot reaction.[1,16,20]

Charcot type Sanders II with acute dislocation needs to be fixated.[23] Occasionally, external fixation is tricky. Internal fixation with locking plates is an option. Historically, bad results are documented. It is believed this is due to fixation: Very rigid and durable fixation along with more hardware than with typical fracture and dislocation types is needed. Titanium locking plates are available in several sizes and shapes. We can use the plates that conform best to the bone (Fig. 11.11).

My favorite plate position is as follows: One plate is applied at the medial arch perpendicular to the weight-bearing surface. A second or more are fixed in a 90° angle to that plate (Fig. 11.11d, e). The aim is a very rigid fixation. In this case, the screws of the plates are crossing each other. If the screws get in contact, we form a titanium-bone cage. Longer fusion distances are first crossed with compression screws. This type of fixation is described later.

The other main point is the length of healing, off-loading, and expected fusion time. It is known the healing time of bone in insensate patients is longer. The fusion site is weaker and again our patients have usually no pain. They cannot control the weight on their feet. Restrictive post-surgical protocol is needed. We use casting, wheelchair, crutches, and a lot of patient education. A lot of individual discussions are needed to explain to patients that even surgeons do not understand what exactly happens with their feet. It helps to get the patient to comply.[24]

The surgical procedure is the same in Charcot Sanders II with involvement of the Naviculo-Cuneiform I–III joints. The Eichenholtz stages 2 and 3 are good options for bony correction and internal fusion. Bony wedges are resected or the bones

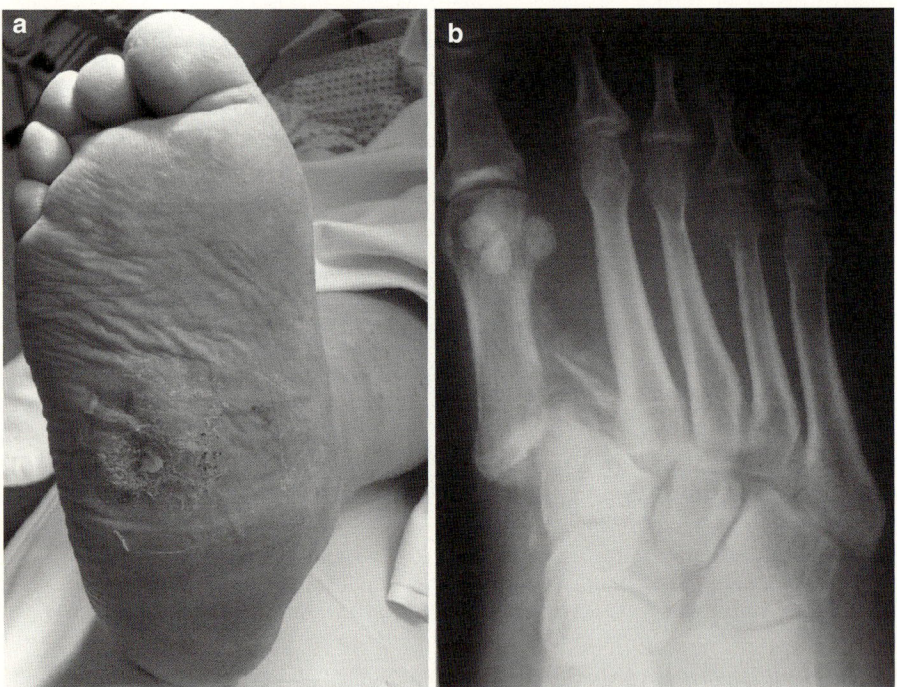

Fig. 11.11 (**a**) Acute dislocation Sanders II in a 52-year-old patient with toxic neuropathy; (**b**) Surgical site with applied plates; (**c**) Reposition and fusion of Lisfranc joint I–III with compression screws and locking plates; (**d**, **e**) Bony fusion after 12 weeks of off-loading, note the formation of new bone dorsal and plantar at fusion site

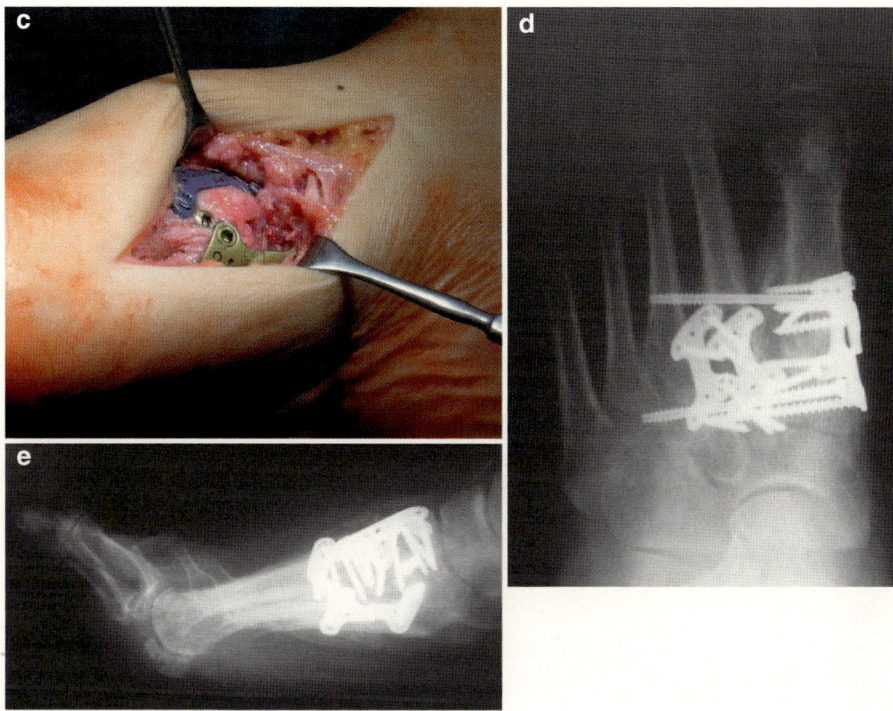

Fig. 11.11 (continued)

repositioned to create and arch or at least a flat foot. A medial approach allows exposing the medial arch with all bones including the talus (Fig. 11.12a–c).

Fixations of the midfoot are stable in most cases. We normally do not stabilize the lateral column. Other surgeons use additional lateral fixation. We avoid incisions laterally if there is no severe dislocation in Sanders II types.

Depending on the rear foot motion, especially in the ankle joint, a lengthening of the Achilles tendon is needed. Every type of equinus position of the heel causes a bending force on the midfoot. There are different reasons for a contracted Achilles tendon: immobilization-restricted joint motion, and diabetes with changes in the structures of joint capsules and tendons due to altered glycosylation.[25] The test is the so-called Silverskjoeld test for gastrocnemius contracture. Extension of the ankle joint is different with straight or bended knee. The lengthening of the gastrocnemius complex with an open or endoscopic technique lengthens the Achilles tendon complex but avoids overlengthening by keeping intact Soleus function. Our aim is at the end of surgery to achieve up to 10° of dorsiflexion at the ankle joint. My favorite technique is a short incision medial side of the calf 12 cm above the medial malleolus. We find gastrocnemius tendon and the distal part of the muscular belly of the Soleus. Separation of tendon and muscle from the Sural nerve is needed. A horizontal incision with a new scalpel blade is made from medial to lateral. Only the tendon

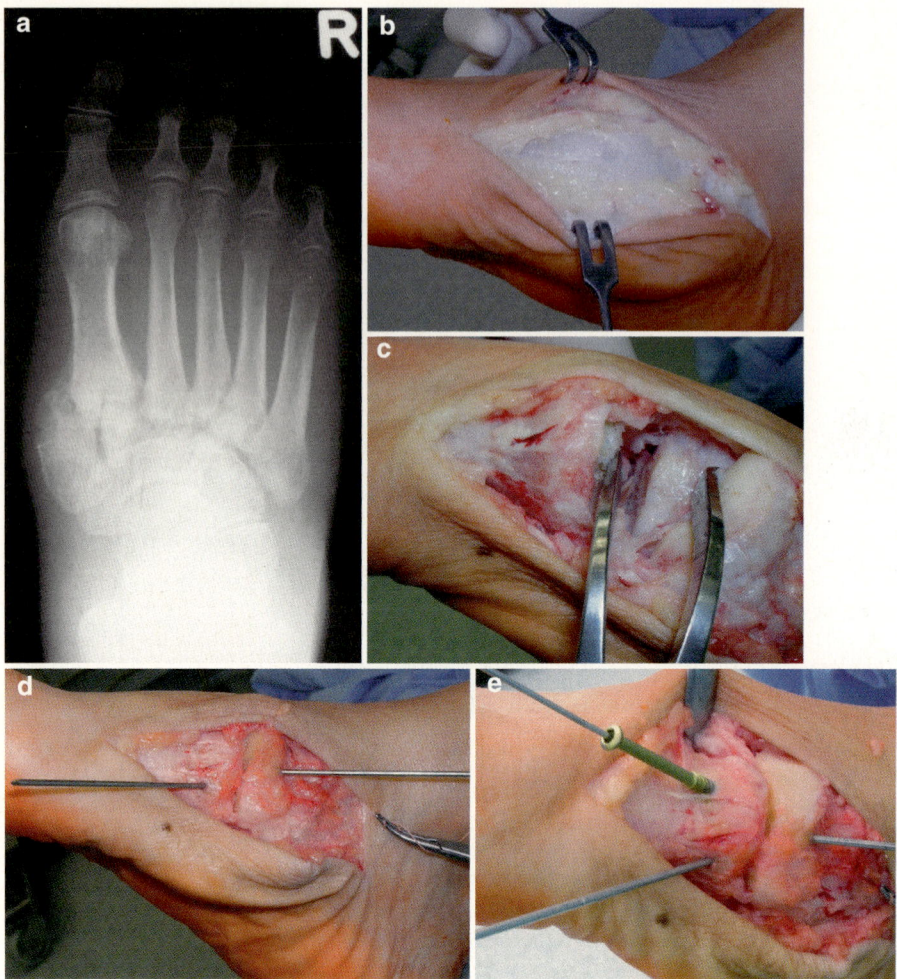

Fig. 11.12 A 72-year-old female Charcot Sanders II, Eichenholtz stage 3, breakdown of the arch; medial exposition of metatarsus I to the Os naviculare; (**a**) X-ray p-d; (**b**) exposure medial approach Metatarsus I to os naviculare; (**c**) removal of cartilage and bony wedges; (**d**) temporary fixation with K- wires; (**e**) compression by shortthreated canulated screws; (**f**) locking plate system applied to the medial arch; (**g, h**) fixation of the medial arch by compression screws, locking plates, titanium systems, X-ray: Saltzmann view and p-p view

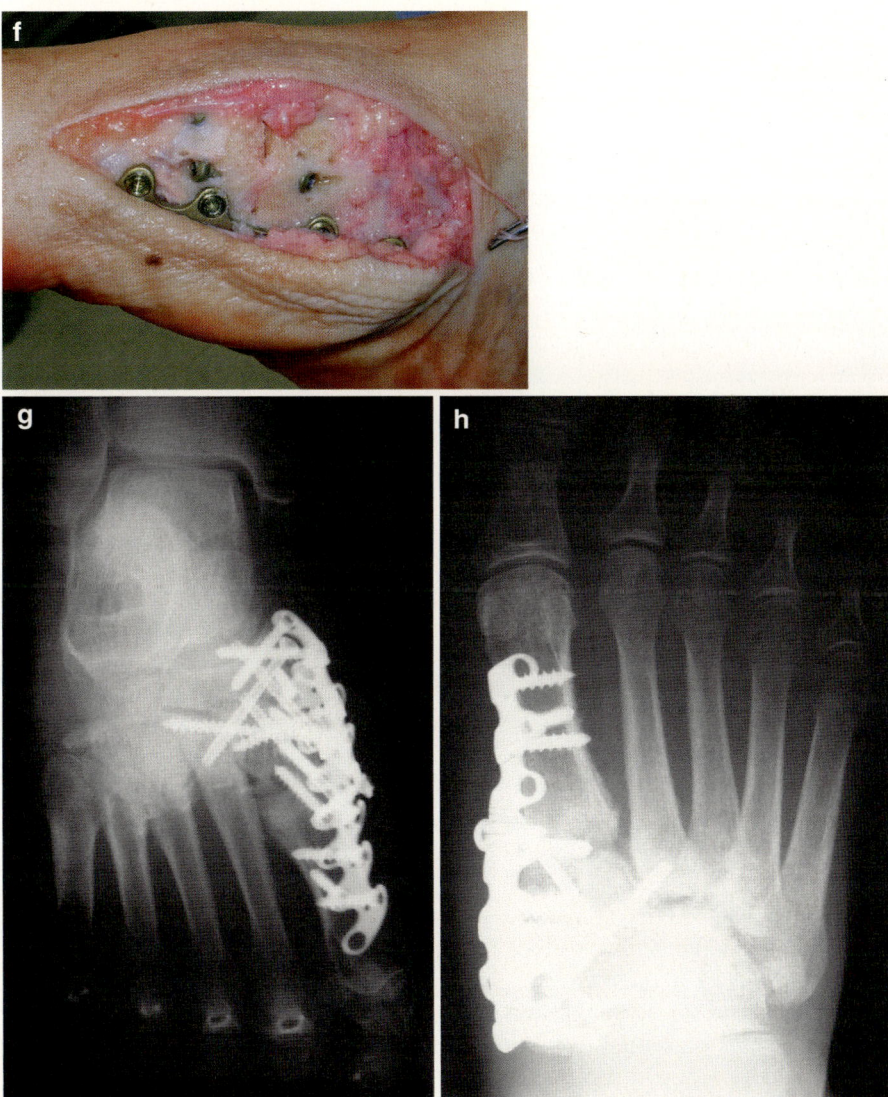

Fig. 11.12 (continued)

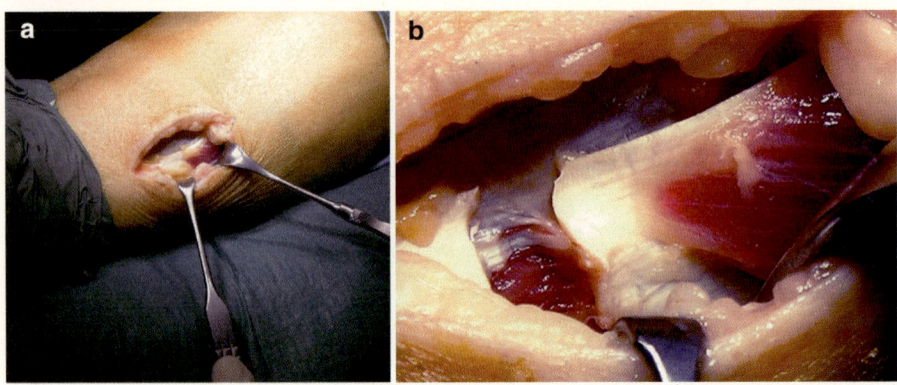

Fig. 11.13 Open gastrocnemius lengthening, medial incision, tenotomy of the gastrocnemius tendon with intact soleus fibers and stretching of the Achilles complex; (**a**) medial incision and exposure of the gastrocenemius complex; (**b**) horizontal incision of the gastrocnemius fibers strechingby dorsiflexion of the ankle joint

fibers of the gastrocnemius muscule are incised. Muscular fibers and intramuscular septae are protected by fingertips to prevent bleedings. Dorsal extension of the ankle shows the effective result of the release (Fig. 11.13).

The treatment of *Charcot feet type Sanders III* often involves not only Chopart's joint, but also other midfoot joints. Plantar dislocation of the Cuboid or Cuneiforms which may become plantar prominent can occur. Excessive peak pressures at those areas are the consequence. Callus formation occurs at the skin; subcutaneous hemorrhage and ulceration are the result. Biomechanical mobility in the Talo-Navicular joint and the small fixation region of the talus are the problems of fixation at Chopart's joint. A severe dislocation of the forefoot and midfoot complex over the rear foot is a typical clinical feature.

Internal fixation in Charcot's type Sanders III is an option. My favorite technique is triple arthrodesis in those cases. Subtalar fusion fixates and stabilizes the subtalar joint. Additional long screw fixation of the lateral column to secure the Calcaneus-Cuboid Complex is useful. Long cannulated double-threaded titanium screws are my favorite devices. Chopart's joint is fixed by compression screws and locking plates. Reposition of the bones and fragments is not easy. Especially formed osteotomes and spreaders of various types are helpful. Preparation at the bone-periosteum level is necessary to protect vascular structures (i.e., avoid periosteum stripping). Sometimes in severely dislocated feet, reposition must be incomplete to protect vital structures. If reposition of bones is impossible, the plantar aspect of the foot is smoothed with saw and chisels. No bony edges or spikes are acceptable (Fig. 11.14).

The stabilization of the medial arch needs a lot of strength. Bending forces have to be neutralized. Because we know of nonunions and fibrotic "fusions," the plates are constantly under pressure. Breakage or fracture of plates or screw heads is possible months and years later. It makes always sense to think about the hardware problems causing pressure and ulceration itself. Consider external fixation as

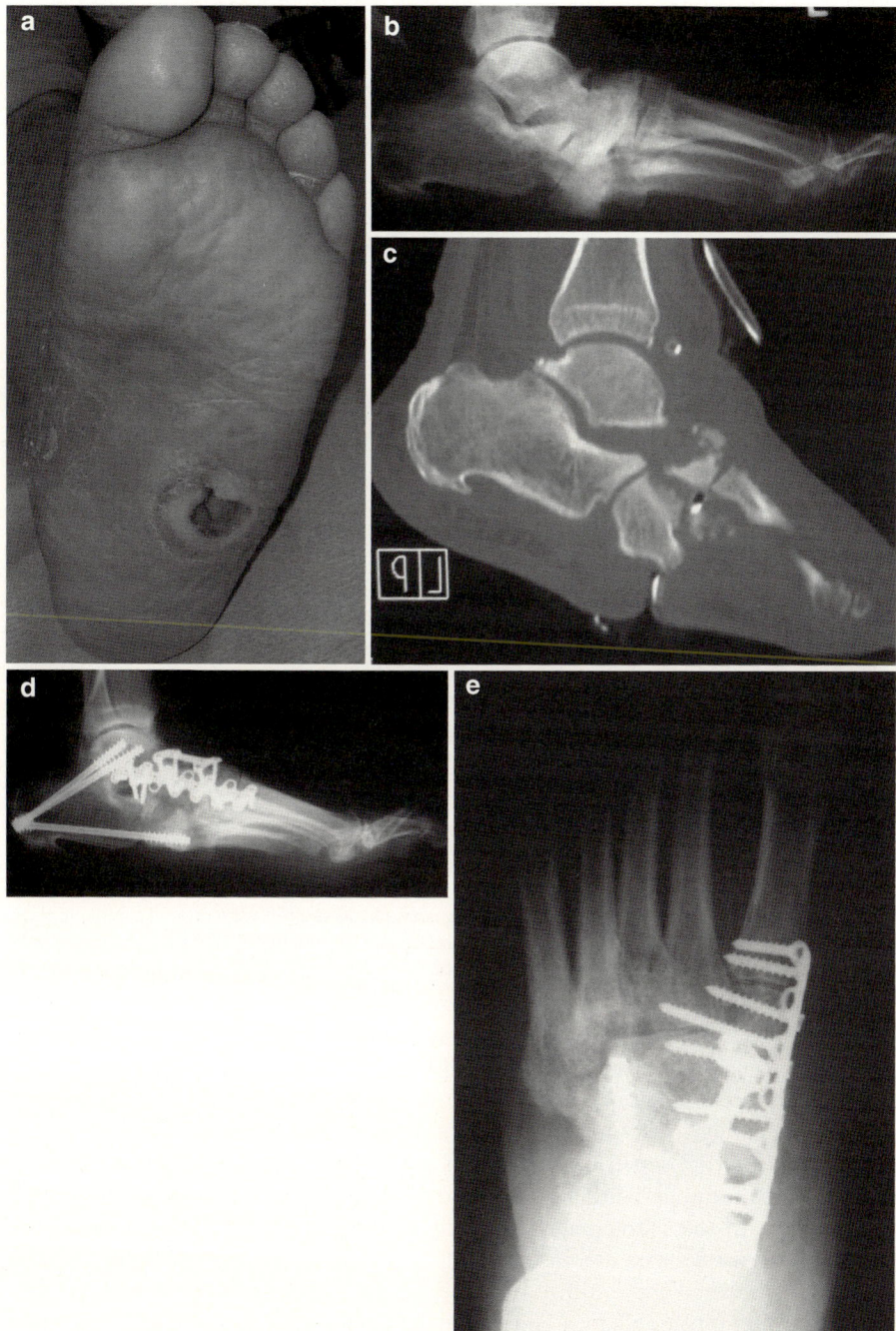

Fig. 11.14 A 48-year-old male, D.M. type II, polyneuropathy, Charcot Sanders III with ulceration, clinical appearance, x-ray, CT scan; (**a**) clinical appearance; (**b**) X-ray lateral view; (**c**) CT scan with contact of the ulceration to os cuboideum; (**d**, **e**) reconstruction with extended triple arthrodesis, lateral and d-p X-ray

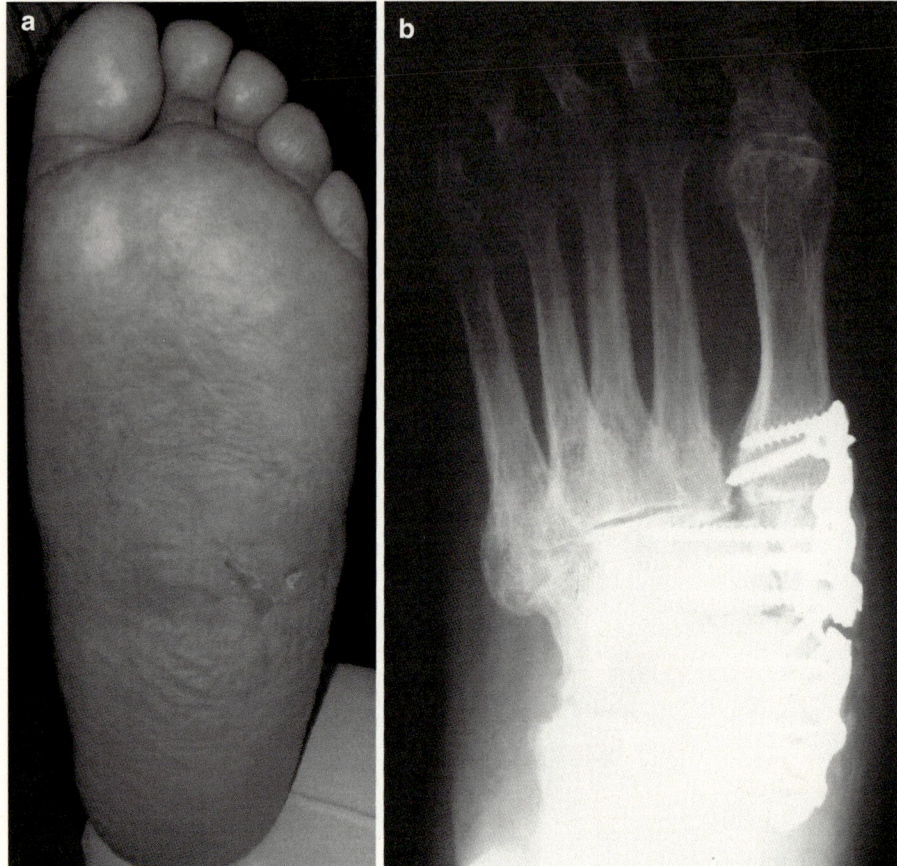

Fig. 11.15 (**a**) Sole of the foot 18 month after surgery. (**b**) X-ray d-p view, note the broken plate, but no loss of correction. Same patient shown in Fig. 11.14, 16 month postmedial plating with broken plate, but no loss of correction. Patient died from sarcoma of the colon 8 months later

option.[21,23] We try to increase the fixation strength by using two or more plates 90° angulated to each other. Second advancement is the fixation of the subtalar joint by long double-threaded screws (Fig. 11.15).

Not all Charcot feet type Sanders III can be treated by internal fixation. Severe dislocations and asymmetric deviation of the midfoot bones need correction and retention with external fixation. In infected cases, this would be of first choice. The aim of all treatments is to create a stabile, plantigrade foot. Shoemakers must have the chance to form shoes and insoles with a harmonic load pattern. Peak loadings have to be smoothed and stabilized.

Charcot feet type Sanders II and III are the common types. Some feet are more or less a combination of both types. The classification of those feet is difficult and may cause some differences in statistics of the frequency. One option to classify midfoot Charcot was published by Schon.[18]

But it is not only the type of Charcot; it is always the stage (activity) to keep in mind. Soft tissue and bones are in very different conditions. Wound infections are more frequent. In doubt is off-loading and casting the safer way. Using the time of casting for further diagnostics and maybe a second opinion makes sense. Clinical pictures, x-rays, and MRI pictures are sent worldwide within seconds today.

Charcot type Sanders IV involves the ankle joint. Destruction of ankle and load axis of the lower limb causes instability, ulcerations, and disability. Often the onset of Charcot is misdiagnosed as simple ankle fracture. The regular fracture treatment will fail. Weak bone, pseudo-arthrosis, loss of correction, and infection are the common complications. Sometimes the role of neuropathy is misunderstood and the cause of complications is assumed in diabetes mellitus.[6,17,26] But there is evidence that diabetes mellitus alone does not interfere with wound and bony healing.[6,26] The neuropathy is the trigger of complications. It is sometimes not easy to decide the causal connection: fracture as a trigger of Charcot reaction, or Charcot reaction and fracture because of the weakened bone. This is an issue with worker's compensation cases.

Charcot type IV or ankle fractures in insensate patients need more stability and longer healing times to avoid pitfalls.[6] The involvement of only the ankle needs fixation of the ankle. The decision to fix the subtalar joint is not easy. Ankle fracture or Charcot type IV is sometimes not easy to distinguish; we mostly solve the problem by primary fusion of the ankle. Soft bone and a lot of fragments are not the good options for AO-type fixations.

One patient had complete recovery after Charcot type II and surgery, off-loading, and custom-made shoes. She felt swelling in the ankle and warmth in the foot but no pain. A week later, she heard a "crack" in the foot followed by axis deviation. We decided for surgery and primary fusion with internal fixation: bilateral approach with locking plates and compression screws (Fig. 11.16).

Failed, infected ankle fusions are a challenge. Removal of all infected tissue and debridement, antibiotic beads, and external fixation is treatment of choice. Stem cells or other growth-increasing factors are options. Often we use "second look" surgeries for repeated debridement and pulsed-lavage.

The restoration of the axis of the leg, calf, ankle, and heel is not easy. Destruction of the talus makes it sometimes impossible to correct heel axis and angulations of the fore foot. The astragalectomy is an option to get the foot in correct alignment. Intramedullary rods are an option for fixation. Some of them are with the option of compression. The use of the dynamic option is possible too. But nails and rods are of metal and may break or cause ulcerations in case of further bony collapse. The problem of casting and shoe wear is axis deviation and instability. The pressure to correct the foot can cause ulceration and infection. Ankle instability with ulceration at the lateral malleolus is a typical clinical appearance of a Charcot type IV. What type of correction and fixation is the best option? In this case, rod fixation failed because of infection. We changed to external fixation and a lot of work including vacuum drainage and maggot therapy were used to heal the wounds (Fig. 11.17).

One of the problems is the talus. Often we see partial or complete necrosis. The removal of the talus, the so-called astragalectomy, is an option. The distal tibia needs to be shaped triangular and fitted between the dorsal facet of the Subtalar joint

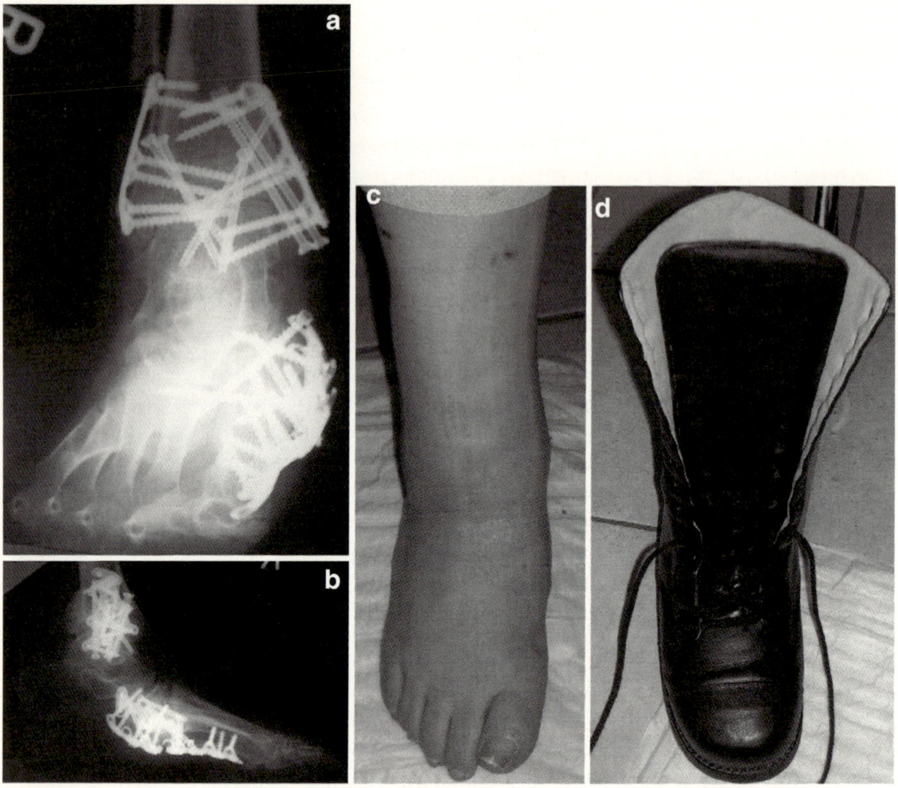

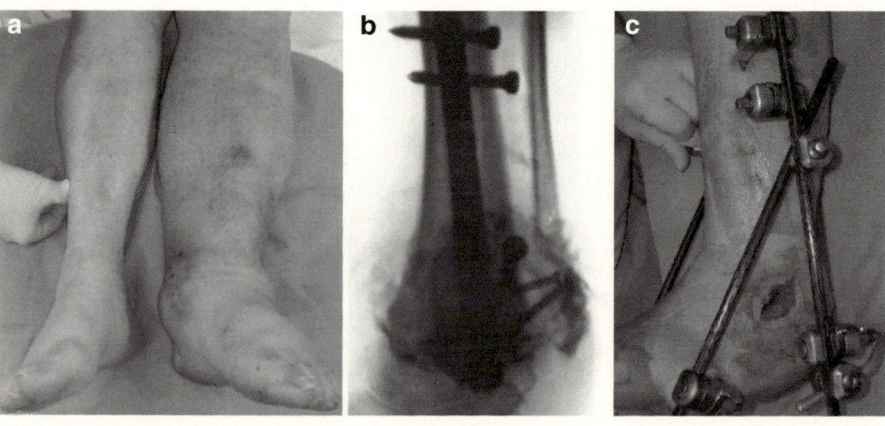

Fig. 11.16 A 36 year old female, D.M. Type I, polyneuropathy, previous Charcot Sanders II, reconstruction with plantar plating two years ago, ankle fracture with Charcot IV, primary ankle fusion, bilateral approach and composite fusion (compression screws and locking plates): (**a**) X-ray ap view, (**b**) X-ray lateral view, (**c**) clinical appearance, (**d**) custom made boot

at the Calcaneus and Navicular bone. Not in every case, bony healing is achievable. But fibrous fixation in patients with neuropathy is an acceptable result as long as we get stability and correct alignment.[23] Subtalar joint has to be cleaned of debris and cartilage if parts of the talus are preserved. We prefer the dynamic implantation of the rod. Fixation to protect rotation is performed by screws in Talus and Calcaneus. Independent of the use of plates or nails, casting in a TCC-like orthotic is an essential part of the postoperative care. Compression of the dynamic situation is given by partial weight-bearing of the patients after 8 weeks of off-loading (Fig. 11.18).

Rare situations may require the so-called Baumgartner amputation. It is a Syme-like amputation with preservation of the midfoot and forefoot.[27] These parts of the foot are docked to the ventral distal Tibia. We did this one time in an MRSA-infected Charcot type V with dead Talus and destroyed Calcaneus. A special luck was needed to place the holes of the previous used nail for fracture still in place with the pins for the external fixator (Fig. 11.19). Inpatient treatment took 128 days and additional 32 days in a second stay. Baumgartner published the book on amputation and prosthetic devices in 2008. It is one of the best books on amputation techniques but only available in German language.[27]

Charcot Foot Sanders Type V with involvement of the Calcaneus is rare. Primary treatment is conservative with off-loading to protect the heel bone from collapsing. Another problem is the pull of the Achilles tendon. The tension of the tendon may fracture and dislocate the calcaneal tuber (Fig. 11.20). Acute Charcot Type V is immobilized with wheelchair and gets a TCC-like orthotic. In late stages with a plantargrade but stabile Calcaneus, in rare cases, the foot loses height. Ulcerations may occur at Chopart's joint. Surgery depends on the stability in that area.

11.5   Author's Experience: Results of Charcot Treatment January 2006–August 2009

The Department of Foot Surgery of the Klinik Dr. Guth, Hamburg, Germany operated on 2,196 patients between January 2006 and August 2009. All types of foot pathologies are included. Within this cohort were 90 patients with all types and stages of Charcot arthropathy. Because of bilateral and reoccurring Charcot, we treated 100 ft. The youngest patient was female and 26 years with D.M. type I and

Fig. 11.17 A 68-year-old female D.M., polyneuropathy, bilateral Charcot, right foot type II with ulceration plantar, left foot with type IV and ankle instability. Contrast x-ray of fistula after intramedullary rod, external fixation and vacuum drainage left foot, simultaneous therapy of Charcot type II and ulceration at the mid foot right foot; (**a**) clinical view; (**b**) internal rod fixation and infection, X-ray detection of the fistula by using contrast fluid; (**c**) removal of the rod and stabilisation with external fixation

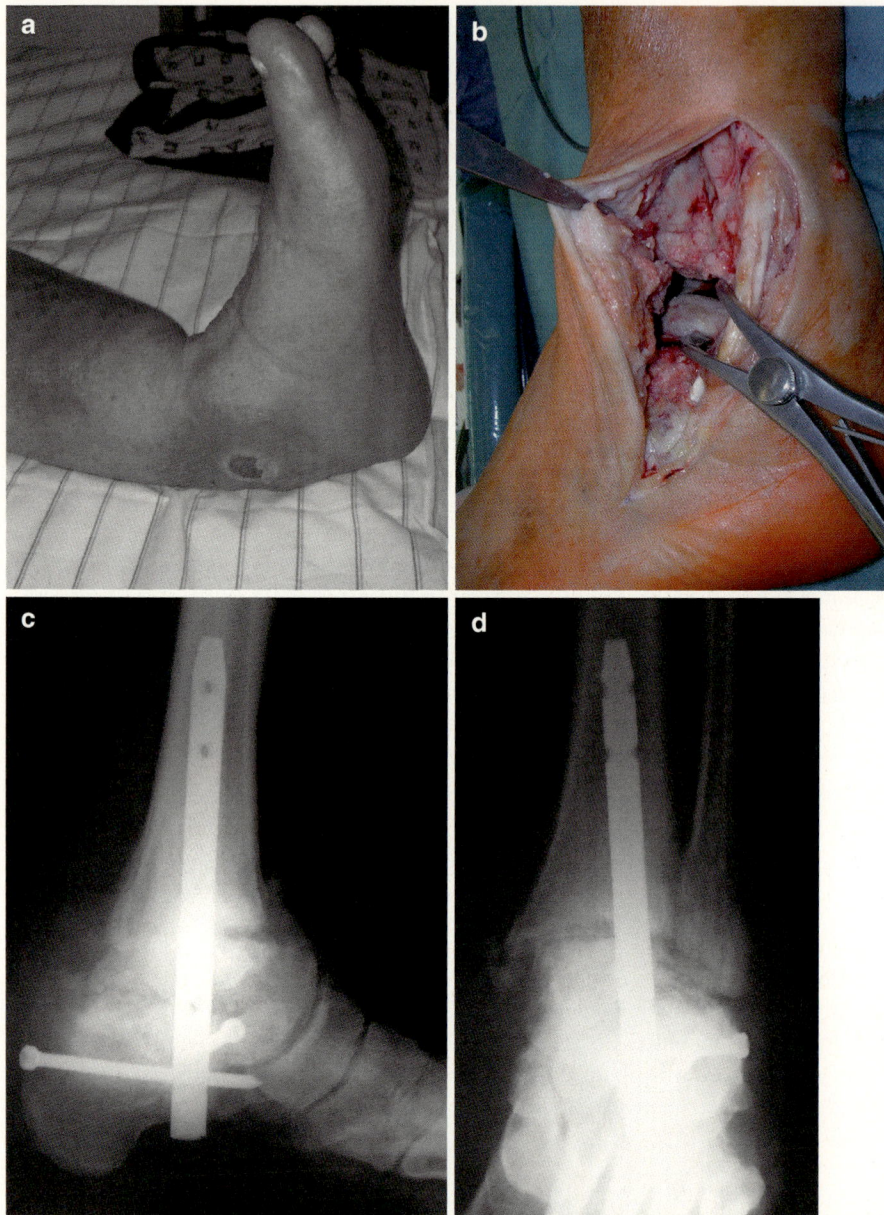

Fig. 11.18 A 67-year-old male D.M., polyneuropathy, Syme's amputation right foot, Charcot type IV left foot, partial resection of talus and dynamic intramedullary rod fixation; (**a**) completely unstable ankle with ulceration at the medial malleolus; (**b**) partial removal of the talus; (**c**, **d**) X-ray lateral and a-p view with dynamic intramedullary rod fixation

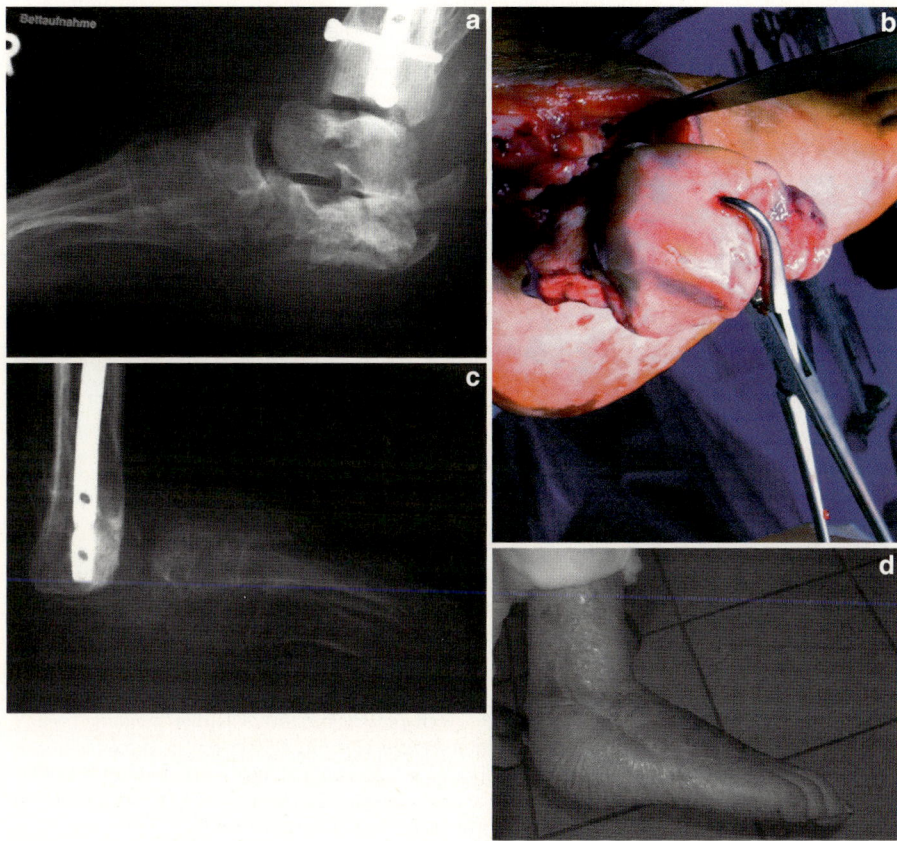

Fig. 11.19 A 42-year-old patient D.M. type I, polyneuropathy, renal failure, Charcot bilateral, MRSA infection and destruction of Calcaneus and avascular Talus. Resection of the Talus: so-called Astragalectomy and the x-ray and clinical appearance of the "Baumgartner" amputation. (**a**) Infection of ankle and subtalar joint; (**b**) astragalectomy (complete resection of the talus); (**c**) lateral X-ray of the so called Baumgartner amputation (internal Syme amputation); (**d**) lateral clinical view of the baumgartner amputation

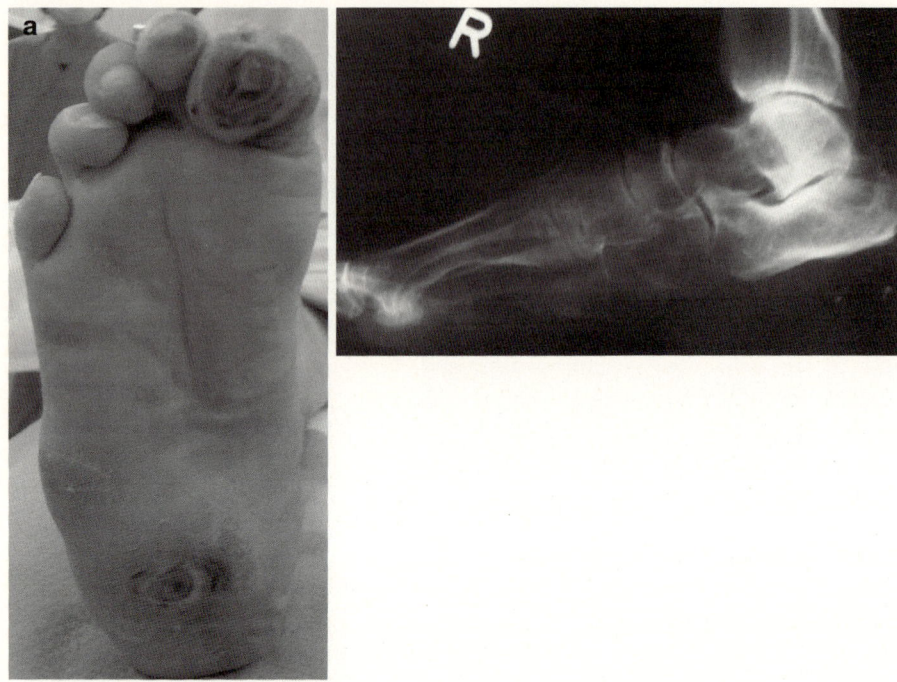

Fig. 11.20 A 37-year-old male, D.M. type I with polyneuropathy, Charcot Sanders Type V, Eichenholtz III. Ulcerations at the Chopart's joint are caused by instability and ulceration at the tip of the great toe by flexion contracture, surgical debridement of both ulcerations, release of the FHL and casting with a TCC- like orthotic, new custom-made shoes with a two-layered insole are required. Note the atrophy of the plantar subcutaneous fat; (**a**) sole of the foot; (**b**) lateral x-ray with functional instability of the Choparts joint

the oldest was a 73-year-old female with neuropathy of unknown origin. The ratio of male to female was 69:21. The age ranged between 26 and 76 years, mean: 55.2 years. The ratio of right to left foot was 52:30, bilateral 8 and 2 patients with different Charcot's on one foot within 3 years.

Ninety patients with Charcot foot were treated within 40 months. Seven out of 90 patients in our series were admitted in a septic condition. All patients had peripheral neuropathy: hereditary with unknown origin: 5 patients, toxic (ethyl) neuropathy: 4 patients, post-polio neuropathy: 1 patient and 80 patients with distal diabetic neuropathy. Ten of them had diabetes mellitus type I. All of our patients had neuropathy. But not all were pain-free.

We observed Charcot arthropathy in 52 left and 30 right feet. Eight patients had bilateral Charcot. Two patients got two different Charcot afflictions on the same foot. According to Eichenholtz, we found 11 ft stage 1; 15 ft stage 2; and 72 ft stage 3. In this series, we did not find a Charcot foot stage 0. The location of the Charcot disease was Sanders type I: 8; Sanders type II: 48; Sanders type III: 27; Sanders type IV: 14; and Sanders type V: 3. Because of the two Charcot at one foot, we treated

100 Charcot feet. Acute dislocation occurred in 3 of our 100 Charcot feet. Acute Charcot dislocation is a rare condition (Koller described 9 out of 103 cases).[28] The follow-up time was 30.2 months.

A lot of complications were noted: 57 patients had severe medical findings at the time of admission. Thirty-eight patients had a plantar ulceration. Seven patients came in a septic situation. Three patients had a major amputation at the opposite leg. Three patients suffered from acute dislocation Charcot. In 3 patients, we determined a postsurgical occurrence of the Charcot.

Thirty-four patients were treated nonsurgically. TCC if needed and custom-made orthopedic boots were used. These shoes are custom-made extra-depth with wide-toed area and molded two-layered insoles. A stiff rocker bottom sole is mandatory. All patients are provided custom-made shoes at the end of therapy. This is a rule secured by the German guidelines for the treatment of diabetic feet (www.leitlinien.de).

We needed a lot of different surgeries depending on the individual situation of the patient. Debridement of the ulceration and bone in 14 cases with additional 4 external fixations; Linck-Witzel internal amputation[29] in 9 cases with 9 additional external fixations; reposition and stabilization with external fixation without open procedure 4 cases; intramedullary rod fixation in 5 cases, ray resection in 2 cases and open reduction and locking plate fixation in 30 patients. Four of this 30 cases got additional external fixation. Forty of all cases were additionally secured with a total contact cast after removing the external fixator for 6–12 weeks.[30] The surgeries ranged from 1 surgical procedure to 23 procedures in a patient while in-patient.

To control the infection and close the ulceration, we utilized a lot of additional techniques: vacuum drainage in 4 cases, maggot therapy in 3 cases, bone marrow aspirate injections in 3 cases, local antibiotic beads and i.v. antibiotics depending on the testing. We avoid mesh grafts at the sole of the foot because of the reduced shear resistance and the hazard of recurrence of ulcerations.

In the time of investigation we noted 16 re-ulcerations. Two of the patients had severe infections. Ten patients healed conservatively with off-loading and improvement of shoes and insoles. Six patients needed revisional surgery. One patient with painful pseudo-arthrosis got a revision with iliac crest interpositional graft and locking plate fixation. Three needed additionally exostosectomy and two a debridement with external fixation.

We treated Charcot patients from entire Germany. We were unable to see all patients for follow-up. Twelve patients were lost from follow-up. One patient died of unrelated causes. Our main success was: No amputation was needed in Charcot patients since January 2006.

11.5.1   Discussion

Charcot arthropathy is still a mysterious disease. We do not know the exact cause of the destruction of bone and joints in the feet. Neuropathy is the main trigger.[2] About 80% of the neuropathies are caused by diabetes mellitus. But other neuropathies

Fig. 11.21 Semmes-
Weinstein-filament, reflex
hammer, tip-therm, tuning
fork (128 Hz)

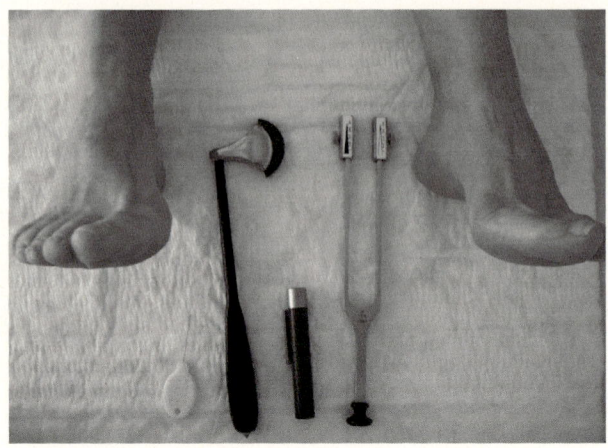

may cause Charcot reaction too.[15] We know about micro fractures, changes in blood flow, different activation of bone metabolism like the RANK-L ligand.[4,5] A lot of other factors are still unknown. When, where, and why a Charcot disease starts and why it ends, typically months later, is not fully understood yet.

The main diagnostic tool is the clinical investigation of the neurology of both legs. We need to investigate, because a lot of patients do not realize their loss of sensation. It is a long slow-onset. We need only few instruments (such as Semmes-Weinstein monofilaments, tuning fork, heat sensors, etc.) and some minutes of time[10] (Fig. 11.21). Neuropathy is the main reason for Charcot reaction. In our opinion, all patients with Charcot joints have a neuropathy. But even this is in debate.

Neuropathy is also taken into account in fracture treatment.[6,16,26] Insensate patients should be treated with a different protocol. Roughly spoken, they need more stable hardware, and a longer postoperative protocol with more off-loading duration is recommended. Sometimes we use additional casting to secure the fractures.

Charcot reaction can be caused by surgery. Trauma is an accepted reason for the onset of Charcot. We have seen Charcot reaction after metatarsal fractures with correct stabilization and K-wire retention, interestingly not at the region of fracture but more proximal. The patient's preoperative consent should include the possibility of onset of Charcot reaction with elective surgery in insensate patients.

Treatment of infection with or without osteomyelitis with or without empyema of joints is a challenge. We need all types of surgery, antibiotics, and additional treatment options. But some patient asked for medical help in a delayed fashion, again because of the insensate situation, the rule "life before limb" is sometimes a difficult decision.

Charcot disease itself is a disease with typical stages. We find a time-dependant course. One of the most used is the Eichenholtz classification 1–3. Today we are able to add the stage 0. It is the onset of the bony destruction marked by bone marrow edema. It is still unknown what happens in the bone. Repeated fatigue fractures are one of the explanations. The best way of treatment would be to detect the patients with stage 0 and bring them to stage 3; off-load the affected foot and protect the skeleton of foot from breakdown. This would not require surgery.[10]

The primary treatment of Charcot disease is nonsurgical.[1,21,23] The aim is a plantigrade and stabile foot. Every patient with Charcot Eichenholtz Stage 3 that has custom-made shoes and a stable situation without any hyperkeratosis or ulcers at the sole of the foot needs only daily inspection of their feet.

Charcot reaction is also divided by the location of joint destruction. The Sanders Types I and V are rare and can mostly be treated nonsurgically. Off-loading the foot is the best primary care. The treatment time depends on the time of reduction of the symptoms. Best marker would be the bone marrow edema. MRI shows the edema prior to x-ray changes. But not only the onset of the disease, also the changes in the bone marrow, reduction of edema, and regained stability of bone are shown by MRI. The question how often a MRI is needed is not answered yet. It is also a question of economic feasibility, at least in Germany, if not in the world.

The Charcot Feet of Sanders Types II, III, and IV show different patterns of bone and joint destruction. Surgical intervention depends on activity, stability, and shape of the sole of the foot. What kind of surgery, fixation of bones and joints, internal or external fixation, grafting with iliac crest or bone marrow, bone growth stimulators, etc. A lot of options are available. The individual treatment depends on experience and the favorite techniques of the surgeon.

A significant influence on the outcome is the postoperative care. Meticulous wound care, antibiotic prophylaxis over the first 5–12 days, and inpatient's treatment until wound healing occurs is our primary protocol. Patient's education is a main point of treatment and affects the outcome.[24] Depending on the healing and the home care situation, we see the patient in the outpatients department every week up to once a month. The patient gets an appointment once a month. This is a must. TCC and x-ray and the off-loading situation is checked. The start of partial weight-bearing and the prescriptions for custom-made shoes are prepared. The shoe-gear controlled by the surgeon is also a must.[17] After the initiation of weight-bearing and the first weeks of weight on the affected foot, the interval of appointments is extended: first to a 3 month period and later on to a 6 month interval. A second pair of shoes is prescribed after the sizing confirms appropriate fit.

One main point in treating Charcot patients is the protection of the opposite foot. As long as we do not know how to prevent it, a Charcot reaction is possible at the opposite side by additional stress caused by off-loading. At the beginning of our treatment, we protect the opposite side with custom-made interim shoes with individual insoles.

Lastly, but a main point, is all patients are in a long-term survey. Twice a year, we look regularly at our Charcot patients or in every acute situation. Most of the patients get complications. Diabetes mellitus, polyneuropathy, and peripheral vascular disease do not disappear.

11.6   Conclusion

Every profession involved in the treatment of Charcot has to take care of the feet: family doctors, physiotherapists, doctors of internal medicine, podiatrists and surgeons. In Germany, so-called Diabetes Mellitus Centers are the key in detecting complications and have the function of referring patients to the medical specialist needed. A lot of simple Charcot diseases are treated by using a TCC-like orthoses and sophisticated wound care within these centers. For this reason, surgical units often only see those cases with complications. Significant infections, chronic ulcerations, or unstable feet are referred to surgeons.

The second situation unique to Germany is the lack of podiatry as a specialty. We do not have specialized foot surgeons. The podiatrists in Germany are not allowed to do surgery. Orthopedic and trauma surgeons normally have little interest in foot surgery. (According to the German Association for Foot & Ankle Surgery, only 100 surgeons in Germany perform 100 or more procedures per year.) So Germany has a small community of surgeons dealing only with feet and even smaller who deal with Charcot foot and ankle disease.

My hope is to find the reason of Charcot disease so that we progress from treating the symptoms to curing the cause. I look forward to seeing this change for the betterment of our patients and the wisdom of those involved in the treatment of Charcot feet.

My bottom line is:

Charcot treatment is a full time job. It is obviously a team approach. Family doctors, the Diabetes centers, neurologists, orthopedic shoemakers, wound care nurses, and sometimes foot surgeons are needed. The surgeon needs to be familiar with all techniques of surgery and needs a huge amount of devices available to have the right answer to deal with all complications of Charcot foot and ankle disease.

References

1. Kessler SB, Kaltheiss TA, Botzlar A. Prinzipien der chirurgischen Behandlung bei diabetisch-neuropathischer Osteoarthropathie. *Internist*. 1999;40:1029-35.
2. Koeck FX, Bobrik V, Fassold A, Grifka J, Kessler S, Straub RH. Marked loss of sympathetic nerve fibers in chronic Charcot foot of diabetic origin compared to ankle joint osteoarthritis. *J Orthop Res*. 2008;27:736-41.
3. Pinzur MS, Sostak J. Surgical stabilization of nonplantigrade Charcot arthropathy of the midfoot. *Am J Orthop*. 2007;36(7):361-5.
4. Jeffcoate WJ. Charcot neuro-osteoarthropathy. *Diabetes Metab Res Rev*. 2008;24(Suppl 1):S62-5.
5. Jeffcoate WJ, Game F, Cavanagh PR. The role of proinflammatory cytokines in the cause of neuropathic osteoarthropathy (acute Charcot foot) in diabetes. *Lancet*. 2005;366:2058-61.
6. Costigan W, Thordarson DB, Debnath UK. Operative management of ankle fractures in patients with diabetes mellitus. *Foot Ankle Int*. 2007;28(1):32-7.
7. Eichenholtz SN. *Charcot joints*. Springfield: Charles C. Thomas; 1966.

8. Sommerey S. Klassifikation des Charcotfußes anhand von klinischen und radiologischen Befunden [Dissertation]. München: LMU; 2004.

9. Sanders LJ, Frykberg RG, The Charcot foot. In: Bowker JH, Pfeifer MA, Levin and O'Neal's The Diabetic Foot, 7th ed., Mosby: Philadelphia; 2008. p. 257-83.

10. Armstrong D, Lavery L, Harkless L. Validation of a diabetic wound classification. Diabetes Care. 1998;21(5):855-9.

11. Laurinaviciene R, Kirketerp-Moeller K, Holstein PE. Exostectomy for chronic midfoot plantar ulcer in Charcot deformity. J Wound Care. 2008;17(2):53-5, 57-8.

12. Zgonis T, Stapleton JJ, Shibuya N, Roukis TS. Surgically induced Charcot neuroarthropathy following partial forefoot amputation in diabetes. J Wound Care. 2007;16(2):57-59.

13. Brodsky JW. The diabetic foot. In: Mann RA, Coughlin M, editors. Surgery of the foot and ankle. St. Louis: CV Mosby; 1994. p. 925-53.

14. de Souza LJ. Charcot arthropathy and immobilization in a weight-bearing total contact cast. J Bone Joint Surg Am. 2008;90(4):754-9.

15. Pinzur MS, Sage R, Kaminsky S, Zmuda A. Treatment algorithm for neuropathic midfoot deformity. Foot Ankle Int. 1993;14:189-7.

16. Springfeld R. Die distale Neuropathie als Wegweiser für die Therapie knöcherner Fußverletzungen. Chirurgenmagazin. 2009;7:46-8.

17. Springfeld R. Eine Facette des diabetischen Fußsyndroms- der sogenannte Charcotfuß. Orthopädieschuhtechnik. 2009;4:28-34.

18. Schon LC, Weinfeld SB, Horton GA, Resch S. Radiographic and clinical classification of acquired midtarsus deformity. Foot Ankle Int. 1998;19(6):394-404.

19. Schon LC, Easley ME, Weinfeld SB. Charcot neuroarthropathy of foot and ankle. Clin Orthop Relat Res. 1998;349:116-31.

20. Sammarco VJ, Sammarco GJ, Walker EW Jr, Guiao RP. Midtarsal arthrodesis in the treatment of charcot midfoot arthropathy. J Bone Joint Surg Am. 2009;91(1):80-91.

21. Zgonis T, Roukis TS, Lamm BM. Charcot foot and ankle reconstruction: current thinking and surgical approaches. Clin Podiatr Med Surg. 2007;24(3):505-17.

22. Fabrin J, Larsen K, Holstein PE. Arthrodesis with external fixation in the unstable or misaligned Charcot ankle in patients with diabetes mellitus. Int J Low Extrem Wounds. 2007;6(2):102-7.

23. Koller A, Hafkemeyer U, Fiedler R, Wetz HH. Rekonstruktive Fußchirurgie bei diabetisch-neuropathischer Osteoarthropathie. Orthopaede. 2004;33:983-91.

24. Zgonis T, Stapleton JJ, Jeffries LC, Girard-Powell VA, Foster LJ. Surgical treatment of Charcot neuropathy. AORN J. 2008;87(5):971-86.

25. Grant W, Sullivan R, Sonenshine D, et al. Electron microscopic evaluation of the effects of diabetes mellitus on the achilles tendon. J Foot Ankle Surg. 1997;36(4):272-8.

26. Ayoub MA. Ankle fractures in diabetic neuropathic arthropathy: can tibiotalar arthrodesis salvage the limb? J Bone Joint Surg Br. 2008;90(7):906-14.

27. Baumgartner R, Botta P. Amputationen und Prothesenversorgung. Stuttgart, New York: Thieme Verlag; 2008.

28. Koller A, Fühner J, Wetz HH. Radiologische und klinische Aspekte der dia-betisch-neuropathischen Osteoarthropathie. Orthopade. 2004;33:972-82.

29. Koller A, Wetz HH. Die Operation nach Link-Witzel beim Diabetiker. Orthopade. 2003;32:231-5.

30. Koller A, Meissner SA, Podella M, Fiedler R. Orthotic management of Charcot feet after external fixation surgery. Clin Podiatr Med Surg. 2007;24(3):583-99.

Chapter 12
Rheumatoid Foot Reconstruction

Andreas Dietze

12.1 General Considerations

Rheumatoid arthritis (RA) is a common chronic immunologic and debilitating disease affecting about 0.5–1% of the population worldwide.[1] It is a systemic disorder involving mainly the peripheral synovial joints in a symmetrical fashion and leads to the progressive destruction of the involved joints.

The treatment of RA patients has dramatically changed during the last decade. Due to the development of biological treatment possibilities like tumor necrosis factor alpha (TNF-α) blockers or interleukin-based medication, both the severity and frequency of the typical destructions in the rheumatoid foot have been changed. Medical treatment has also changed the clinical situation for most of the patients in a direction of better physical health. In former years the typical RA patient was an elderly woman bounded to a wheelchair without any demand for outdoor activities. In contrast, many RA patients today are fully active in social and working life and have the same demand to physical activities as others. At the same time, advantages in total knee and hip arthroplasty have placed increased importance on the preservation or improvement of foot and ankle function of RA patients. This means that most of the traditional surgical techniques are modified due to increased demand of physical function from the patients.

The Clayton resection (Fig. 12.1), which implicates the resection of the whole metatarsal phalangeal (MTP) joint from a plantar approach is a procedure which is

A. Dietze, M.D., Ph.D.
Department of Orthopaedic Surgery,
Sykehuset i Vestfold – Tønsberg,
H. Wilhelmsers Allee, Tønsberg 3103, Norway
e-mail: andreas.dietze@siv.no

A. Saxena (ed.), *Special Procedures in Foot and Ankle Surgery*,
DOI 10.1007/978-1-4471-4103-7_12, © Springer-Verlag London 2013

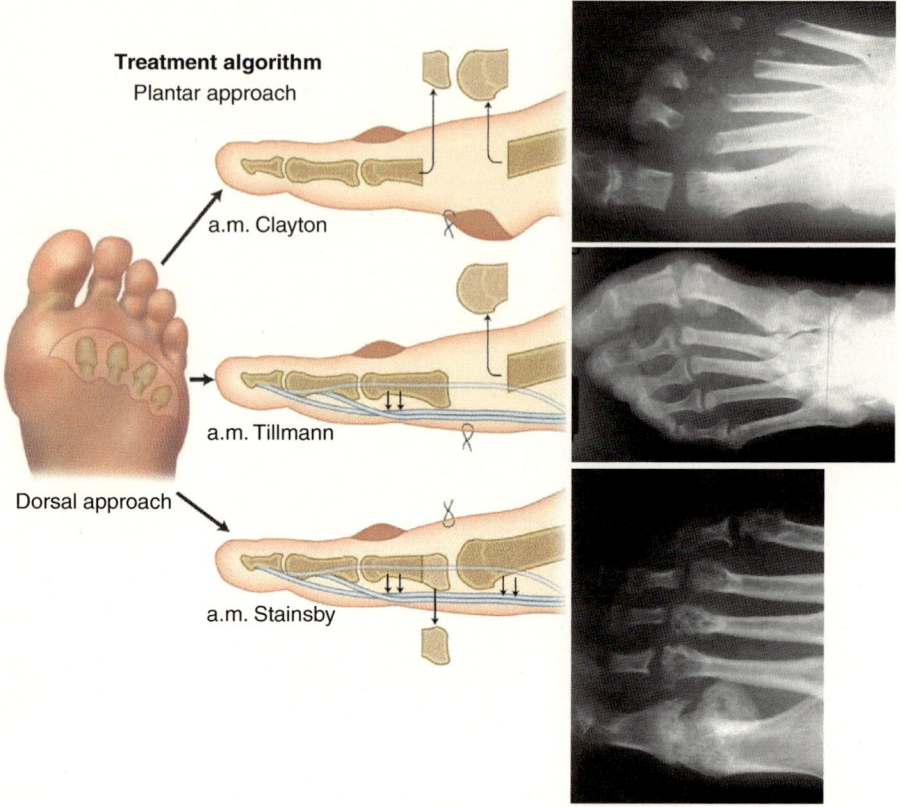

Fig. 12.1 Treatment algorithm for the rheumatoid forefoot. The Clayton resection is shown only for historical reasons and is not recommended by the author. The x-rays show the typical picture following the resection of the particular parts of the lesser MTPJ. Both Tillmann and Stainsby underline the importance of relocating the flexor apparatus to the plantar site of the metatarsus

described as a "functional forefoot amputation." It would not reestablish a reasonable gait for the patients in the long run. It was a considerable operation in the 1970s, but the functional result would be hard to accept for most of RA patients in 2009. Therefore, we do not recommend the Clayton procedure as a standard procedure any longer. Although the recently introduced immunomodulatory and biological treatment of RA patients has given remarkable results, about 30% of the patients suffer from severe oligo- or polyarthritis due to a lack of response to the medication or side effects which leads to discontinuation of the treatment. A special understanding of the pathogenesis and clinical presentation of this group of patients allows a dedicated treatment with the goals of preserving function, delaying disease progression, and correcting a deformity at the appropriate time.

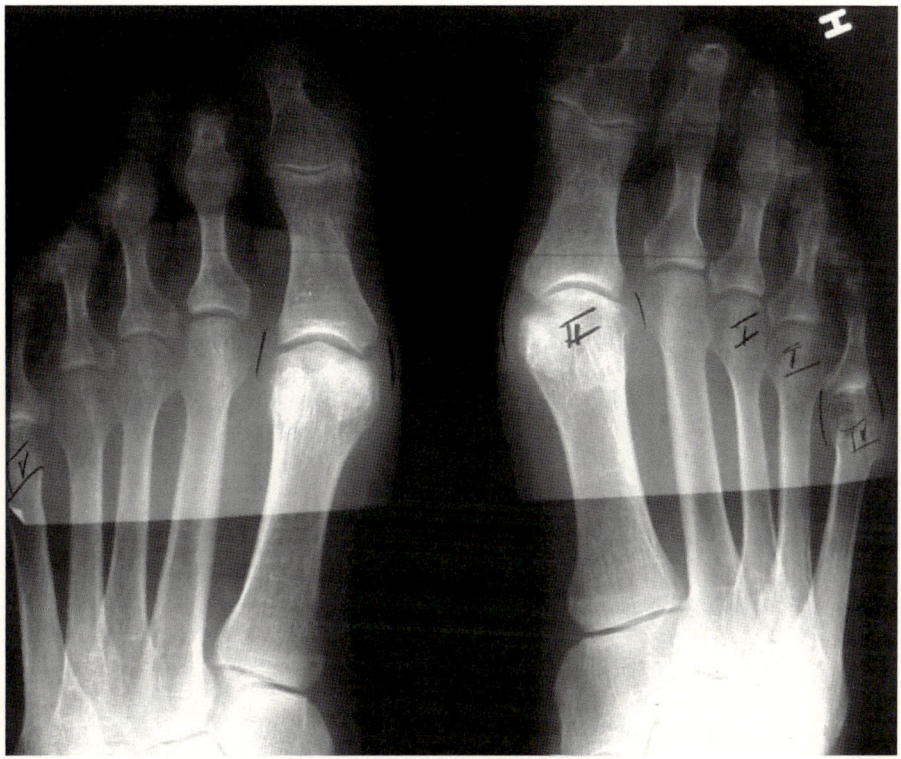

Fig. 12.2 Forefeet with Larsen-Dale-Eek (LDE) staging. The numbering is for the staging of the particular joint and the pericapsular fat streaks are marked

12.2   Radiographic Examination

The radiographic changes of the rheumatic foot are not pathognomonic and they appear rather late, mainly after 5–7 years after the debut.[2,3] Effusion and synovial swelling lead in early stages to a protrusion of the pericapsular fat streaks, later on to subchondral ersosions (due to pannus) and destruction of the joint surfaces. Ultrasound techniques visualize such changes at an early stage and in addition with the duplex technique the method is very sensitive. MRI with contrast is also of high sensitivity and specificity to detect synovitis in the joints. The progression of rheumatic destruction can be evaluated by various methods. Larsen described a widely used staging by standard X-rays.[4] This method is easy to adopt by the foot and ankle surgeon (Figs. 12.2 and 12.3). X-rays should be taken bilaterally and ideally for the purpose of staging with the corresponding views on one film. Forefeet should be investigated in a dorsoplantar and lateral view in weight-bearing position.

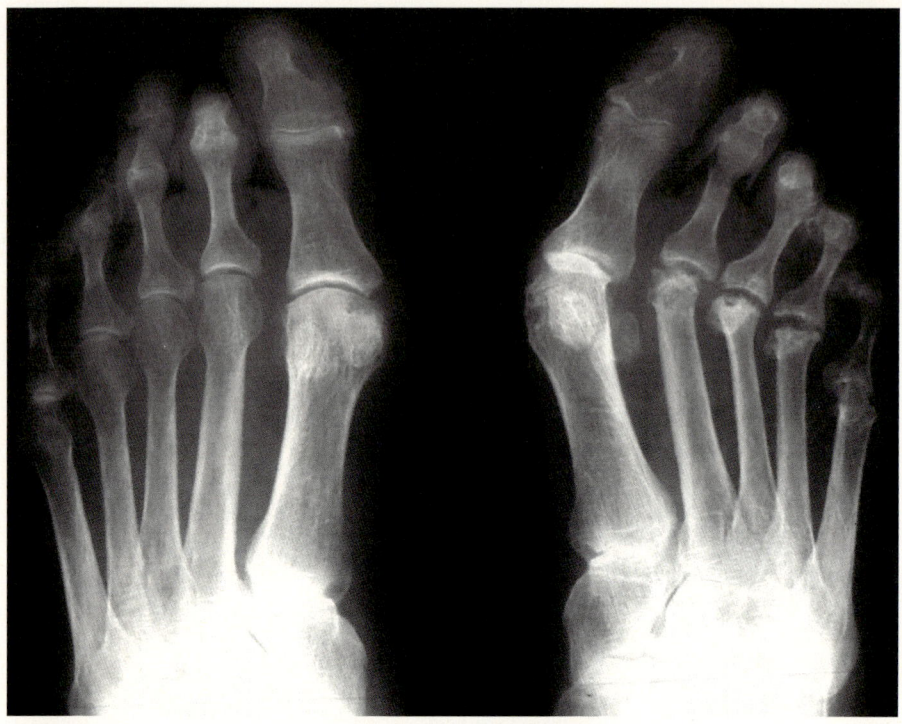

Fig. 12.3 Same patient as in Fig. 12.2. at 5 y FU. The left foot was treated with synovectomy of the MTP joints and the right foot by pan-metatarsal head resection. Notice the beginning bone apposition in the resection area which may lead to revision surgery

12.3   Rheumatoid Forefoot Reconstruction

12.3.1   Surgical Treatment

When nonoperative management is inefficient and the treatment with insoles, custom-molded shoe and occupational therapy is not solving the patient's problems, surgery might prevent the total breakdown of the foot. Surgical procedures in the rheumatic foot imply a certain amount of complications. Disturbance of wound healing due to long-term cortisone use, methotrexate, or biological treatments is possible but can be avoided by a meticulous surgical technique. In our hands only the biological treatment (e.g., anti TNF) have to be stopped 2 weeks before surgery and should not be started before complete wound healing is achieved. All surgery is performed under a tourniquet in a bloodless field. Intraoperatively, hemostasis should be obtained by the use of bi-polar diathermia. Skin incisions proposed for the access to the forefoot are numerous and are reported both for plantar and dorsal approaches. Tillmann and Kates[5,6] advocated for the transverse plantar approach

Fig. 12.4 (**a**) Plantar approach to the metatarso-phalangeal joint line and (**b**) its reconstruction

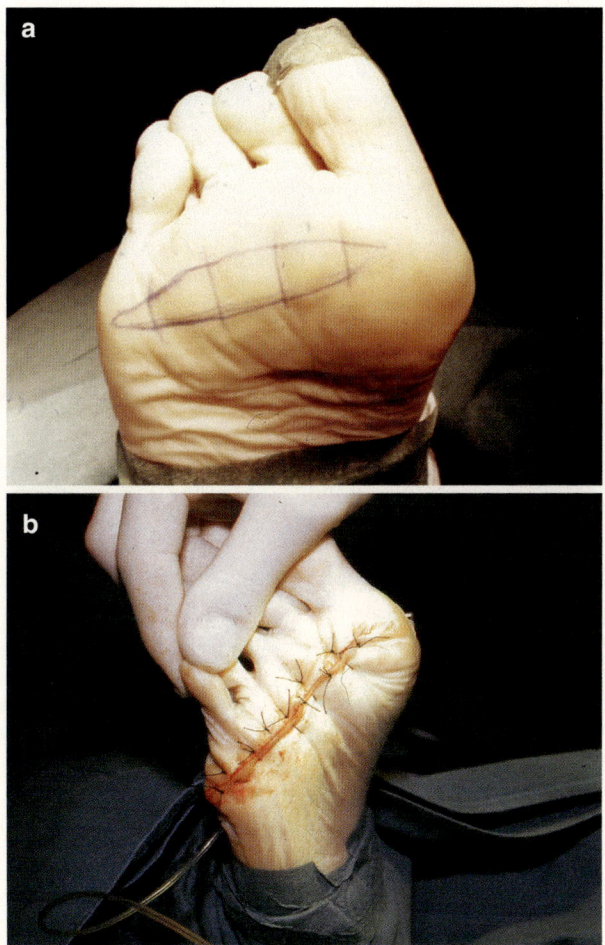

with oval resection of hypertrophic skin, callus, and bursae (Fig. 12.4) while Clayton, Marmor and Fowler[6-8] did the transverse dorsal incision. During the recent years, we have used a dorsal straight or z-shaped incision modified with respect to the procedures on the joints (Figs. 12.5 and 12.6).

12.3.2 Synovitis and Synovectomy

Isolated synovitis with wet proliferation of the synovial tissue might cause both pain and functional impairment in all MTP joints. In spite of good response to medical treatment, some joints remain swollen and painful. In these early stages without subluxation or destruction of cartilage, synovectomy is in our hands a reasonable possibility to obtain long-lasting pain relief and to preserve the cartilage and joint

Fig. 12.5 Intermetatarsal approach which gives access to the adjacent MTP joints

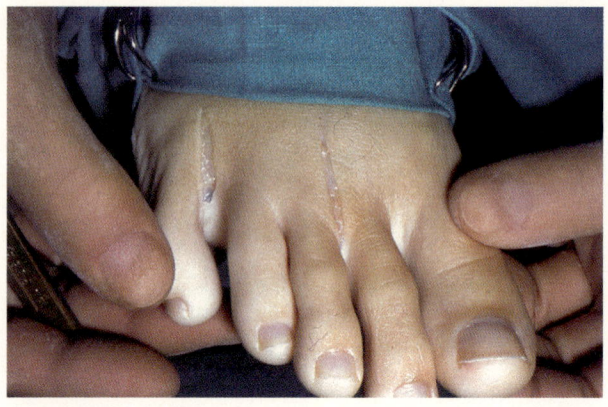

functions. Especially in adolescence with RA and patients with psoriatic arthropathy, this procedure might be indicated.

12.3.2.1 Surgical Technique

For the approach to the lesser toe, we use a straight dorsal skin incision in the middle of the 2nd and 3rd metatarsus and the 4th and 5th metatarsus to address the adjacent joint through one incision (Fig. 12.5). If necessary the tendon is cut and the joint capsule opened. If possible to use, the Mc Glamary elevator is a useful instrument to visualize the lateral and plantar parts of the joint and to mobilize the fat pad. All synovial tissues are removed carefully with special attention paid to the pannus tissue which normally is adherent at chondro-bone junction (Fig. 12.7). Careful examination of the plantar pad will identify bursae which should be removed without additional incisions. The capsule is left open and the wound is closed only by adapting skin sutures.

For the big toe, a standard dorso-medial skin incision is suitable and gives access to the whole joint, both medial and laterally (Fig. 12.6). The sesamoids should be inspected. Total resection of a subcutaneous medial bursa or noduli is not advisable due to the skin which is at risk. Both bursas and callosities disappear in a reasonable time after surgery.

Postoperatively, elevation is advised as for all kinds of forefoot surgery. If the wound healing and edema is reasonable, weight-bearing is allowed in a stiff shoe of any kind.

12.3.3 Rheumatoid Splayfoot

Due to the involvement of the joint capsules and ligaments into the inflammation, a progressive collapse of the longitudinal arch is flattening the foot over time. This leads to a lengthening of the foot sole and a serious disturbance of the tendon balance in the foot. Lateralization of the extensor hallucis longus and brevis, and flexor hallucis longus and brevis are forcing the 1st metatarsal bone into varus position,

Fig. 12.6 Stainsby procedure at 2yFU. (**a**) Plantar view of the foot sole at without any signs of callosities. (**b**) Dorsal view of the Z-shaped skin incision for the lateral toes and the dorso-medial incision for the great toe

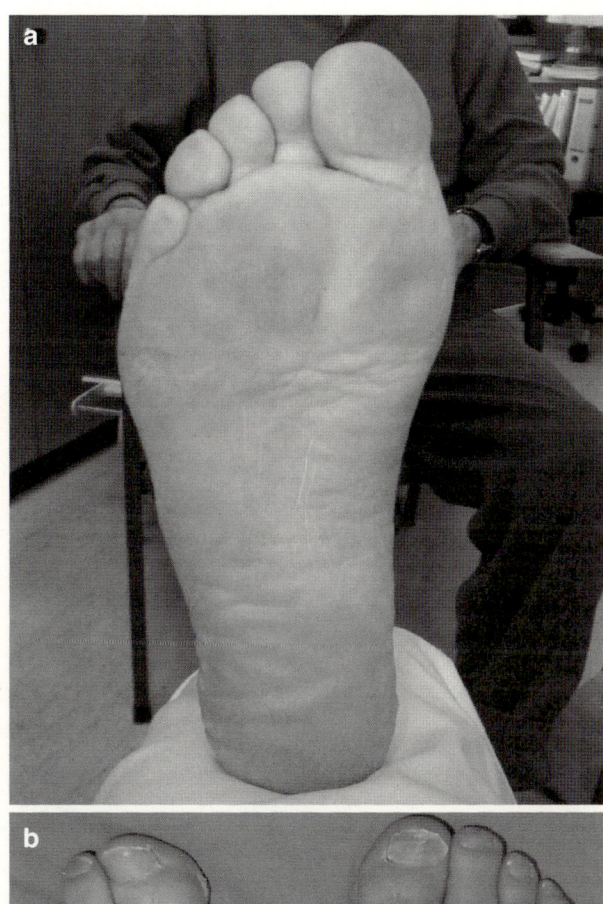

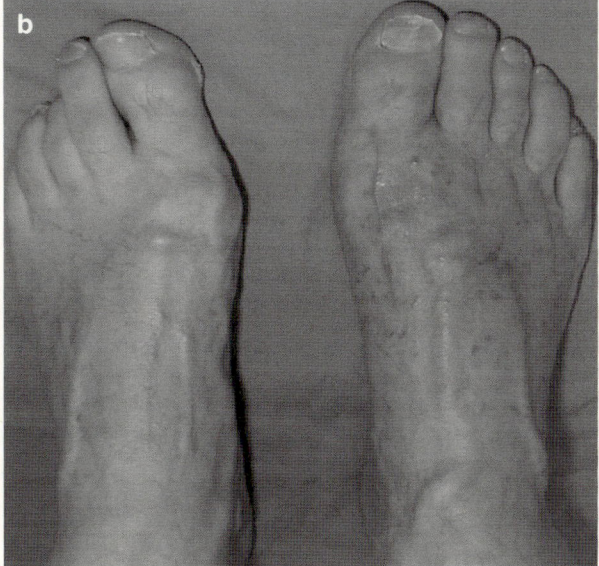

Fig. 12.7 Removal of synovial tissue from the chondro-bony junction during synovectomy of MTP joints

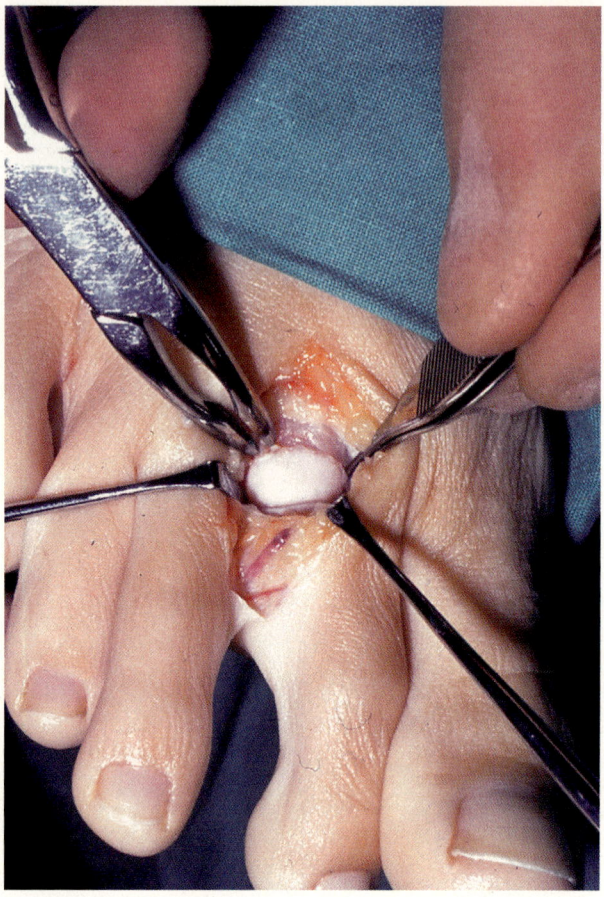

whereas the medialization of the extensor digitorum for the 5th toe together with its pronation leads to a valgus deformity of the 5th metatarsus. At the end, this might be the pathology which explains the development of the typical rheumatoid splay-foot deformity.[9] Hallux valgus is often the most obvious clinical sign together with fixed or flexible hammertoes and plantar callosities (Fig. 12.8). Studies by Stainsby and colleagues[10] have shown that the longitudinal arch and the splay of the forefoot during gait is also controlled by a longitudinal and transverse tie-bar system which correspond with the deep layer of the plantar fascia. This is also described by Hicks[11,12] who stated that the windlass mechanism controls the plantar fascia.

The treatment options for the rheumatoid splayfoot deformity are various and the goal should be the restoration of anatomy and thereby function of the foot.

12.3.3.1 Forefoot Reconstruction

Based on the theory that the skeleton of the foot is to a great extent controlled by a ligamentous tie-bar system and that defects in this system result in deformities like

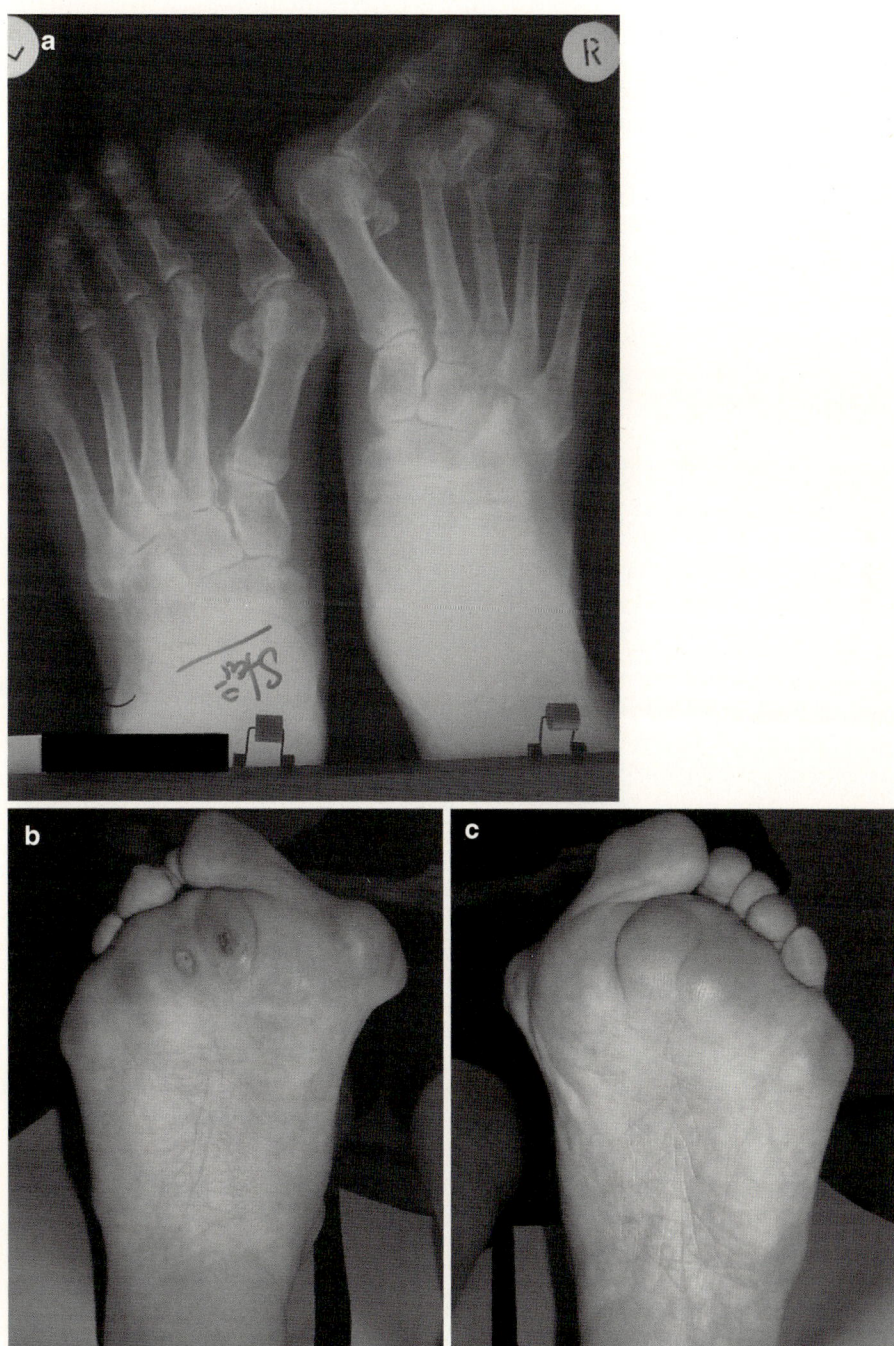

Fig. 12.8 A typical picture of a rheumatoid splay foot. Notice the excessive callosities on plantar pedis. The subluxation of the MTPJ which is obvious in the X-ray (**a**) of the right foot causes excessive callosities on the plantar skin (**b**, **c**)

claw toes, hammer toes, and hallux valgus to different extent, the repair of these tie-bar defects should correct the deformity.

Stainsby reported a resection arthroplasty in 1997[10] where he describes the removal of the parts of the proximal phalanx combined with the replacement of the plantar plate and the plantar fat pad (Fig. 12.9).

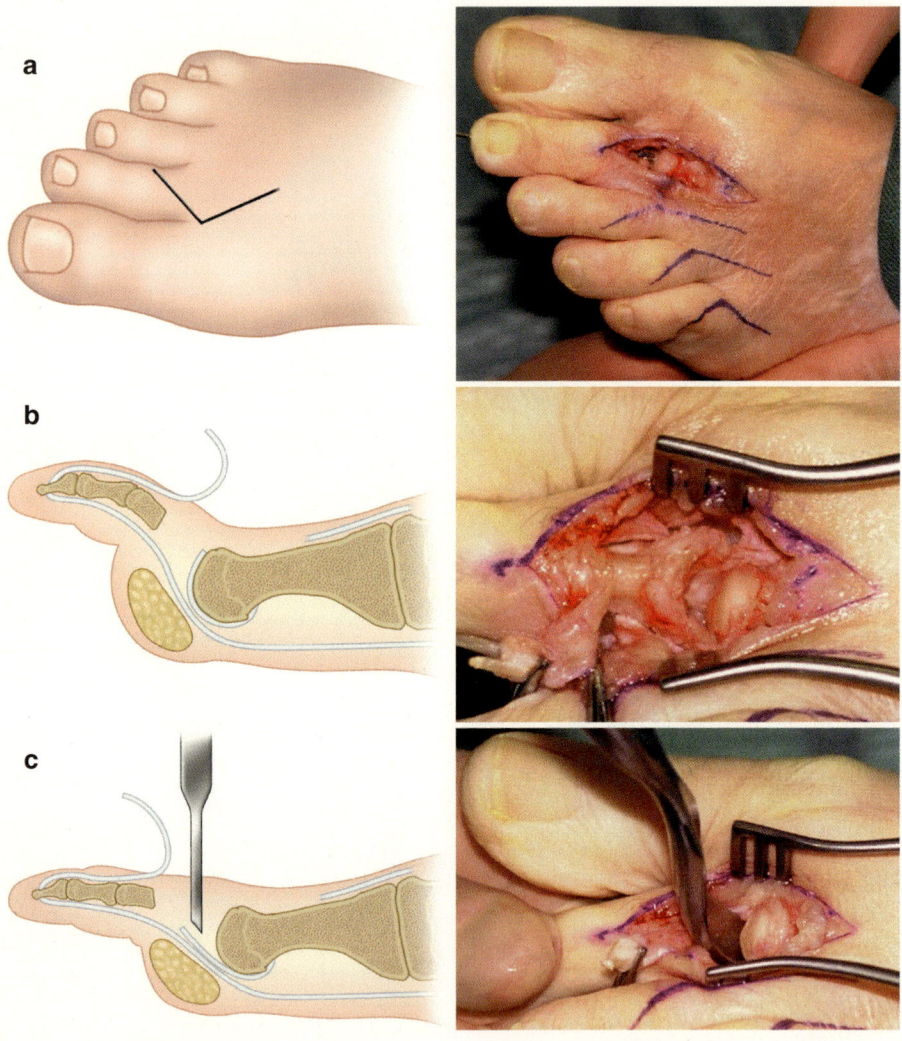

Fig. 12.9 Stainsby resection arthroplasty. (**a**) Z-shaped skin incision for each toe. (**b**) Extendor tendon is divided and reflected distally. Joint capsule is resected and a synovectomy performed. The proximal phalanx is resected. (**c**) Relocation of the plantar plate by using a capsule and McGlamry elevator. (**d**) Fixation of the reflected part of the extensor tendon to the plantar plate and temporary fixation by a K-wire. (**e**) Wound closure by simple suture technique. Notice the straightened incisions due to a relatively lengthening of the forefoot as a result of the surgery. Too high tension on the closure should be avoid by leaving small gaps between the sutures

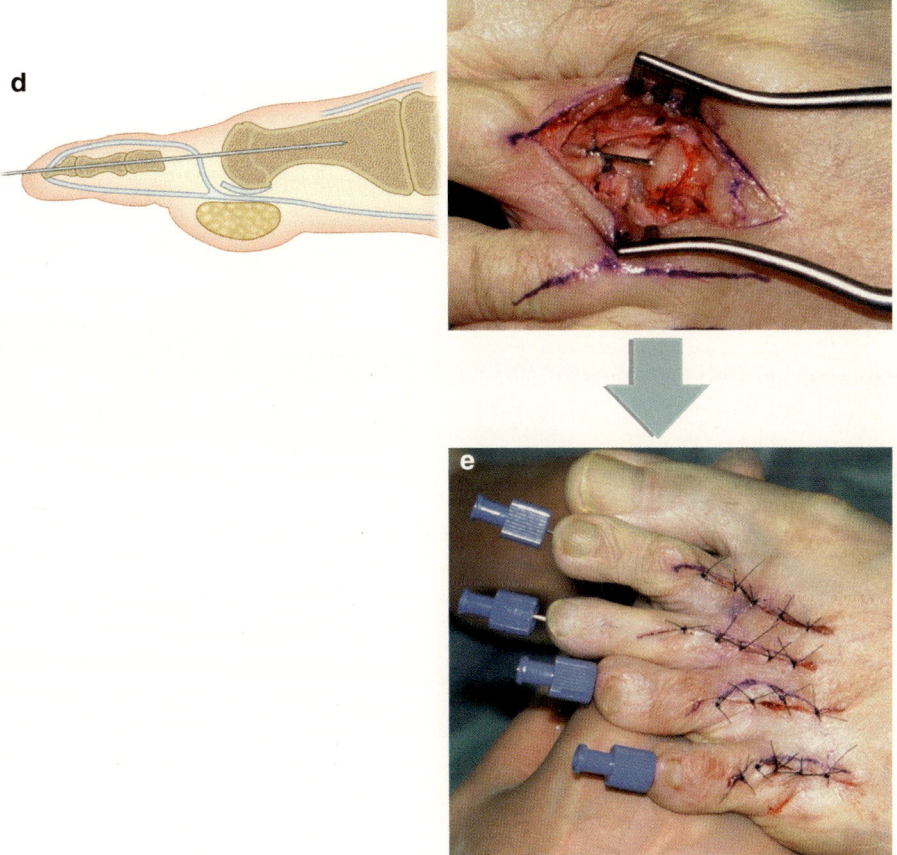

Fig. 12.9 (continued)

12.3.3.2   Hammertoe and Claw Toe Deformity

According to Hicks[11] and Stainsby,[10] the tie-bar system is fixed to the metatarsal heads and a distal and dorsal displacement of the plantar plate is one of the key pathologies (plunger effect) explaining the development of the dorsal dislocation of the proximal phalanges of the lesser toes. The plantar fat pad is following the phalanges. A subluxation or luxation of the proximal phalanges riding on the dorsal aspect of the metatarsal head is often seen in the RA foot (Fig. 12.10). Erosions of the cortical bone in that area are frequent findings. Instead of resection of the metatarsal head to gain space, Stainsby advocates for the resection of the proximal phalanges.[10] This resection arthroplasty keeps the tie-bar system intact and strengthens the foot function when the plantar plate is reduced into its original position. The procedure stands in contrast with other technique, where the metatarsal head is

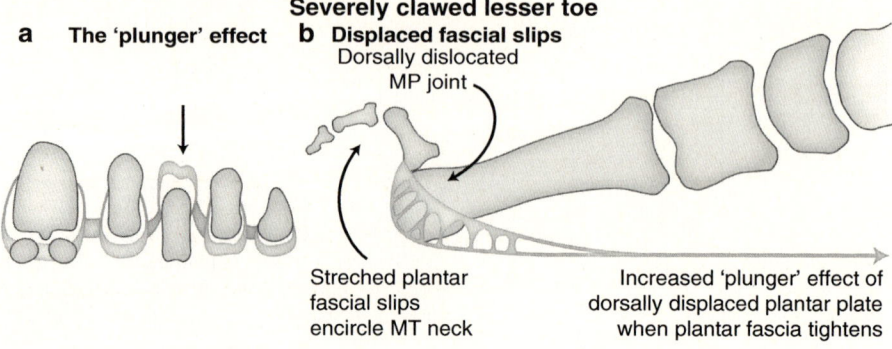

Fig. 12.10 (a) The displaced plantar plate causes severely clawed toes. (b) The plunger effect enhances the pressure on the metatarsal head during gait

resected (pan-metatarsal head resection or Tillmann procedure) to obtain the reduction of the metatarsal (MT) joints. In our hands, the Stainsby procedure gains several advantages compared with other techniques. First, the lever arm of the foot is preserved in its original length which results in a better balance of the patients in standing phase. Second, it allows the possibility to correct only affected toes while leaving unaffected toes untouched. This is an important advantage in the view of current medical treatment options and the fact that destructive arthritic changes are more and more controlled by these. Third, the procedure is easily done through a dorsal approach even if severe plantar bursitis should be addressed. Concerns about skin healing problems are understandable and should remind the surgeon to operate a-traumatic and handle the tissue with care. The reduction of fixated claw toes leads to a relative elongation of the toes and therefore this could give some stress on the skin sutures, especially when all 4 lesser toes have to be corrected. The procedure has been performed by the author since 1999 without severe complications. The correction of a hammertoe deformity in the proximal interphalangeal (PIP) joint is done simultaneously and before resecting the proximal phalanx. It can be done either by manual manipulation of the fixed joint or by all other resection arthroplasty techniques. We prefer to achieve an arthrodesis in the corrected PIP joint.

12.3.3.3 Surgical Technique Ad Modum Stainsby

The patient is in supine position, and the procedure is done in a bloodless field. The surgeon is sitting at the end of the table with both feet in front of him. A Z-shaped skin incision is made for each joint which should be addressed (Fig. 12.9a). The option of two dorsal longitudinal incisions in the second and fourth web spaces is available. Although I have used that approach mainly for synovectomy (Fig. 12.5), it is possible to address the MPJ for resection purpose through that incision. The advantage of larger skin bridges between the incisions is greatly diminished by over-retraction of the soft tissue which frequently leads to bruising and ecchymosis.

The extensor tendon is divided approximately 1 cm proximal to the joint space. A subluxation of the joint is reduced if possible. With a McGlamry elevator, the plantar adhesions are liberated and the fat pad comes into its original position. The tendon is reflected distally. A hammertoe deformity should be considered and eventually addressed at that stage. Otherwise that might get difficult after shortening the proximal phalanx significantly by the following steps (Fig. 12.9b, c).

In the next step, the proximal phalanx is resected in a way that a gap of 1–1.5 cm is created. The resection is done with a high frequency saw because other techniques might crush the soft bone with unwanted short- and long-term ossification effects. In serious cases, the whole phalanx might get resected to gain enough space for the reduction of the fixed hammer and claw toe deformity. At that stage, it is important to preserve the plantar plate and to replace it beneath the metatarsal head. If necessary, plantar bursae are removed through the same approach. The toe is now stabilized with a k-wire which is introduced intramedullarily, and the distal part of the extensor tendon is sutured to the plantar plate and the flexor apparatus. This is a very important part of the procedure because it is creating a soft tissue inter-positioning which secures the stability of the toe and avoids direct bone-to-bone contact (Fig. 12.9c). Finally, the wire is driven retrograde through the extensor tendon across the MPJ into the metatarsal head to secure the position of the toe and the healing of the resection arthroplasty for about 3–4 weeks. The wound is closed with deep skin sutures. Attention has to be paid on the skin traction when two or more lesser toes are corrected. Postoperatively, the patient can ambulate in a stiff shoe with respect to other simultaneous procedures which might need to off-load the foot (Fig. 12.9d, e).

12.3.3.4   Forefoot Reconstruction Ad Modum Tillmann

Based on the understanding that a flattening of the medial arch results in the lengthening of the foot sole, Tillmann in 1977[5] reported a pan-metatarsal resection arthroplasty which modified the original Hoffmann procedure (Fig. 12.1).

Through a curved plantar incision, the MTP joints 2–5 are addressed by opening the plantar plate via a longitudinal cut to prevent damage on the vessels and nerves (Fig. 12.4). The metatarsal heads are removed by a bone cut from proximal plantar to distal dorsal to avoid plantar spurs. Synovectomy of the remaining joint is mandatory. The procedure could also be carried out using 2 dorsal longitudinal skin incisions similar to what is described above. The resection should not be done on single toes since this will disturb the forefoot alignment and cause an overload of the neighboring toes.

12.3.4   Hallux Valgus Deformity

The RA big toe is treated in accordance to the treatment option for hallux valgus deformity in general and the same algorithms are valuable. If reasonable bone stock is left, an osteotomy could be preformed after a meticulous synovectomy. If the joint destruction is severe or the intermetatarsal angle large, arthrodesis of the MPJ is a good treatment option. This stabilizes the medial column and gives a long-lasting correction of the splay foot. As for all arthrodesis in that joint, no lateral release should be performed to preserve the tie-bar system and the self-reducing forces of the adductor system.

A Keller or Mayo resection is reserved for patients who are low-demand or housebound. If a Keller resection is performed (bunionectomy and resection of 1/3 of the proximal phalanx), it should be done with precaution not to produce a mallet toe. Dividing the short flexor tendons, without reconstructing them or addressing the long flexor tendon, produces a hyper-dorsiflexion in the MPJ and a plantarflexion contracture in the IP joint. Keller and later Mann[13,14] described the technique with the reinsertion of the FHB tendons to the proximal phalanx.

Silastic implants have been widely used for the correction of a rheumatoid hallux valgus. Implant failure by fracture of the silastic stem and recurrence of the deformity in combination with reports of inflammatory synovitis due to silastic particles limits the use of the implant to low demanding patients.

12.3.4.1 Metatarso-Cuneiform Joint Arthrodesis (Lapidus Procedure)

In cases with severe plano-valgus deformity combined with a high IM angle and reasonable MPJ left, a Lapidus procedure could restore both the longitudinal arch and joint function (technique see Lapidus). This procedure in combination with the Stainsby procedure is a favorable combination for forefoot reconstruction. It is recommended to use a locking plate system for the fixation of the TMT 1 arthrodesis to secure an uneventful bony healing. Synovectomy and the reduction of sesamoids under the MT head should be carried out.

12.4   Rheumatoid Midfoot and Hindfoot Reconstruction

The typical involvement of the hindfoot leads to progressive and destructive changes in all joints of the foot. Arthritis affects the capsule and ligamentous structures and causes instability of the subtalar joint which results in a severe valgus position of the calcaneus. Affection of the talo-navicular joint causes a breakdown of the longitudinal arch and causes the planus position of the foot. Arthritis of the hindfoot might be combined with tenosynovitis of the posterior tibial tendon and the peroneal tendons. Insufficient tendon strength and weakened muscle power support the development of the typical pes plano-valgus position of the RA foot.

12.4.1 Surgical Treatment

The tendons should be inspected carefully and an open tenosynovectomy should be performed if any clinical signs are detected. Triple arthrodesis is a reliable procedure to correct the plano-valgus deformity and to restore foot function over time. Two incisions are recommended to obtain sufficient overview on the medial aspect of the foot and to minimize the deterioration of the soft tissues by extensive use of retractors. Generally, the procedure is performed as described in Chap. 6. Isolated arthrodesis of the joints in the midfoot and hindfoot is possible and should be considered in younger patients. Synovectomy of the joints in the hindfoot is rarely indicated and is not considered as a standard treatment.

12.5 Ankle Joint

The ankle joint is frequently involved and effected by RA. With a longer duration of the disease, the involvement is up to 50% of the patient with RA. Severe synovitis with effusion of the joint is painful and reduces the function. Due to the anatomical construction of the joint, instability is not very often the major problem. If it occurs, a valgus deviation of the talus is the most frequent one.

12.5.1 Surgical Treatment

In an early stage, it could be recommended to perform an arthroscopic synovectomy, if necessary in combination with open tenosynovectomy. In the latter cases, the posterior part of the ankle joint can be reached through the open approach for the tendons. Otherwise the posterior standard ports for ankle arthroscopy are used.

Recent results for ankle arthroplasty are encouraging[15-17] although long-term follow-up studies reported severe complications and revision rates up to 35% of the cases.[18] In cases with relevant valgus deformity, a triple arthrodesis could be performed in preparation of ankle joint prosthesis. Some authors recommend a 6-month period between the triple and the implantation of the prosthesis, while others will prefer 6–8 weeks.[19,20]

Arthrodesis of the ankle joint still is the most frequently used treatment option.[21] It is a reliable method to restore alignment and function in the lower extremity with a reasonable treatment time and long-term results.[22-24] Several methods of ankle arthrodesis are described and we are recommending internal fixation with screws in primary surgery and retrograde nailing for revision surgery. In cases with subtalar involvement, a pantalar arthrodesis is indicated as primary surgery.

References

1. Alamanos Y, Drosos AA. Epidemiology of adult rheumatoid arthritis. Autoimmun Rev. 2005;4:130-6.
2. Tillmann K. Recent advances in the surgical treatment of rheumatoid arthritis. Clin Orthop Relat Res. 1990;258:62-72.
3. Vainio K. Surgery of rheumatoid arthritis. Surg Annu. 1974;6:309-35.
4. Larsen A, Dale K, Eek M. Radiographic evaluation of rheumatoid arthritis and related conditions by standard reference films. Acta Radiol Diagn (Stockh). 1977;18:481-91.
5. Tillmann K. The rheumatic foot and its treatment. Fortschr Med. 1977;95:1699-705.
6. Kates A, Kessel L, Kay A. Arthroplasty of the forefoot. J Bone Joint Surg Br. 1967;49:552-7.
7. Clayton ML. Surgery of the forefoot in rheumatoid arthritis. Clin Orthop Relat Res. 1960;16:136-40.
8. Fowler AW. A method of forefoot reconstruction. J Bone Joint Surg Br. 1959;41-B:507-13.
9. Tillmann K. Surgical treatment of the foot in rheumatoid arthritis. Reconstr Surg Traumatol. 1981;18:195-204.
10. Stainsby GD. Pathological anatomy and dynamic effect of the displaced plantar plate and the importance of the integrity of the plantar plate-deep transverse metatarsal ligament tie-bar. Ann R Coll Surg Engl. 1997;79:58-68.
11. Hicks JH. The mechanics of the foot. II. The plantar aponeurosis and the arch. J Anat. 1954;88:25-30.
12. Hicks JH. The foot as a support. Acta Anat (Basel). 1955;25:34-45.
13. Keller W. The surgical treatment of bunions and hallux valgus. N Y Med J. 1904;80:741-2.
14. Mann RA, Horton GA. Management of the foot and ankle in rheumatoid arthritis. Rheum Dis Clin North Am. 1996;22:457-76.
15. DiDomenico LA, Treadwell JR, Cain LZ. Total ankle arthroplasty in the rheumatoid patient. Clin Podiatr Med Surg. 2010;27:295-311.
16. Kofoed H. Scandinavian total ankle replacement (STAR). Clin Orthop Relat Res. 2004;424:73-9.
17. Valderrabano V, Hintermann B, Dick W. Scandinavian total ankle replacement: a 3.7-year average followup of 65 patients. Clin Orthop Relat Res. 2004;424:47-56.
18. SooHoo NF, Zingmond DS, Ko CY. Comparison of reoperation rates following ankle arthrodesis and total ankle arthroplasty. J Bone Joint Surg Am. 2007;89:2143-9.
19. Helm R, Stevens J. Long-term results of total ankle replacement. J Arthroplasty. 1986;1:271-7.
20. Su EP, Kahn B, Figgie MP. Total ankle replacement in patients with rheumatoid arthritis. Clin Orthop Relat Res. 2004;424:32-8.
21. Trieb K. Management of the foot in rheumatoid arthritis. J Bone Joint Surg Br. 2005;87:1171-7.
22. Sammarco VJ. Ankle arthrodesis in rheumatoid arthritis: techniques, results, and complications. Foot Ankle Clin. 2007;12:475-95, vii.
23. Nagashima M, Tachihara A, Matsuzaki T, Takenouchi K, Fujimori J, Yoshino S. Follow-up study of ankle arthrodesis in severe hind foot deformity in patients with rheumatoid arthritis using an intramedullary nail with fins. Mod Rheumatol. 2005;15:269-74.
24. Cracchiolo A III, Cimino WR, Lian G. Arthrodesis of the ankle in patients who have rheumatoid arthritis. J Bone Joint Surg Am. 1992;74:903-9.

Chapter 13
Total Ankle Arthroplasty: The US Experience

Andrew Haskell

13.1 Introduction

Ankle arthritis severely disables those it affects. Most commonly, it presents after ankle trauma, though instability, deformity, and inflammatory arthropathy are other common causes. Quality of life is affected to a degree similar to hip arthritis.[1] A variety of surgical treatment options are available including ankle debridement, distraction arthroplasty, interposition arthroplasty, arthrodesis, allograft replacement, and total joint arthroplasty, each with its own limitations and benefits.[2] Knowledge of these techniques allows the surgeon to tailor treatment of ankle arthritis based on patient needs, expected benefits, and risks.

Ankle fusion has a long history and demonstrated clinical success. However, there is growing understanding of the limitations of ankle fusion. Clinical results degrade with time, primarily because of progressive hindfoot arthritis.[3] Gait analysis reveals the functional abnormalities associated with fusion. The cost-effectiveness of ankle replacement over fusion has not been demonstrated, though incorporation of newer data showing improved functional outcome after replacement could alter this balance in favor of replacement.[4]

Total ankle replacement remains an evolving technology. The US experience has been shaped by both domestic innovation and imported knowledge. Improved understanding of patient selection, surgical technique, management of complications, and refinement of implant technology have led to improved outcome and more general acceptance of total ankle replacement as an alternative to ankle fusion.

A. Haskell, M.D.
Department of Orthopaedic Surgery, University of California,
San Francisco, CA, USA

Department of Orthopedics, Palo Alto Medical Foundation,
795 El Camino Real, Palo Alto, CA 94010, USA
e-mail: haskela@pamf.org

A. Saxena (ed.), *Special Procedures in Foot and Ankle Surgery*,
DOI 10.1007/978-1-4471-4103-7_13, © Springer-Verlag London 2013

13.2   Currently Available Designs in the United States

The US experience with total ankle replacement has been shaped by what implants have been made available by the Food and Drug Administration (FDA). In the 1970s, implants were approved based on a two-component, cemented design. Most of these went on to fail for a variety of reasons.[5] Overly constrained designs placed excessive stress at the bone–metal interface. Designs with limited inherent stability relied on the ankle's intrinsic stability and failed if this was not adequate. For many years, the US experience with ankle replacement was largely based on a single two-component design. However, over the last few years, a number of new designs have been made available here. The remainder of this section will review implant design features of ankle replacement systems widely available or largely based in the United States.

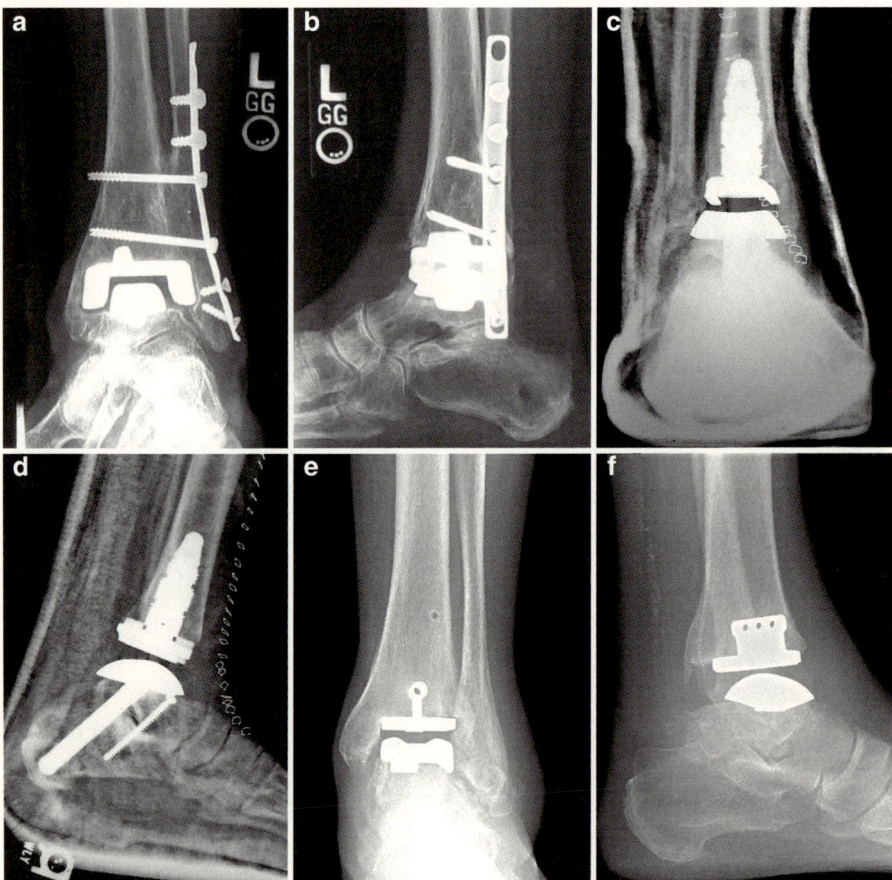

Fig. 13.1 Anteroposterior (*AP*) and lateral radiographs of the Agility (**a, b**), InBone (**c, d**), Salto Talaris (**e, f**), and STAR (**g, h**) total ankle replacements

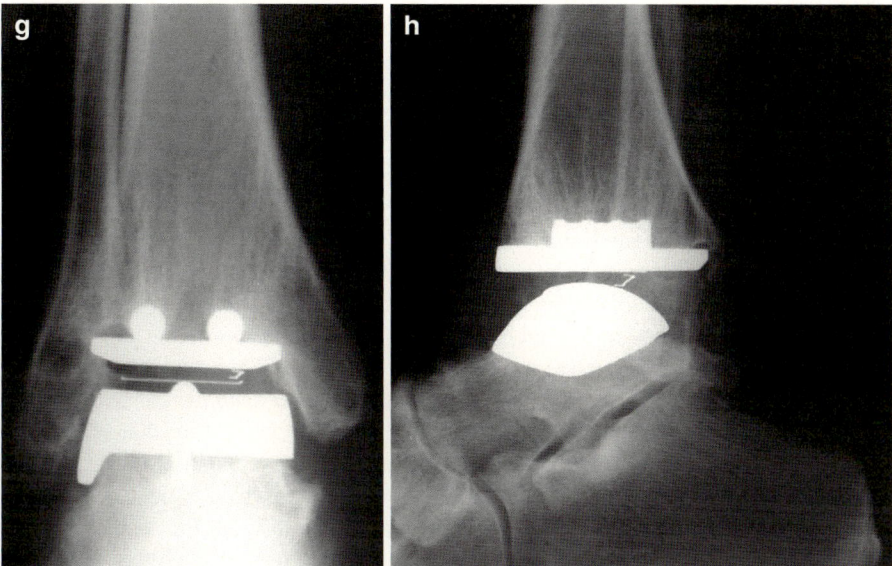

Fig. 13.1 (continued)

The Agility (Depuy) ankle replacement (Fig. 13.1a, b) is a two-component design released in 1993 that relies on successful fusion of the syndesmosis to provide a strong bony base to prevent the tibial subsidence seen in earlier designs.[6] The components are titanium and cobalt-chrome with an ultrahigh molecular weight polyethylene bearing fixed to the tibial component. The tibial and talar cuts are made using a single block cutting guide with the assistance of external fixation to hold the ankle position still. The tibial cuts resurface the inner aspects of the medial and lateral malleoli and have a fin for stability. The talar component is slightly incongruent to allow some motion in multiple planes. The talar component resurfaces the superior surface as well as medial and lateral facets using a flat cut. A wider talar component is available to address issues with talar subsidence. In the United States, it is approved for cemented use but typically is used as an uncemented implant. A newly introduced custom peg from the talar component may facilitate complex reconstruction or revision cases.

The InBone (Wright Medical) ankle replacement (Fig. 13.1c, d), released in 2005, is a two-component, titanium and cobalt-chrome design with a unique insertion mechanism that allows construction of a modular tibial stem and implantation with axial compression by drilling a hole through the plantar calcaneus and talus into the ankle joint. An external jig holds the foot and leg, and fluoroscopy is used to align the cuts prior to incision. The polyethylene is fixed to the tibial component and has a congruent saddle shape to articulate with the talus. The talus component resurfaces the superior talus and medial/lateral facets using a flat cut surface and has a short stem. Long stems to traverse the subtalar joint may be beneficial when talar avascular necrosis or subtalar pathology is present, but these are not yet approved by the FDA. In the United States, the implant is approved for cemented use but typically is used as an uncemented implant.

The Salto Talaris (Tornier) ankle replacement (Fig. 13.1e, f) was introduced in 2006 as a two-component, cobalt-chrome redesign of a three-component mobile-bearing device in use outside the United States.[7] The tibial component is fixed with a single anterior-to-posterior peg and does not resurface the inner edges of the malleoli. The ultra high molecular weight polyethylene bearing is fixed to the tibial surface and has a bipolar, slightly incongruent interface with the talar component, allowing micro-motion in multiple planes. The talar implant resurfaces the superior talus and the lateral facet using an apex superior angled cut and has a central hollow peg for stability. There are left and right talar components to match the different curvature of radius of the native medial and lateral talus. This was based on measurement of cadaveric ankle morphology and strives to recreate the cut cone axis of rotation of the ankle. The insertion technique has a unique feature that allows for rotation of the tibial component to match placement of the talus before fixation in an effort to recreate the transverse plane motion of a three-component design and provide fixation in a position that will minimize implant bone interface forces. In the United States, the implant is approved for cemented use but typically is used as an uncemented implant with titanium plasma spray bony ingrowth surfaces.

The Scandinavian Total Ankle Replacement (Fig. 13.1g, h), or STAR (Small Bone Innovations), is a three-component, mobile-bearing, cobalt-chrome implant with titanium plasma spray porous ingrowth surfaces. It was released in Europe in 1986 as a three-component redesign of a two-component system and was upgraded to an uncemented design in 1990. It recently has been approved after extensive study by the FDA in the United States. It has a tibial component fixed with two anterior-to-posterior pegs and a flat articular surface. An ultrahigh molecular weight polyethylene mobile-bearing component has a flat superior surface and a cylindrical, congruent inferior surface with a small groove. The talar component is cylindrical with a sagittal ridge to match the groove in the mobile bearing. The talar component resurfaces both the medial and lateral sides of the talus. The talus is cut with a superior flat surface, and anterior and posterior chamfer cuts, with a central fin for stability. The device is approved for uncemented use.

The Buechel-Pappas (Endotec) was initially designed in the early 1980s in the United States. While it has not been approved for wide release in the United States, it has been used abroad. It incorporates a bony ingrowth tibial component with a stem inserted through a slot in the anterior distal tibia. There is a mobile-bearing polyethylene component with a flat superior surface. A wedged biconcave inferior surface fits into a groove in the talar component. The talar component resurfaces the superior talus but not the medial or lateral talar facets.

The Mobility (DePuy) is similar to the Buechel-Pappas in design and is currently under study by the FDA in the Unites States and in use abroad. It consists of a bony ingrowth tibial component placed through a slot in the anterior distal tibia, a mobile-bearing polyethylene component with congruent, biconcave inferior surface, and a cylindrical talar cap.

13.3   Insertion Technique

Total ankle replacements are implanted with the goal of restoring ankle alignment to provide the ideal environment for implant longevity. The nuances of ligament balancing and limits of bony deformity that can be corrected with total ankle replacement are not as well-defined as in the knee or hip. Unfortunately, there is limited data to correlate implant position with longevity or clinical outcome.[8] The remainder of this section will examine issues related to sagittal, coronal, and axial plane alignment. The order of presentation is based on how many of the implant designs approach implantation. Others devices approach alignment en-block with a single cutting jig that links tibial and talar cuts. External alignment jigs or external fixation also may be used to hold alignment and distraction with certain implant designs.

A few definitions are needed. The *anatomic axis of the tibia* is a mid-diaphyseal line of the tibia extended to the ankle joint. The *mechanical axis of the tibia* is a line from the center of the knee to the center of the ankle plafond. The *mechanical axis of the lower extremity* is a line from the center of the femoral head to the center of the ankle plafond.

13.3.1   Tibial Coronal Alignment

Placement of the tibial component in the coronal plane typically relies on instrumentation that approximates a perpendicular to the anatomic axis of the tibia (Fig. 13.2). In most patients, this equals the mechanical axis of the lower extremity. The native tibial plafond is approximately perpendicular to this axis in the coronal plane. Placing the implant perpendicular to the mechanical axis of the lower extremity recreates the native plafond position and should disperse bone–implant contact pressures evenly.

Deformity above the ankle will change the mechanical axis of the lower extremity and may result in coronal plane malalignment if not recognized. Long leg films will demonstrate the true mechanical axis of the lower extremity and help identify and plan for these deformities. Minor, isolated tibial deformity, particularly when close to the joint, may be addressed with implant positioning (Fig. 13.3). Alternatively, larger deformities and those farther from the ankle joint may need to be corrected preoperatively to allow appropriate soft tissue balancing of the ankle with the implant perpendicular to the mechanical axis of the lower extremity.

One common situation is ipsilateral knee osteoarthritis and ankle arthritis. The ankle may be neutrally aligned in the coronal plane (perpendicular) relative to the tibial shaft, but may be malaligned relative to the mechanical axis of the lower extremity because of deformity at the knee. In these situations, it is advantageous to

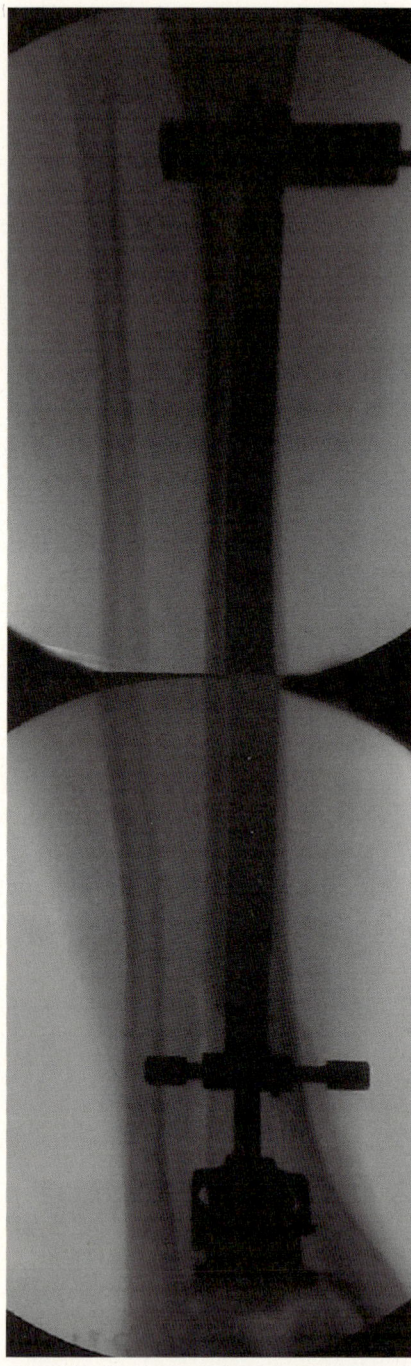

Fig. 13.2 AP fluoroscopic image of the Salto Talaris tibial alignment jig. Notice the rod sits directly over the mid-diaphysis of the tibia recreating the anatomic axis

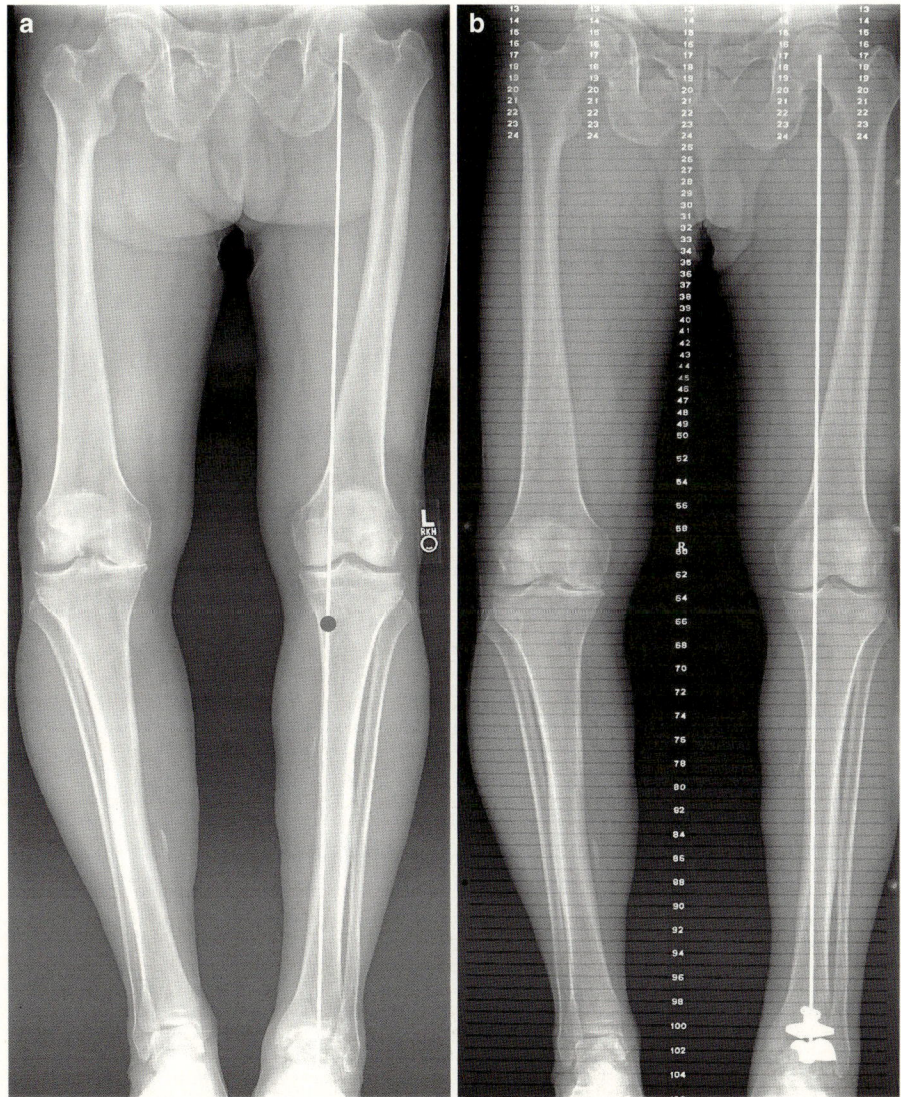

Fig. 13.3 Preoperative (**a**) and postoperative (**b**) long leg standing alignment films showing a mild varus alignment of the lower extremity (*white line*). The gray dot in the preoperative film shows where to set the proximal end of the tibial alignment rod to place the ankle component perpendicular to the mechanical axis of the lower extremity. For larger deformities above the ankle, knee replacement or corrective osteotomy may be needed

the ankle surgeon to have the knee deformity addressed first with knee arthroplasty or periarticular osteotomy. This realigns the anatomic axis of the tibia to the mechanical axis of the lower extremity and allows for a straightforward ankle replacement.

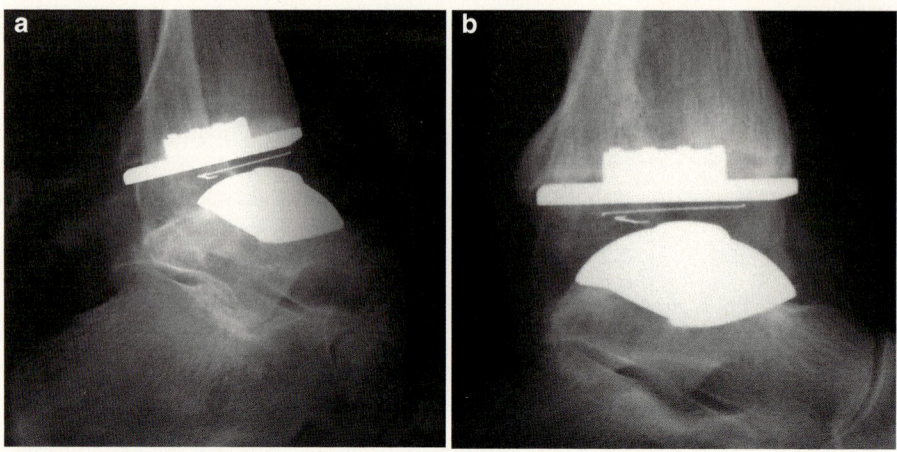

Fig. 13.4 Postoperative lateral radiographs showing options for talar sagittal slope. Slope may match the native posterior slope of approximately 10° (**a**), be set perpendicular to the tibial anatomic axis (**b**), or somewhere in between

13.3.2 Tibial Sagittal Alignment

The tibial component placement in the sagittal plane varies from perpendicular to the tibial anatomic axis to posteriorly sloped to match the slope of the native tibial plafond. Issues involving this decision include effect on sagittal plane motion and tibial component subsidence, but are not completely understood. The native tibial plafond is sloped posteriorly allowing dorsiflexion of the ankle without impingement of the talar neck on the anterior distal tibia. Spurs on the anterior distal tibia and/or talar neck can cause bony impingement, limiting ankle dorsiflexion and causing pain.

One strategy is to make the distal tibial cut parallel to a line drawn from the anterior-to-posterior tibial plafond on a lateral x-ray, or approximately 10° of posterior slope (Fig. 13.4a). This recreates the native anatomy and should prevent talar neck impingement. However, in order to make a flat cut, the cut is moved proximally so the roof of the plafond is included in the cut. The farther proximal the cut is made, the weaker the bone becomes, raising concern for subsidence. In addition, the limit to dorsiflexion after total ankle arthroplasty is not typically from talar neck impingement on the anterior distal tibia but rather from tight posterior structures and joint capsule stiffness. Leaving the posterior plafond more distal may accentuate this posterior tightness. The other extreme is to make the distal tibial cut parallel to the anatomic axis of the tibia, that is, parallel to the floor (Fig. 13.4b). This has the advantage of evenly distributing the bone-implant pressure during stance. Finally, the difference can be split and a flat cut with slight anterior slope can be used. Attention should be given to the manufacturers' recommendations as stemmed tibial components may not insert correctly if the surgeon deviates from the suggested sagittal alignment.

Tibial sagittal translation must also be appreciated. Since anterior tibial subsidence is more common, there may be benefit in placing the tibial component on the anterior tibial cortex to provide additional restraint to anterior tibial subsidence. However, placement of the tibial component at the center of the tibial plafond minimizes abnormal stresses on surrounding ligamentous structures.[9]

13.3.3 Tibial Rotational Alignment, Shear Stress, and Height

Rotational stresses are placed on the tibial component during ambulation for a number of reasons. Normal hindfoot kinematics at heel strike involves tibial internal rotation linked to calcaneal eversion. Later in gait, external rotation of the pelvis and leg is linked to hindfoot inversion. This rotational linkage occurs through the oblique axis of the subtalar joint but by necessity is transmitted through the ankle joint.

Abnormal rotational stresses may occur as well. Cylindrical implant designs do not take into account the differential curvature of radius of the medial and lateral talus and may put rotational stress on the implant during ankle motion. Malpositioning of the implant in relation to the rotational axis of the ankle or malpositioning of the tibial implant in relation to the talar implant may result in rotational stresses as well. The magnitude of these rotational stresses and their clinical significance is unknown. However, in contrast to vertical load, which compresses bone–implant interface, rotational forces and side-to-side shear forces do not contribute to implant stability and may lead to implant loosening, polyethylene wear, or strain on surrounding ligaments.

This rotational stress has been addressed in a number of ways. Three-component designs have a flat interface between the tibial component and the polyethylene insert that rotates freely in the axial plane. This allows the talar component to find its natural position as dictated by the surrounding collateral ligaments. Minor rotational malpositioning of the tibial component is unlikely to lead to excess stress on the bone–implant interface and may contribute to the success of three-component designs where older two-component designs failed. Even if one of the interfaces stops moving over time, the bone–implant interface has been protected from rotational stresses for the initial period of bony ingrowth.

Rotational alignment of the tibial component is more important for two-component designs since all rotational stress is imparted to the implants. Many of these prosthesis designs incorporate a partially congruent polyethylene-bearing surface that allows some rotational and translational motion between the tibial and talus.[10,11] Placing the components in a malrotated position however will accentuate the rotational stresses. Instrument design can also allow the implant position to self-select rotational position before final implantation. That is, the trial implants are taken through a range of motion, the tibial implant adjusts its rotation to the talar component, and final tibial preparation sets this self-selected position. How much this protects the tibial component from rotational stresses is unknown.

Tibial resection height is a function of the thickness of the implant plus polyethylene, with the goal of maintaining joint line position. The thicker the components, the more bone must be resected. Tibial bone strength is greatest closest to the subchondral bone and declines moving proximally into the metaphyseal bone. Minimizing tibial bone cut height places the tibial implant on stronger bone, but risks overstuffing the joint with resulting increased stress on the surrounding ligaments and potential loss of motion. Designs that minimize the thickness of the tibial component plus polyethylene thickness may cause excessive internal stress and premature failure of the polyethylene.

13.3.4 Talar Coronal Alignment

The talar component should be placed in the coronal plane so that the upper surface is parallel to the tibial component with the foot plantigrade. Care should be taken to avoid medial or lateral translation or coronal plane tilt as this will lead to edge-loading, asymmetric joint contact pressure, and early failure. A variety of implant-specific instrumentation strategies help facilitate this intraoperatively.

Careful consideration should be given to patients with a preoperative coronal plane deformity.[12] Ankles in which the talus is tilted over 10° relative to the tibial plafond in the coronal plane (incongruent joints) are more likely to have a progressive postoperative coronal plane tilt than an ankle with a congruent coronal plane deformity.[13] Some consider deformity greater than 15° to be a contraindication to ankle replacement.[14]

When evaluating an ankle with a congruent coronal plane deformity (also known as an extra-articular deformity), evaluation of the center of rotational deformity should be made with long leg films using standard techniques. If the deformity is small or close to the ankle joint, the deformity may be correctable with the tibial and talar cuts. If the deformity is farther from the ankle joint or large, it may need to be addressed with osteotomy or knee replacement. The subtalar and transverse tarsal joints should be evaluated to be sure a rigid compensatory deformity has not developed that would leave the foot non-plantigrade when the ankle deformity is corrected.

Incongruent coronal plane deformity at the ankle typically comes in the form of a tibial plafond perpendicularly aligned to the anatomic axis of the lower extremity and a talus tilted in varus or valgus relative to the plafond. The most common forms of this are a varus-aligned talus from chronic lateral ankle ligament instability and a valgus-aligned talus from stage-IV posterior tibial tendon dysfunction. Attention to the hindfoot alignment, compensatory forefoot alignment, and ligament integrity is paramount in these situations when considering total ankle replacement. Simply holding the foot in a neutral position when implanting the talar component will likely lead to early recurrence of deformity, edge-loading of the implant, and early failure. Correction of an incongruent coronal plane deformity when the source of deformity is distal to the plafond necessitates correction of the deformity below the ankle and possibly augmentation of the surrounding ligamentous structures.

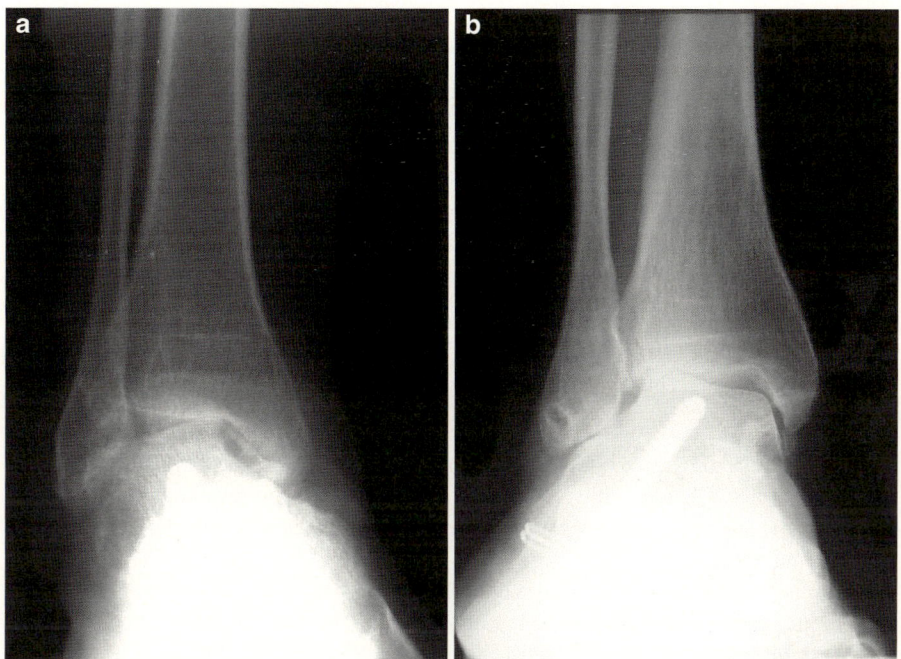

Fig. 13.5 Preoperative incongruent coronal plane deformity is defined as an angle of 10° or greater between the tibial plafond and the talar dome in the coronal plane. This may be a varus (**a**) or valgus (**b**) deformity, and is a risk factor for progressive postoperative coronal plane deformity

A varus incongruent deformity (Fig. 13.5a) often involves laxity of the lateral ankle ligament complex, erosion of the medial gutter, so the talus rides in a rut worn into the medial plafond, and contraction of the deltoid ligament. Correction should correct the bony erosion with well-aligned bone cuts, and must address the ligament imbalance.[14] Often a medial release will be required. Depending on the implant design, the deep deltoid may be released with the medial talar cut. Further deltoid release can be taken as a periosteal sleeve off the medial malleolus from the midline anterior incision. Alternatively a medial malleolar oblique osteotomy can be made and allowed to slide into a balanced position.[15] If there is any hindfoot varus, a calcaneal osteotomy that shifts the weight-bearing axis of the hindfoot laterally should be added, such as a Dwyer lateral closing wedge, lateral slide, or hybrid type osteotomy. With severe or fixed varus, a hindfoot fusion may be needed. If there is a rigid cavus deformity, this may need to be corrected as well. Standard lateral ligament repair or reconstruction procedures can be useful tools as well to help maintain coronal alignment, but care should be given to insure the medial ligaments are balanced and the hindfoot is in mild valgus. Fibular shortening may be employed as well.

A valgus incongruent deformity (Fig. 13.5b) often involves laxity of the deltoid ligament and erosion of the lateral gutter so that the talus rides in a rut worn into the lateral corner of the plafond and the fibula. Correction should address the bony erosion with well-aligned bone cuts.[16] Deltoid imbrication or reconstruction may be required. Finally, hindfoot deformity must be corrected with osteotomy or fusion. Medial slide calcaneal osteotomy may restore the calcaneus under the mechanical axis of the lower extremity, tending closer to neutral than 5° of valgus in this circumstance. With severe hindfoot valgus or inflexible compensatory forefoot varus, a triple arthrodesis may be indicated.

An incongruent coronal plane deformity of the ankle less frequently results from a chronic deformity above the level of the ankle with a compensatory deformity below the plafond to keep the foot plantigrade. Attention to the mechanical axis of the lower extremity must be given to be sure that, while the plafond is perpendicular to the anatomic axis of the tibia, it is also perpendicular to the mechanical axis of the lower extremity. When the subtalar joint complex cannot adequately compensate for a lower extremity malalignment, the ankle joint may become incongruently aligned, with the talus perpendicular to the mechanical axis of the lower extremity and the tibial plafond tilted relative to the mechanical axis of the lower extremity. Correction of the deformity above the ankle, placement of components perpendicular to the corrected mechanical axis of the lower extremity, ligament balancing around the implant as described above, and possible osteotomy or fusion of the hindfoot to achieve slight valgus may be needed. Alternatively, placement of the tibial component perpendicular to the mechanical axis of the lower extremity but tilted relative to the anatomic axis of the tibia can be used for mild deformity, but runs the risk of placing components in softer bone farther from the subchondral surface, intraoperative fracture, and progression of deformity. Also, the ankle implants will be malpositioned if the deformity above the ankle is corrected in the future.

In rare circumstances, the talus is tilted in the coronal plane, and the subtalar joint is tilted in the opposite direction to compensate and keep the foot plantigrade. This makes correction difficult because any techniques that correct the talar tilt accentuate the subtalar deformity. For a successful ankle arthroplasty, the subtalar joint may need to be fused in a corrected position of slight valgus. Alternatively, the implant can be placed in-situ, with an oblique cut of the talus and acceptance of the talus position and hindfoot compensation. This runs the risk of talar placement in softer bone farther from the subchondral surface and progression of deformity.

13.3.5   Talar Sagittal Alignment

Placement of the talus in the sagittal plane involves both tilt and anterior–posterior translation. The talar component is tilted such that it articulates with the polyethylene with the ankle ranged from full dorsiflexion to full plantarflexion. Generally this is based off the anatomic axis of the tibia in the sagittal plane, but may be based off the tibial implant position, depending on specific implant manufacturers' designs.

Anterior-to-posterior positioning of the talar component should recreate the central position of the talus under the anatomic axis of the tibia in the sagittal plane. Depending on the implant manufacturer's design, this position is set during chamfer cuts of the talus. Malpositioning of the talus component in the sagittal plane may put abnormal stresses on the bone–implant interface as well as on the polyethylene given the ankle's fixed axis of rotation and ligamentous constraints.[9,17]

Anterior translation of the talus is common in arthritic ankles and can be difficult to correct during total ankle replacement. During implantation, a bump should be under the distal calf to allow the calcaneus to float off the operating table, preventing iatrogenic anterior translation. Mild translation can be corrected by placing the talar component slightly posterior on the talus, centering it under the tibial component, but runs the risk of losing some talar bone stock and placing the center of rotation slightly off the ankle's axis of rotation. Three-component designs and designs that allow slight anterior-to-posterior translation in the talus-polyethylene may accommodate this discrepancy between rotational axes, but this has not been proven. Alternatively, release of bone and soft tissue in the medial and lateral gutters may allow the talus to fall back to a neutral position, but may lead to pain and bony exostoses, especially in implant designs that do not resurface the medial and/or lateral talar facets. Finally, if the talus slides anteriorly with dorsiflexion, tightness of the Achilles may need to be addressed, possibly with lengthening procedures, downsizing the polyethylene component, or moving the tibial cut proximally. However, making the polyethylene component too thin may lead to abnormal intra-polyethylene stresses and failure, and moving the tibial cut proximally increases the risk of malleolar fracture and alters the joint line.

13.3.6 Talar Rotational Alignment

The talar component should line up with the long axis of the talus allowing the rotational axis of the component to match as closely as possible the rotational axis of the native ankle. While some implant designs allow the talus rotation to be set when making the talar cuts, others fix the talus rotation to the tibial implant rotation. Three-component designs allow rotation at the tibia polyethylene interface minimizing transfer of rotational stress from slight rotational mismatch. Some two-component designs allow a small amount of rotation to occur by way of an incongruent polyethylene talus interface. The Salto Talaris allow the tibial rotation to be set to match the talar rotation after cuts are made but before implants are placed. With more congruent designs, matching the tibia and talar component rotations theoretically becomes increasingly important.

13.3.7 Sizing

Sizing of the tibial component is typically based on placing the largest appropriate implant maximizes bone–implant contact and pressure distribution. It helps avoid undersizing in the anteroposterior direction. Oversizing, however, may lead to leaving too thin a bone bridge at the malleoli and fracture.

Sizing of the talus is typically based on the medial to lateral size of the talus. Placing the largest appropriate implant maximizes bone–implant contact and pressure distribution and helps avoid undersizing in the anteroposterior direction. Oversizing, however, may lead to overstuffing the medial and lateral gutters depending on implant design. Component design may also place constraints on what talar sized match with a certain tibial component size and polyethylene insert.

Polyethylene insert thickness is chosen to allow adequate ligament tension without over-tensioning the soft tissues resulting in stiffness.[18] Little is known in the ankle about minimum acceptable polyethylene thickness as it relates to polyethylene wear, though many of the polyethylene inserts for ankles are thinner than those considered acceptable for total knee replacement. Polyethylene fracture is another concern, though this has not been directly linked to polyethylene thickness. Three-component designs have the added risk of polyethylene mobile bearing dislocation if the soft tissue envelope tension is inadequate.

13.3.8   Syndesmosis Fusion

The Agility total ankle replacement is unique in that it relies on syndesmosis fusion to provide a stable base for tibial component placement. Failure of syndesmosis fusion leads to early failure.[8,19] A number of techniques have been advocated to improve the rate of fusion. Techniques include a single screw, two screws, and two screws and a plate. An oblique osteotomy of the fibula above the fusion site may minimize micro-motion from the fusion site. Bone grafting from the bone removed during ankle replacement may assist with fusion. Autologous concentrated growth factors may substitute for bone graft to assist syndesmosis fusion.[20,21]

13.3.9   Computer Navigation

Computer-assisted navigation to assist with intraoperative alignment has been promoted for total knee replacement and may minimize variability in implant position, though the clinical benefit has yet to be shown worth the additional intraoperative time needed. Translation of this technology to the total ankle replacement has been attempted in computer simulations and cadaver models.[22,23]

13.4   Results

When considering the results of total ankle replacement, a number of factors must be taken into consideration.[24] Patient satisfaction, pain relief, functional improvement, longevity of results, and ability to salvage or revise failures, all will impact the decision to replace an ankle. In the case of knee or hip replacement, there is no debating the efficacy of total joint replacement. Total ankle replacement, however, must be compared to the results of ankle fusion to determine its overall success, and both techniques should be considered for individual patients on a case-by-case basis.

13.4.1 Brief History

When interpreting the results of currently available total ankle implants, it is important to look to the history of ankle replacement for perspective. A variety of implant designs were abandoned with disappointing intermediate-term results.[25-27] During this period, cementation was abandoned for uncemented designs.[28,29] Some felt the procedure was best reserved for lower demand, elderly, and rheumatoid patients.[30] Perhaps most telling is the Mayo Clinic experience that found reasonable short-term results only to abandon the procedure when intermediate-term results were reviewed.[31,32] Because of this experience, short- or intermediate-term results may not necessarily reflect long-term outcome and should be viewed skeptically.

During the 1990s, early results from modern implant designs were encouraging.[8,33-36] Longer-term follow-up of these designs became available encouraging a wider acceptance.[37-39] Joint registry data has also become available.[40-42] These prospective, longitudinal, or comparative clinical studies have provided an accurate picture of the current state of ankle arthroplasty and allow an educated decision as to the best treatment for individual patients.

13.4.2 Survival of the Implants

Overall implant survival is an important measure of the success of total ankle replacements and useful information for patients and providers deciding among treatment options. Intermediate-term results are available for a variety of implant designs. The Agility implant has 80% 5-year survival, 89% in patients over 54 years old.[43] The Buechel-Pappas has 84% 8-year survival in ankles replaced for rheumatoid arthritis.[44] The Scandinavian total ankle replacement has 93% 5-year survival, 80% 10-year survival,[37] and 72–75% 14-year survival.[45] A randomized, prospective comparison of 200 total ankles at 6 years found a strong trend toward better survival in the STAR group than the Buechel-Pappas group (94% vs. 79%, $p = 0.09$).[46]

13.4.3 Clinical Results

Total ankle replacement reliably improves pain and function. Clinical scales are consistently improved in a variety of studies. AOFAS (American Organization of

Foot and Ankle Surgeons) scores improved from 34 to 84 in 38 patients 45 months after Agility total ankle replacement.[47] A modified Foot Function Index improved from 59 to 35 after STAR implantation in 29 ankles at 28 months postoperatively.[48] The Kofoed score improved from 39 points to 70 points after ankle replacement in 51 ankles at 52 months postoperatively.[49,50] In 147 patients 2 years after ankle replacement, range of motion improved from 21° to 35°.[51]

A prospective comparison between 606 ankle replacements and 66 fusion patients at 24 months showed that ankles treated with the STAR ankle replacement had better function and equivalent pain relief as ankles treated with fusion. Ankle replacement was associated with a higher rate of complications and secondary procedures, though a learning curve effect was noted.[52]

Activity scores improve after ankle replacement, and subjectively patients' sports ability improves.[53] Before surgery, 36% of 152 arthritic ankles were active in sports, increasing to 56% after ankle replacement.[51] Participation most commonly included hiking, biking, gym workouts, and swimming. Patients who reported participation in sports had better functional scores than those who do not participate.[51]

13.4.4 Gait Analysis, Kinematics, and Kinetics

Gait analysis is one method of measuring functional results of total ankle replacement and may reveal functional differences from ankle fusion. Parameters such as stride length and speed are easily obtained estimates of global function. More detailed analysis of hindfoot kinematics, ground reaction forces, and force distribution on the foot may provide data for finite element modeling and reveal the benefits and limitations of replacement and fusion compared to normal ankles.[54]

Patients after both total ankle replacement and fusion have shorter stride lengths and reduced speed of ambulation compared to control. Ankle replacement restored gait symmetry to a greater degree than fusion, but restored stride length and speed to a lesser extent.[55] Measurements of gait improve between 3 months and 1 year after surgery.[56]

Ankle kinematics after total ankle replacement more closely match normal controls than after ankle fusion.[55] Radiographic sagittal plane range of motion is improved by an average of 5°.[57] However, all ankle and foot segments display diminished range of motion after ankle replacement compared to the contralateral side.[58] Knee kinematics are similar to controls after ankle replacement.[59]

Rotation in the sagittal plane is the primary motion seen with walking and stepping; however, there are smaller rotational and translational movements that may affect polyethylene loading and bone–metal interface stresses.[10,11] These non-sagittal plane motions cause a hysteresis effect, such that the component position is dependent on the direction of movement for any given sagittal plane rotation.[60] Proper placement of the tibial and talar components and proper sizing of the polyethylene thickness minimize atypical stresses on the surrounding soft tissue.[9,17] Implant design affects joint kinematics.[61-63] Implant size also affects kinematics, with smaller implant size leading to larger forces experienced by the implant and polyethylene.[64]

The altered energy expenditure at the whole body level and at the ankle caused by the stiff, antalgic gait of ankle arthritis is improved after total ankle replacement. Ground reaction forces after total ankle replacement more closely match normal controls than after ankle fusion.[55] In vitro studies of kinetics show increased translational forces and torque;[65] however, in vivo measures show internal forces at the ankle after replacement are similar to controls.[66] Total ankle replacement has a beneficial effect on vertical center of mass displacement, restoring more normal gait pattern and reducing overall energy expenditure.[67]

13.4.5 Proprioception, Muscle Recovery, and Bone Density

Change occur to the nerve, muscle, and bone around the ankle after total ankle replacement. Understanding these processes may influence timing and intensity of rehabilitation and weight-bearing. Bone mineral density around a total ankle implant increases over time, and the increase is correlated with clinical results, though this is unlikely to be causative.[68,69] Proprioception is not altered after total ankle replacement when compared to the opposite side.[70] Muscle function improves significantly after total ankle replacement as measured by peak dorsiflexion and plantarflexion force as well as by electromyographic (EMG) intensity.[71,72] However, at 1 year after surgery, this still does not normalize with the opposite side.

13.4.6 Specific Clinical Situations

13.4.6.1 Rheumatoid Arthritis

Inflammatory arthropathy such as rheumatoid arthritis can lead to painful end-stage ankle arthritis. A number of studies describe good results with total ankle replacement in patients with rheumatoid arthritis.[73,74] A large retrospective study of 93 ankles replaced for rheumatoid arthritis found improvement in pain and motion, and an 8-year implant survival of 84%.[44] Given the poor bone quality in these patients, care should be given to avoid fractures and undersizing should be avoided to prevent subsidence. Early loosening has been described in early case series.[75] However, no difference in clinical outcome or long-term survivorship was found when comparing results of a large series of ankles replaced for rheumatoid arthritis or osteoarthritis.[45]

13.4.6.2 Hemophilia

Hemophilia-related arthropathy can also lead to end-stage ankle arthritis. If conservative measures and controlling intra-articular bleeds fail to relieve symptoms, ankle replacement can be considered.[76,77] A number of case reports describe good results with short-term follow-up and small numbers of patients.[78,79]

13.4.6.3 Coronal Plane Deformity

Patients with a preoperative coronal plane deformity have a greater risk of complications including edge-loading, need for revision, or failure.[46] Incongruent deformities, when the talus is tilted but the tibia is neutrally aligned, have the worse prognosis.[13] Care should be given to patients with varus or valgus deformity greater than 10–15°, and consideration of adjuvant or alternative treatments should be given.[44]

13.4.6.4 Takedown of Arthrodesis

There has been recent interest in converting ankle fusion to total ankle replacement. Patients with identifiable sources of pain, such as subtalar joint arthritis, do better with conversion, and patients with prior malleolar resection do worse.[80] Short-term results in small series have been encouraging, though likely not as good as with a primary total ankle replacement.[81]

13.5 Complications

Adverse events after total ankle replacement are varied, ranging from minor inconveniences to implant or limb-threatening events.[43,82,83] Close follow-up, prompt recognition of deviations from an expected postoperative course, and appropriate treatment can minimize the effect of many complications and return patients toward a desirable outcome. Learning from others' complications helps prevent the occurrence or propagation of adverse events.[84-87] Comparison of complications after total ankle replacement and ankle fusion based on hospital readmission data over a 10-year period in California reveals major reoperation rates at 5 years post-surgery of 23% and 11%, and subtalar fusion rates of 0.7% and 2.8%, respectively.[88] This data does not reflect advances in implant design now available in the United States, and lack of randomization may lead to selection bias.

13.5.1 Learning Curve

Each new operation we as surgeons perform is an incremental advance on the body of knowledge and surgical skills we have acquired. Some procedures, however, are more complicated or more distinct from the types of things we see and do on a day-to-day basis. New operations may not have been included as part of our training. When deciding to include a new operation into your practice, we must weigh the potential risks and benefits of the procedure and be cognizant of the fact that the risks may be higher when first starting to do the operation. This experience-dependent effect on risk is termed the learning curve. It measures the time over which experience is gained and risk decreases to a more stable, sustainable rate. Learning curve may be affected by complexity of the procedure, overall surgeon experience, and surgeon education with the new procedure.

The importance of the learning curve of newer generation total ankle replacements has been confirmed in a number of ways. The outcome measured is typically short-term complication rate, given its ease of measurement and shorter study period than, say, survivorship or long-term outcome. The effect of surgeon experience on early complication rate using the Agility was studied by stratifying based on type of experience[89] and by single surgeon experience.[90] The STAR learning curve was measured by comparing short-term complication rate for the first ten implants and a later set of implants for ten experienced foot and ankle surgeons. Despite an initial training period, a significant effect of individual experience with the STAR implant was noted on total number of complications and wound complications.[91] This effect was noted as well for the Hintegra implant, with complications decreased from the first to second group of 25 inserted.[92]

13.5.2   Soft Tissue Healing and Infection

Wound healing complications can ruin an otherwise successful ankle replacement. The risk of deep infection persists until the skin is healed. Wound problems typically present early, but can develop over the first 6 weeks. Prevention is the best treatment, and begins with patient selection. Patients with peripheral vascular disease, diabetes, poor skin from prior trauma or incisions, venous stasis, and history of smoking are all at increased risk. Thorough patient counseling and consideration of alternative treatments is required.

The ankle soft tissue is unforgiving, and intraoperative factors may play a role as well in wound healing complications. Incorporate prior incisions when possible. Sharp dissection and full-thickness flaps preserve blood supply to the skin. Self-retaining retractors should be avoided in favor of handheld retraction. Place retractors deep to avoid pressure necrosis at the wound edges. Try to keep a soft tissue layer over the tibialis anterior and extensor hallucis longus tendons, and frequently irrigate to avoid desiccation. Drain use may help the wound seal. Multilayer closure will help limit the depth of exposure if there is superficial wound dehiscence.

Fig. 13.6 Postoperative AP radiograph showing internal fixation of an intraoperative medial malleolus fracture

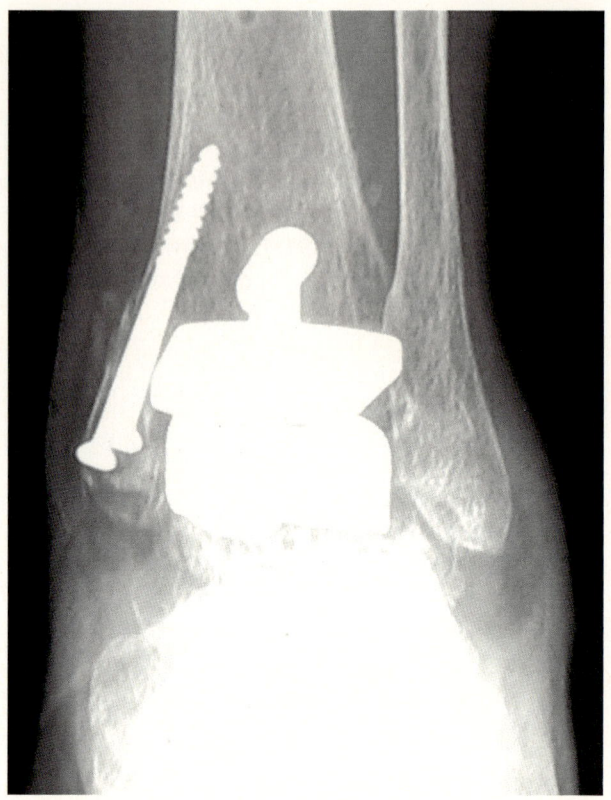

If wound problems occur, aggressive treatment may be indicated to avoid conversion to a deep infection. Wounds well away from the joint without exposed bone or tendon may be amenable to dressing changes and watchful waiting. Larger wound dehiscence or wounds over the joint may need debridement, dressing changes, or vacuum-assisted wound closure. Alternatively, fasciocutaneous or free flap coverage may be required.[93]

Superficial wound infection should be treated with debridement and antibiotics. Deep infection should be ruled out with lab tests including white blood cell count, erythrocyte sedimentation rate, and c-reactive protein level. Joint aspiration should be performed if the superficial infection is near the joint, there is joint swelling or erythema, or lab markers suggest deep infection.

Treatment of deep infection is largely based on data from the hip and knee replacement literature, though small series in the ankle have been reported.[94] Consideration of incision, debridement, and liner exchange, and intravenous antibiotics can be made for early or hematogenous infection with non-virulent organisms. Late presentation of infection or aggressive organisms are more likely to need explantation, thorough debridement, and placement of antibiotic-impregnated cement spacer.

13.5.3   Fracture

Fractures of the medial or lateral malleolus may occur intraoperatively or postoperatively (Fig. 13.6). Intraoperative fractures may be a result of poor bone quality, inadequate bone bridge, component over-sizing, poor cutting technique, retractor placement, bony impingement, and component design.[95] When recognized, these should be fixed with standard techniques and the patient immobilized until fracture healing is achieved. Results typically are not compromised.

Postoperative fractures may represent unrecognized intraoperative fractures or stress fractures that develop after surgery. Scrutiny of postoperative radiographs should include ruling out these fractures. Non-displaced postoperative fractures with stable components may be treated with casting. Displaced fractures should undergo open reduction and internal fixation to avoid implant loosening.

Insufficiency fractures of the distal tibial metaphysis or talar body will often result in component subsidence and may require revision if component position has changed substantially. Finally, stress fractures around the tibial metaphysis or diaphysis may result from placement of the pins to hold tibial cutting jigs.

13.5.4   Subsidence

Component subsidence may result from poor bone quality, osteolysis-related bone loss, or poor component positioning (Fig. 13.7). Early subsidence of a millimeter or less may represent settling of the components into a stable position and does not portend failure of the implants. Measurement of implant position is dependent on true implant position as well as on limb position during the radiograph, and variation may make measurement of small changes in position difficult on standard radiographs.[96,97] Radiostereometric analysis (RSA) allows for measurement of submillimeter changes in implant position in vivo. RSA study of 15 rheumatoid patients who underwent Buechel-Pappas total ankle replacement demonstrated that tibial components tend to subside into dorsiflexion, valgus, and proximally by less than a millimeter during the first 3 months, and stabilize by 6 months.[98] Similar results were found for the STAR implant.[99] Since most designs do not allow axial impaction of the components, this settling may represent the implant finding a stable position as weight-bearing is allowed. Patients with severe osteoporosis or avascular necrosis may not have strong enough bone to support the placement of a total ankle replacement.

A number of factors affect risk of subsidence. Initial implant positioning may contribute to subsidence. Subsidence tends to occur in the anterior distal tibia, dorsiflexing the tibial component, or in the anterior talus or posterior talus. Anterior translation of the talar component or excessive dorsiflexion of the tibial component should be avoided to prevent overloading the bone in these at risk areas. Another

Fig. 13.7 Postoperative lateral radiograph showing subsidence and subsequent loosening of the tibial component into the anterior distal tibia

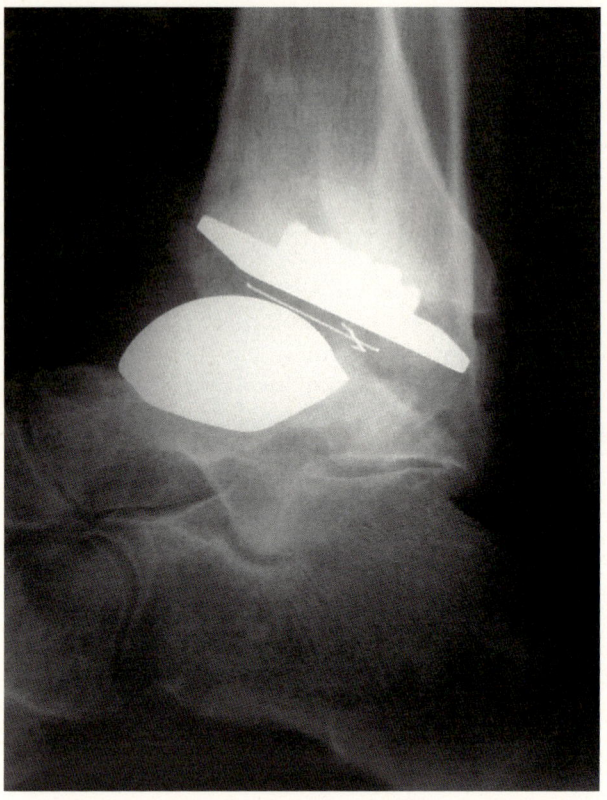

situation may arise specifically with the Agility device with subsidence related to failure of syndesmosis fusion (Fig. 13.8). Late subsidence related to osteolysis is more concerning. Sudden change in implant position in the setting of osteolysis signifies loss of supporting bone. Revision or explantation and fusion may be necessary.

13.5.5 Polyethylene Fracture

The mechanics of the polyethylene insert are at risk for complications as well. Mobile bearing total ankle replacement designs may have complications related to the mobility of the polyethylene insert. These include polyethylene extrusion and fracture.[100] Malalignment and progressive edge-loading may place the polyethylene insert at risk for failure.[101] The risk of implant fracture related to polyethylene thickness has not been defined. Fixed polyethylene designs may dislodge if the locking mechanism is not engaged appropriately. Care must be taken to insure secure locking during component assembly.

Fig. 13.8 Postoperative AP radiograph showing subsidence of the tibial component into the distal tibia as a result of failure of syndesmosis fusion. This is a complication unique to the Agility implant

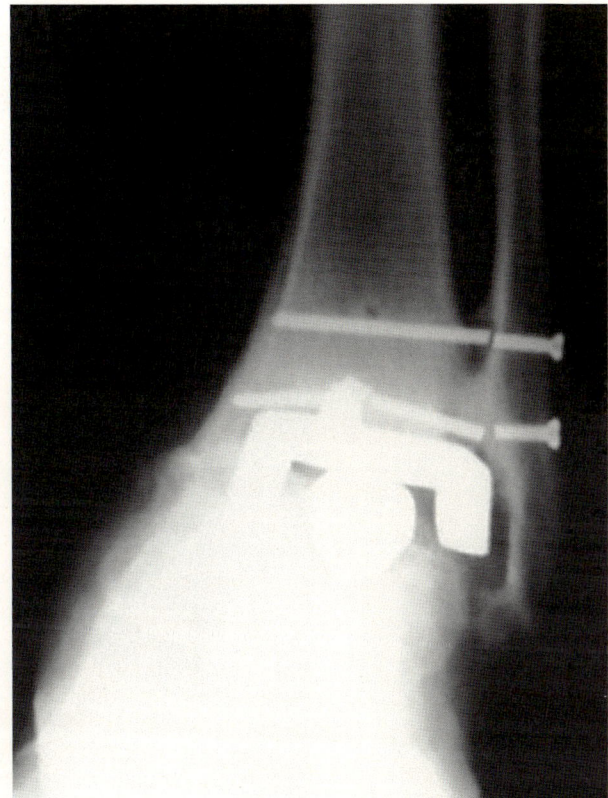

13.5.6   Osteolysis

The by-products of frictional wear between the metal and polyethylene components of joint replacements lead to peri-prosthetic bone resorption. This process is named osteolysis and can result in subclinical or significant bone loss, loss of implant stability, subsidence, and implant failure. Osteolysis has been studied extensively related to hip and knee replacements, but factors such as polyethylene composition and thickness, implant stability, two- vs. three-component designs, alternative bearing surfaces, and component design related to total ankle replacement have not been thoroughly defined.

Polyethylene wear can be measured in vivo and in vitro. Measurement of particle size and morphology after successful ankle replacement shows similarities to total knee wear production.[102] Ankle motion simulators try to match the forces and motion experienced by an ankle implant, but accelerate the cycle rate to condense years of natural wear to days or weeks.[103] In this way, comparison of wear characteristics between implant designs can be measured.[104]

Early recognition, monitoring, and treatment of progressive peri-prosthetic osteolysis may prevent loss of implant stability. Screening radiographs at regular

Fig. 13.9 Postoperative
lateral radiograph showing
development of osteophytes
along the anterior ankle joint

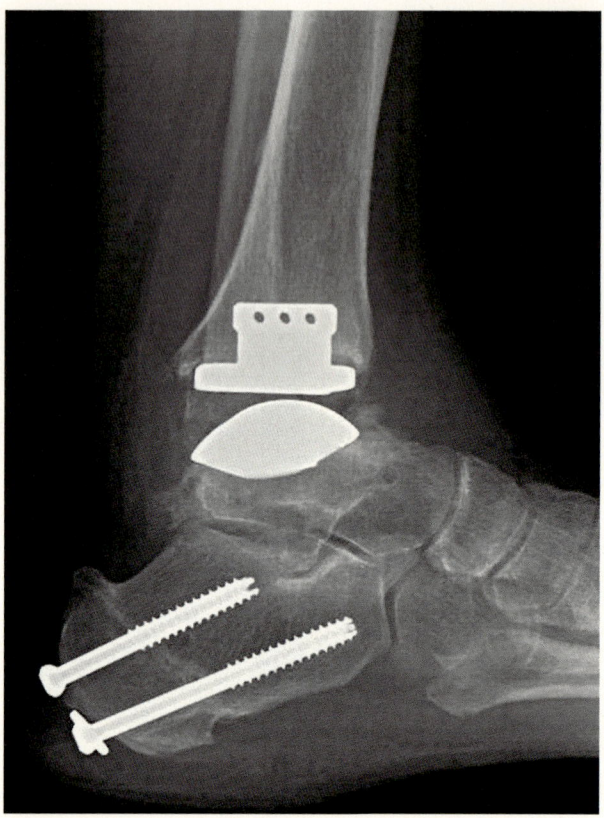

intervals in patients with stable, painless, well functioning ankle replacements may demonstrate early osteolytic lesions. Computed tomography (CT) scans may help define the lesion size and find lesions not seen on standard radiography.[105] Debridement of the cyst and grafting, correction of malalignment if present, and polyethylene exchange may arrest progressive osteolysis and should be performed before implant failure.

13.5.7 Impingement

Development of postoperative periarticular ossification can lead to pain and stiffness after total ankle replacement (Fig. 13.9). Gutter pain can develop in 25% of patients.[106] Debridement of soft tissue and bony impingement may be required. Little is known about relative risk of impingement based on implant design and degree of medial and lateral talar facet coverage. Attention should be given intraoperatively to be sure arthritic osteophytes are not impinging after implant placement. Adjuvant treatment with nonsteroidal anti-inflammatory medication or radiation has not been studied in the setting of total ankle replacement.

13.5.8 Progressive Edge-Loading

Progressive edge-loading refers to instability of the post-ankle replacement talus leading to joint line incongruity between the tibial component and the talar component (Fig. 13.10). Preoperative joint line incongruity is a risk factor for progressive postoperative joint line incongruity and edge-loading, even if the initial deformity is corrected during implant placement.[13] Patients with a preoperative incongruent coronal plane deformity should be assessed for bony deformity and loss of soft tissue stability above and below the ankle and steps taken to address these issues as described in section 43.3.

Progressive postoperative edge-loading should be recognized and treated aggressively to minimize the risk of implant failure. Scrutiny of bony alignment above and below the implant with long leg standing radiographs and heel alignment radiographs may reveal deviation from a neutral mechanical axis. Physical examination of ankle stability may reveal loss of medial or lateral soft tissue restraint. Patients with generalized ligament laxity may not have adequate ligament strength. The factors leading to progressive edge-loading should be corrected to rebalance the mechanical axis around the implant. Soft tissue correction alone is likely to be insufficient to maintain this correction, and consideration of osteotomy or fusion should be given. Soft tissue reconstruction of the medial or lateral ligament complexes may be needed as well. Polyethylene exchange is typically performed as well, since the edge-loading leads to abnormal polyethylene wear and may lead to osteolysis.

13.5.9 Nerve and Vessel Damage

The incision for total ankle replacement places a number of nerves at risk. The superficial peroneal nerve leaves the lateral compartment of the leg near the superior aspect of the incision and travels distal-medially, sending sensory branches to the dorsomedial distal leg and foot in the subcutaneous tissue. These branches are frequently encountered and protected during dissection, but sharp or compressive injury can occur leading to loss of sensation of portions of the dorsal leg or foot, but typically no loss of function. Patients should be counseled about this possibility preoperatively.

The deep peroneal nerve travels with the tibialis anterior/dorsalis pedis vascular bundle deeper in the dissection between the tibialis anterior and extensor hallucis longus tendons. It should be identified and protected during dissection to avoid numbness in the first interspace and possible vascular compromise to the foot. If the artery is injured, vascular consultation should be considered. The tourniquet will need to be deflated prior to closure to be sure there is adequate circulation to the foot, and the artery may be tied off or repaired as needed.

The posteromedial neurovascular bundle is generally safe during an anterior approach, but can be injured during bone cuts or compressed by implant placement, leading to tarsal tunnel syndrome or vascular compromise.[107] Some implant

Fig. 13.10 Postoperative AP radiograph showing progressive deformity of the talus resulting in edge-loading of the polyethylene

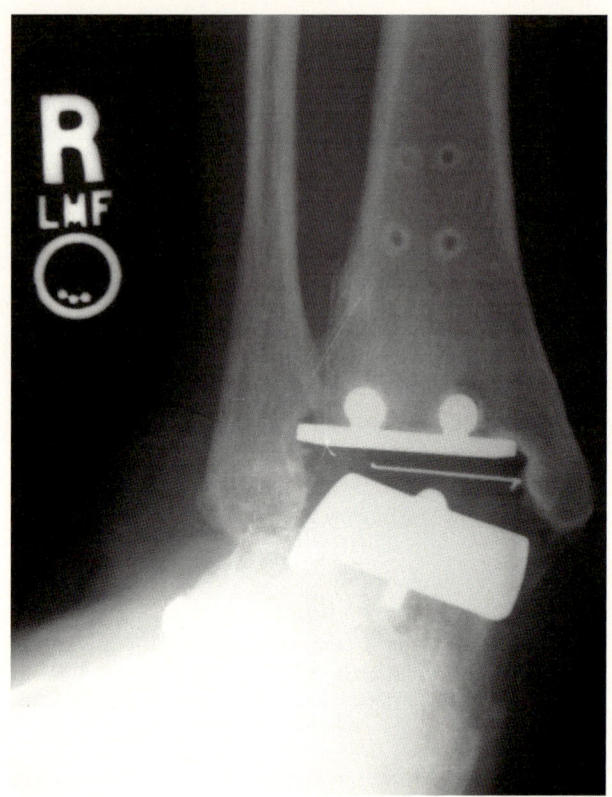

instrumentation protects these structures with pins at the edge of the saw cuts or malleable retractors placed in the medial gutter. However, care must still be given to proper saw technique to avoid posteromedial injury. Recognition of the full saw excursion and avoiding pulling the blade to the edge of the cutting block will help prevent this injury. Avoiding malrotation or placement of the tibial component beyond the posteromedial tibial cortex will prevent implant impingement on the posteromedial neurovascular bundle.

13.6   Treatment of Total Ankle Replacement Failure

Total ankle replacements may fail for any of the reasons listed in the complications section above. When the decision is made that further efforts to salvage the existing implant are not warranted, the goal of restoring a painless, plantigrade, stable,functional limb remains. While in cases of life-threatening sepsis, non-reconstructable soft tissue defects, or patient preference, this may mean below-knee amputation,[43] ankle fusion or revision replacement are more commonly chosen.

Conversion to ankle fusion is the typical salvage for failed total ankle replacement.[108,109] Ankle fusion in this setting is more difficult than primary fusion because of the bone loss predicated by ankle replacement explantation. When choosing a treatment plan, consideration must be given to host factors such as tobacco use, medical comorbidities, and ability to remain non-weight-bearing; to local factors such as soft tissue coverage, vascular supply, and bone quality; and to disease-specific factors such as degree of bone loss and presence of infection. Soft tissue defects may require free flap coverage. Deep infections will need serial debridement and possible antibiotic-impregnated spacer placement along with intravenous antibiotics prior to definitive salvage procedures.

The first technical consideration in fusion after ankle replacement is to restoring leg length versus shortening and primary fusion. Interposition of structural or cancellous graft can lead to successful bridging of bone from the distal tibia to talus while maintaining leg length. Interposition of bone graft with allograft femoral head,[110] tricortical iliac crest autograft,[111] or fibular autograft can lead to good results in aseptic failure.[112] Use of a metal cage and autologous bone graft has not been as successful.[113] Circular wire external fixation can be used, but results may not be as predictable.[114,115]

Fusion in the setting of infection is best carried out with a two-stage process to debride all infected tissue, place antibiotic-impregnated bone cement, and return for later fusion. Fusion may be carried out with primary bone apposition after malleolar ostectomy or with interposition grafting when there is no concern of indolent infection.

A variety of fixation methods have been proposed for fusion after ankle replacement. Intramedullary fixation from the calcaneus into the distal tibia has been successful.[110,112] Traditional internal fixation methods spanning the fusion site may be used as well.[111] Posteriorly applied blade plate fixation can be used to bridge the calcaneus to the tibia.[116] Compression screw fixation of the tibiotalar joint can be successful in cases with minimal bone destruction.[117]

Fusion rates after failed ankle replacement depend on patient and surgical factors. A series of 38 fusions with 8-year follow-up had fusion rate of 89%.[118] One series reports 17 of 23 successful fusions.[117] Another reports 9 of 9 successful fusions.[94] Use of external fixation may be needed based on poor soft tissue or active infection, but fusion is achieved in only 80% of cases.[114]

Revision total ankle replacement may be considered in select cases with adequate bone remaining after explantation of the initial prosthesis.[119] Custom implants or conversion to a larger device may make up for bone loss.[120,121] Reports are limited to case reports and small series.[122]

13.7 Conclusion

Total ankle replacement is a challenging procedure that requires attention to patient selection, proper alignment, meticulous technique, and vigilance for complications. Clinical results show comparable pain relief and improved functions compared to ankle fusion. A variety of implants are now available with good intermediate-term survival, but more information on long-term survival is needed. The learning curve required to reach proficiency with the procedure must be considered when considering embarking on performing total ankle replacement.

References

1. Glazebrook M, Daniels T, Younger A, et al. Comparison of health-related quality of life between patients with end-stage ankle and hip arthrosis. J Bone Joint Surg Am. 2008;90:499-505.
2. Chou LB, Coughlin MT, Hansen S Jr, et al. Osteoarthritis of the ankle: the role of arthroplasty. J Am Acad Orthop Surg. 2008;16:249-59.
3. Coester LM, Saltzman CL, Leupold J, Pontarelli W. Long-term results following ankle arthrodesis for post-traumatic arthritis. J Bone Joint Surg Am. 2001;83-A:219-28.
4. SooHoo NF, Kominski G. Cost-effectiveness analysis of total ankle arthroplasty. J Bone Joint Surg Am. 2004;86-A:2446-55.
5. Cracchiolo A 3rd, Deorio JK. Design features of current total ankle replacements: implants and instrumentation. J Am Acad Orthop Surg. 2008;16:530-40.
6. Cerrato R, Myerson MS. Total ankle replacement: the Agility LP prosthesis. Foot Ankle Clin. 2008;13:485-94, ix.
7. Bonnin M, Judet T, Colombier JA, Buscayret F, Graveleau N, Piriou P. Midterm results of the Salto Total Ankle Prosthesis. Clin Orthop Relat Res. 2004;(424):6-18.
8. Pyevich MT, Saltzman CL, Callaghan JJ, Alvine FG. Total ankle arthroplasty: a unique design. Two to twelve-year follow-up. J Bone Joint Surg Am. 1998;80:1410-20.
9. Saltzman CL, Tochigi Y, Rudert MJ, McIff TE, Brown TD. The effect of agility ankle prosthesis misalignment on the peri-ankle ligaments. Clin Orthop Relat Res. 2004;(424):137-42.
10. Leszko F, Komistek RD, Mahfouz MR, et al. In vivo kinematics of the salto total ankle prosthesis. Foot Ankle Int. 2008;29:1117-25.
11. Conti S, Lalonde KA, Martin R. Kinematic analysis of the agility total ankle during gait. Foot Ankle Int. 2006;27:980-4.
12. Coetzee JC. Management of varus or valgus ankle deformity with ankle replacement. Foot Ankle Clin. 2008;13:509-20, x.
13. Haskell A, Mann RA. Ankle arthroplasty with preoperative coronal plane deformity: short-term results. Clin Orthop Relat Res. 2004;(424):98-103.
14. Hennessy MS, Molloy AP, Wood EV. Management of the varus arthritic ankle. Foot Ankle Clin. 2008;13:417-42, viii.
15. Cornelis Doets H, van der Plaat LW, Klein JP. Medial malleolar osteotomy for the correction of varus deformity during total ankle arthroplasty: results in 15 ankles. Foot Ankle Int. 2008;29:171-7.
16. Bluman EM, Chiodo CP. Valgus ankle deformity and arthritis. Foot Ankle Clin. 2008;13:443-70, ix.
17. Tochigi Y, Rudert MJ, Brown TD, McIff TE, Saltzman CL. The effect of accuracy of implantation on range of movement of the Scandinavian total ankle replacement. J Bone Joint Surg Br. 2005;87:736-40.
18. McIff TE, Alvine FG, Saltzman CL, Klaren JC, Brown TD. Intraoperative measurement of distraction for ligament tensioning in total ankle arthroplasty. Clin Orthop Relat Res. 2004;(424):111-7.
19. Knecht SI, Estin M, Callaghan JJ, et al. The Agility total ankle arthroplasty. Seven to sixteen-year follow-up. J Bone Joint Surg Am. 2004;86-A:1161-71.

20. Coetzee JC, Pomeroy GC, Watts JD, Barrow C. The use of autologous concentrated growth factors to promote syndesmosis fusion in the Agility total ankle replacement. A preliminary study. Foot Ankle Int. 2005;26:840-6.
21. Barrow CR, Pomeroy GC. Enhancement of syndesmotic fusion rates in total ankle arthroplasty with the use of autologous platelet concentrate. Foot Ankle Int. 2005;26:458-61.
22. Adams SB Jr, Spritzer CE, Hofstaetter SG, et al. Computer-assisted tibia preparation for total ankle arthroplasty: a cadaveric study. Int J Med Robot. 2007;3:336-40.
23. Leardini A, Rapagna L, Ensini A, Catani F, Cappello A. Computer-assisted preoperative planning of a novel design of total ankle replacement. Comput Methods Programs Biomed. 2002;67:231-43.
24. Pena F, Agel J, Coetzee JC. Comparison of the MFA to the AOFAS outcome tool in a population undergoing total ankle replacement. Foot Ankle Int. 2007;28:788-93.
25. Kirkup J. Richard Smith ankle arthroplasty. J R Soc Med. 1985;78:301-4.
26. Bolton-Maggs BG, Sudlow RA, Freeman MA. Total ankle arthroplasty. A long-term review of the London Hospital experience. J Bone Joint Surg Br. 1985;67:785-90.
27. Jensen NC, Kroner K. Total ankle joint replacement: a clinical follow up. Orthopedics. 1992;15:236-9.
28. Unger AS, Inglis AE, Mow CS, Figgie HE 3rd. Total ankle arthroplasty in rheumatoid arthritis: a long-term follow-up study. Foot Ankle. 1988;8:173-9.
29. Kofoed H. Scandinavian total ankle replacement (STAR). Clin Orthop Relat Res. 2004;(424):73-9.
30. McGuire MR, Kyle RF, Gustilo RB, Premer RF. Comparative analysis of ankle arthroplasty versus ankle arthrodesis. Clin Orthop Relat Res. 1988;226:174-81.
31. Kitaoka HB, Patzer GL, Ilstrup DM, Wallrichs SL. Survivorship analysis of the Mayo total ankle arthroplasty. J Bone Joint Surg Am. 1994;76:974-9.
32. Kitaoka HB, Patzer GL. Clinical results of the Mayo total ankle arthroplasty. J Bone Joint Surg Am. 1996;78:1658-64.
33. Buechel FF, Pappas MJ, Iorio LJ. New Jersey low contact stress total ankle replacement: biomechanical rationale and review of 23 cementless cases. Foot Ankle. 1988;8:279-90.
34. Kofoed H. Cylindrical cemented ankle arthroplasty: a prospective series with long-term follow-up. Foot Ankle Int. 1995;16:474-9.
35. Buechel FF, Pappas MJ. Survivorship and clinical evaluation of cementless, meniscal-bearing total ankle replacements. Semin Arthroplasty. 1992;3:43-50.
36. Alvine FG. Total ankle arthroplasty: new concepts and approaches. Contemp Orthop. 1991;22:397-403.
37. Wood PL, Prem H, Sutton C. Total ankle replacement: medium-term results in 200 Scandinavian total ankle replacements. J Bone Joint Surg Br. 2008;90:605-9.
38. Hurowitz EJ, Gould JS, Fleisig GS, Fowler R. Outcome analysis of agility total ankle replacement with prior adjunctive procedures: two to six year followup. Foot Ankle Int. 2007;28:308-12.
39. San Giovanni TP, Keblish DJ, Thomas WH, Wilson MG. Eight-year results of a minimally constrained total ankle arthroplasty. Foot Ankle Int. 2006;27:418-26.
40. Hosman AH, Mason RB, Hobbs T, Rothwell AG. A New Zealand national joint registry review of 202 total ankle replacements followed for up to 6 years. Acta Orthop. 2007;78:584-91.
41. Henricson A, Skoog A, Carlsson A. The Swedish ankle arthroplasty register: an analysis of 531 arthroplasties between 1993 and 2005. Acta Orthop. 2007;78:569-74.
42. Fevang BT, Lie SA, Havelin LI, Brun JG, Skredderstuen A, Furnes O. 257 ankle arthroplasties performed in Norway between 1994 and 2005. Acta Orthop. 2007;78:575-83.
43. Spirt AA, Assal M, Hansen ST Jr. Complications and failure after total ankle arthroplasty. J Bone Joint Surg Am. 2004;86-A:1172-8.
44. Doets HC, Brand R, Nelissen RG. Total ankle arthroplasty in inflammatory joint disease with use of two mobile-bearing designs. J Bone Joint Surg Am. 2006;88:1272-84.

45. Kofoed H, Sorensen TS. Ankle arthroplasty for rheumatoid arthritis and osteoarthritis: prospective long-term study of cemented replacements. J Bone Joint Surg Br. 1998;80:328-32.
46. Wood PL, Sutton C, Mishra V, Suneja R. A randomised, controlled trial of two mobile-bearing total ankle replacements. J Bone Joint Surg Br. 2009;91:69-74.
47. Kopp FJ, Patel MM, Deland JT, O'Malley MJ. Total ankle arthroplasty with the Agility prosthesis: clinical and radiographic evaluation. Foot Ankle Int. 2006;27:97-103.
48. Schutte BG, Louwerens JW. Short-term results of our first 49 Scandanavian total ankle replacements (STAR). Foot Ankle Int. 2008;29:124-7.
49. Anderson T, Montgomery F, Carlsson A. Uncemented STAR total ankle prostheses. J Bone Joint Surg Am. 2004;86-A(Suppl 1):103-11.
50. Anderson T, Montgomery F, Carlsson A. Uncemented STAR total ankle prostheses. Three to eight-year follow-up of fifty-one consecutive ankles. J Bone Joint Surg Am. 2003;85-A: 1321-9.
51. Valderrabano V, Pagenstert G, Horisberger M, Knupp M, Hintermann B. Sports and recreation activity of ankle arthritis patients before and after total ankle replacement. Am J Sports Med. 2006;34:993-9.
52. Saltzman CL, Mann RA, Coughlin MJ. Prospective controlled trial of STAR ankle replacement vs. ankle fusion: initial results. Annual Meeting of the American Academy of Orthopaedic Surgeons; 2009; Las Vegas.
53. Naal FD, Impellizzeri FM, Loibl M, Huber M, Rippstein PF. Habitual physical activity and sports participation after total ankle arthroplasty. Am J Sports Med. 2009;37:95-102.
54. Reggiani B, Leardini A, Corazza F, Taylor M. Finite element analysis of a total ankle replacement during the stance phase of gait. J Biomech. 2006;39:1435-43.
55. Piriou P, Culpan P, Mullins M, Cardon JN, Pozzi D, Judet T. Ankle replacement versus arthrodesis: a comparative gait analysis study. Foot Ankle Int. 2008;29:3-9.
56. Valderrabano V, Nigg BM, von Tscharner V, Stefanyshyn DJ, Goepfert B, Hintermann B. Gait analysis in ankle osteoarthritis and total ankle replacement. Clin Biomech (Bristol, Avon). 2007;22:894-904.
57. Coetzee JC, Castro MD. Accurate measurement of ankle range of motion after total ankle arthroplasty. Clin Orthop Relat Res. 2004;(424):27-31.
58. Muller S, Wolf S, Doderlein L. Three-dimensional analysis of the foot following implantation of a HINTEGRA ankle prosthesis: evaluation with the Heidelberg foot model. Orthopade. 2006;35:506-12.
59. Doets HC, van Middelkoop M, Houdijk H, Nelissen RG, Veeger HE. Gait analysis after successful mobile bearing total ankle replacement. Foot Ankle Int. 2007;28:313-22.
60. Michelson JD, Schmidt GR, Mizel MS. Kinematics of a total arthroplasty of the ankle: comparison to normal ankle motion. Foot Ankle Int. 2000;21:278-84.
61. Valderrabano V, Hintermann B, Nigg BM, Stefanyshyn D, Stergiou P. Kinematic changes after fusion and total replacement of the ankle: part 1: range of motion. Foot Ankle Int. 2003;24: 881-7.
62. Valderrabano V, Hintermann B, Nigg BM, Stefanyshyn D, Stergiou P. Kinematic changes after fusion and total replacement of the ankle: part 2: movement transfer. Foot Ankle Int. 2003;24:888-96.
63. Valderrabano V, Hintermann B, Nigg BM, Stefanyshyn D, Stergiou P. Kinematic changes after fusion and total replacement of the ankle: part 3: talar movement. Foot Ankle Int. 2003;24: 897-900.
64. Nicholson JJ, Parks BG, Stroud CC, Myerson MS. Joint contact characteristics in agility total ankle arthroplasty. Clin Orthop Relat Res. 2004;(424):125-9.
65. Richter M, Zech S, Westphal R, Klimcsch Y, Gosling T. Robotic cadaver testing of a new total ankle prosthesis model (German Ankle System). Foot Ankle Int. 2007;28:1276-86.
66. Houdijk H, Doets HC, van Middelkoop M, Dirkjan Veeger HE. Joint stiffness of the ankle during walking after successful mobile-bearing total ankle replacement. Gait Posture. 2008;27:115-9.
67. Detrembleur C, Leemrijse T. The effects of total ankle replacement on gait disability: analysis of energetic and mechanical variables. Gait Posture. 2009;29(2):270-4.

68. Zerahn B, Kofoed H. Bone mineral density, gait analysis, and patient satisfaction, before and after ankle arthroplasty. Foot Ankle Int. 2004;25:208-14.
69. Zerahn B, Kofoed H, Borgwardt A. Increased bone mineral density adjacent to hydroxy-apatite-coated ankle arthroplasty. Foot Ankle Int. 2000;21:285-9.
70. Conti SF, Dazen D, Stewart G, et al. Proprioception after total ankle arthroplasty. Foot Ankle Int. 2008;29:1069-73.
71. Valderrabano V, Nigg BM, von Tscharner V, Frank CB, Hintermann B. J. Leonard Goldner Award 2006. Total ankle replacement in ankle osteoarthritis: an analysis of muscle rehabilitation. Foot Ankle Int. 2007;28(281):291.
72. Valderrabano V, Hintermann B, von Tscharner V, Gopfert B, Dick W, Nigg BM. Muscle biomechanics in total ankle replacement. Orthopade. 2006;35:513-20.
73. Wood PL, Crawford LA, Suneja R, Kenyon A. Total ankle replacement for rheumatoid ankle arthritis. Foot Ankle Clin. 2007;12:497-508, vii.
74. Lachiewicz PF, Inglis AE, Ranawat CS. Total ankle replacement in rheumatoid arthritis. J Bone Joint Surg Am. 1984;66:340-3.
75. Helm R, Stevens J. Long-term results of total ankle replacement. J Arthroplasty. 1986;1:271-7.
76. Radossi P, Bisson R, Munari F, et al. Total ankle replacement for end-stage arthropathy in patients with haemophilia. Haemophilia. 2008;14:658-60.
77. Scholz R, Scholz U. The total ankle replacement for severe arthropathy in haemophilia. Hamostaseologie. 2008;28(Suppl 1):S40-4.
78. van der Heide HJ, Novakova I, de Waal Malefijt MC. The feasibility of total ankle prosthesis for severe arthropathy in haemophilia and prothrombin deficiency. Haemophilia. 2006;12:679-82.
79. Davies MB, Saxby T. Ankle arthropathy of hemochromatosis: a case series and review of the literature. Foot Ankle Int. 2006;27:902-6.
80. Greisberg J, Assal M, Flueckiger G, Hansen ST, Jr. Takedown of ankle fusion and conversion to total ankle replacement. Clin Orthop Relat Res. 2004;(424):80-8.
81. Hintermann B, Barg A, Knupp M, Valderrabano V. Conversion of painful ankle arthrodesis to total ankle arthroplasty. J Bone Joint Surg Am. 2009;91:850-8.
82. Liao X, Gao Z, Huang S, Yang S. Prevention and treatment of perioperative period complication of total ankle replacement. Zhongguo Xiu Fu Chong Jian Wai Ke Za Zhi. 2008;22:40-3.
83. Schuberth JM, Patel S, Zarutsky E. Perioperative complications of the Agility total ankle replacement in 50 initial, consecutive cases. J Foot Ankle Surg. 2006;45:139-46.
84. Raikin SM, Myerson MS. Avoiding and managing complications of the Agility total ankle replacement system. Orthopedics. 2006;29:930-8.
85. Stamatis ED, Myerson MS. How to avoid specific complications of total ankle replacement. Foot Ankle Clin. 2002;7:765-89.
86. Conti SF, Wong YS. Complications of total ankle replacement. Foot Ankle Clin. 2002;7:791-807, vii.
87. Conti SF, Wong YS. Complications of total ankle replacement. Clin Orthop Relat Res. 2001;391:105-14.
88. SooHoo NF, Zingmond DS, Ko CY. Comparison of reoperation rates following ankle arthrodesis and total ankle arthroplasty. J Bone Joint Surg Am. 2007;89:2143-9.
89. Saltzman CL, Amendola A, Anderson R, et al. Surgeon training and complications in total ankle arthroplasty. Foot Ankle Int. 2003;24:514-8.
90. Myerson MS, Mroczek K. Perioperative complications of total ankle arthroplasty. Foot Ankle Int. 2003;24:17-21.
91. Haskell A, Mann RA. Perioperative complication rate of total ankle replacement is reduced by surgeon experience. Foot Ankle Int. 2004;25:283-9.
92. Lee KB, Cho SG, Hur CI, Yoon TR. Perioperative complications of HINTEGRA total ankle replacement: our initial 50 cases. Foot Ankle Int. 2008;29:978-84.
93. Fukui A, Tanaka Y, Inada Y, et al. Turndown retinacular flap for closure of skin fistula after total ankle replacement. Foot Ankle Int. 2008;29:624-6.

94. Kotnis R, Pasapula C, Anwar F, Cooke PH, Sharp RJ. The management of failed ankle replacement. J Bone Joint Surg Br. 2006;88:1039-47.
95. McGarvey WC, Clanton TO, Lunz D. Malleolar fracture after total ankle arthroplasty: a comparison of two designs. Clin Orthop Relat Res. 2004;(424):104-10.
96. Tochigi Y, Suh JS, Amendola A, Pedersen DR, Saltzman CL. Ankle alignment on lateral radiographs. Part 1: sensitivity of measures to perturbations of ankle positioning. Foot Ankle Int. 2006;27:82-7.
97. Tochigi Y, Suh JS, Amendola A, Saltzman CL. Ankle alignment on lateral radiographs. Part 2: reliability and validity of measures. Foot Ankle Int. 2006;27:88-92.
98. Nelissen RG, Doets HC, Valstar ER. Early migration of the tibial component of the buechel-pappas total ankle prosthesis. Clin Orthop Relat Res. 2006;448:146-51.
99. Carlsson A, Markusson P, Sundberg M. Radiostereometric analysis of the double-coated STAR total ankle prosthesis: a 3–5 year follow-up of 5 cases with rheumatoid arthritis and 5 cases with osteoarthrosis. Acta Orthop. 2005;76:573-9.
100. Dahabreh Z, Gonsalves S, Monkhouse R, Harris NJ. Extrusion of metal radiological marker from a total ankle replacement insert: a case report. *J Foot Ankle Surg*. 2006;45:185-9.
101. Assal M, Al-Shaikh R, Reiber BH, Hansen ST. Fracture of the polyethylene component in an ankle arthroplasty: a case report. *Foot Ankle Int*. 2003;24:901-3.
102. Kobayashi A, Minoda Y, Kadoya Y, Ohashi H, Takaoka K, Saltzman CL. Ankle arthro-plasties generate wear particles similar to knee arthroplasties. *Clin Orthop Relat Res*. 2004;(424):69-72.
103. Affatato S, Leardini A, Leardini W, Giannini S, Viceconti M. Meniscal wear at a three-com-ponent total ankle prosthesis by a knee joint simulator. *J Biomech*. 2007;40:1871-6.
104. Bell CJ, Fisher J. Simulation of polyethylene wear in ankle joint prostheses. *J Biomed Mater Res B Appl Biomater*. 2007;81:162-7.
105. Hanna RS, Haddad SL, Lazarus ML. Evaluation of periprosthetic lucency after total ankle arthroplasty: helical CT versus conventional radiography. *Foot Ankle Int*. 2007;28:921-6.
106. Kurup HV, Taylor GR. Medial impingement after ankle replacement. *Int Orthop*. 2008;32:243-6.
107. Bejjanki NK, Moulder E, Al-Nammari S, Budgen A. Tarsal tunnel syndrome as a complica-tion of total ankle athroplasty: a case report. *Foot Ankle Int*. 2008;29:347-50.
108. Wapner KL. Salvage of failed and infected total ankle replacements with fusion. *Instr Course Lect*. 2002;51:153-7.
109. Myerson MS, Miller SD. Salvage after complications of total ankle arthroplasty. *Foot Ankle Clin*. 2002;7:191-206.
110. Thomason K, Eyres KS. A technique of fusion for failed total replacement of the ankle: tibio-allograft-calcaneal fusion with a locked retrograde intramedullary nail. *J Bone Joint Surg Br*. 2008;90:885-8.
111. Culpan P, Le Strat V, Piriou P, Judet T. Arthrodesis after failed total ankle replacement. *J Bone Joint Surg Br*. 2007;89:1178-83.
112. Schill S. Ankle arthrodesis with interposition graft as a salvage procedure after failed total ankle replacement. *Oper Orthop Traumatol*. 2007;19:547-60.
113. Carlsson A. Unsuccessful use of a titanium mesh cage in ankle arthrodesis: a report on three cases operated on due to a failed ankle replacement. *J Foot Ankle Surg*. 2008;47:337-42.
114. Zarutsky E, Rush SM, Schuberth JM. The use of circular wire external fixation in the treat-ment of salvage ankle arthrodesis. *J Foot Ankle Surg*. 2005;44:22-31.
115. Carlsson AS, Montgomery F, Besjakov J. Arthrodesis of the ankle secondary to replacement. *Foot Ankle Int*. 1998;19:240-5.
116. Ritter M, Nickisch F, DiGiovanni C. Technique tip: posterior blade plate for salvage of failed total ankle arthroplasty. *Foot Ankle Int*. 2006;27:303-4.
117. Hopgood P, Kumar R, Wood PL. Ankle arthrodesis for failed total ankle replacement. *J Bone Joint Surg Br*. 2006;88:1032-8.
118. Kitaoka HB, Romness DW. Arthrodesis for failed ankle arthroplasty. *J Arthroplasty*. 1992;7:277-84.

119. Gould JS. Revision total ankle arthroplasty. *Am J Orthop*. 2005;34:361.
120. Myerson MS, Won HY. Primary and revision total ankle replacement using custom-designed prostheses. *Foot Ankle Clin*. 2008;13:521-38, x.
121. Assal M, Greisberg J, Hansen ST Jr. Revision total ankle arthroplasty: conversion of New Jersey Low Contact Stress to Agility: surgical technique and case report. *Foot Ankle Int*. 2004;25:922-5.
122. DiDomenico LA, Williams K. Revisional total ankle arthroplasty because of a large tibial bone cyst. *J Foot Ankle Surg*. 2008;47:453-6.

Chapter 14
Tumors and Tumor-Like Lesions of the Foot and Ankle: Diagnosis and Treatment

Hans Gollwitzer, Andreas K. Toepfer, Ludger Gerdesmeyer, Reiner Gradinger, and Hans Rechl

14.1 Introduction

Bone and soft tissue tumors of the foot and ankle are not rare in the foot special-ist's practice. Although masses are usually seen early with early symptoms due to compact anatomy with thin soft tissue coverage (e.g., pain on weight-bearing), diagnosis is often delayed. Diagnostic errors are more common than in other regions, since neoplasia is often not considered. Tumor size is a major prognostic factor for recurrence-free survival, and delayed diagnosis finally results in under-treatment or overtreatment with serious consequences. Thus, if early diagnosis is compelled, prognosis is generally improved.

H. Gollwitzer, M.D., C.C.R.P. (✉)
Klinik für Orthopädie und Sportorthopädie, Klinikum rechts der Isar,
Technische Universität München,
Ismaninger Str. 22, Munich 81675, Germany
e-mail: gollwitzer@bone-and-joint.org

A.K. Toepfer, M.D.
Klinik für Orthopädie und Unfallchirurgie, Technische Universität München,
Munich, Germany

L. Gerdesmeyer, M.D.
Department of Orthopaedic and Trauma Surgery, Mare Klinikum Kiel,
Kiel-Kronshagen, Germany

R. Gradinger, M.D.
Clinic for Orthopaedics and Traumatology, Klinikum rechs der Isar,
Technische Universität München, Munich, Germany

H. Rechl, M.D., D.V.M.
Klinik für Orthopädie und Unfallchirurgie, Technische Universität München,
Munich, Germany

A. Saxena (ed.), *Special Procedures in Foot and Ankle Surgery*,
DOI 10.1007/978-0-85729-609-2_14, © Springer-Verlag London 2013

283

14.2 Epidemiology

Suspicion is warranted in investigating any foot mass, including especially those with an apparently indolent course. Several investigations have shown that malignancy rates are much higher at the foot and ankle than previously thought. The foot and ankle, which represents approximately 3% total body mass, is also the site of 3% of osseous neoplasms.[1] Even more important, 5% of malignant and 8% of all benign soft-tissue tumors occur at the foot and ankle region.[2] In larger case series, 3.4–12.8% of the treated foot and ankle tumors in referral centers have been reported as malignant.[3-5]

14.3 Diagnosis

Benign and indolent soft tissue masses are common at the foot, and failure of suspicion can substantially delay diagnosis of neoplasia. Patient age and location of tumor can be useful in determining possible diagnoses. A detailed history of risk factors, prior malignancy, and metastatic disease especially in patients older than 50 years (e.g., lung or genitourinary tract) should raise the index of suspicion toward malignancy. Furthermore, especially preexisting painless masses that suddenly start growing should be followed by further diagnostic measures to rule out neoplasia. Fractures mandate the question for adequate trauma. Hence, fractures following inadequate trauma should not be accepted without ruling out underlying bone disease.

14.3.1 Physical Exam

Physical exam confirming the presence of a mass must analyze whether the tumor is fixed to or can be moved against the underlying tissue. Pain is generally unspecific; however, sharp electrifying pain or tingling at palpation with positive Hofmann-Tinel sign can point toward nerve entrapment by the mass or peripheral nerve tumors. Thorough diagnostics should be initiated with pigmented lesions of the skin, since malignant melanoma is quite common in the foot and ankle region.[6] In any case of suspicion, a biopsy is mandatory to confirm or rule out melanoma. Transillumination is still helpful to confirm the presence of a cystic lesion, although further diagnostic measures have to be taken if there is any doubt of a completely cystic mass or if therapeutic measures are to be taken.

14.3.2 Ultrasound

Ultrasound is an appropriate tool for differentiation of solid and cystic tumors (e.g., ganglion). Additionally, ultrasound can be used to guide needle aspiration or biopsy.[7]

Table 14.1 Lodwick classification of bone tumors

Grade	Destruction	Margin	Cortex penetration	Sclerotic rim	Expanded cortical shell
IA	Mandatory geographic	Regular, lobulated, or multicentric	None or partial	Thick	Optional, ≤1 cm
IB	Mandatory geographic	Regular, lobulated, or multicentric	None or partial	Optional	Optional, >1 cm
IC	Mandatory geographic	Regular, lobulated, or multicentric	Mandatory total	Optional	Optional
II	Moth-eaten or geographic	Irregular, poorly defined	Total	Optional but unlikely	Optional but unlikely
III	Mandatory permeated	Any edge	Total	Optional but unlikely	Optional but unlikely

However, specific diagnosis based on ultrasound alone is generally not sufficiently accurate, which commonly results in further diagnostic steps like magnetic resonance imaging (MRI) and biopsy.[8]

14.3.3   X-Rays

Radiographic workup is initiated to differentiate bone tumors with soft tissue masses from soft tissue tumors. High-quality dorsoplantar, oblique, and lateral radiographs should be taken so as not to miss subtle osseous lesions. X-rays should especially be analyzed for localization of the tumor (epiphyseal, metaphyseal, or diaphyseal), morphology of the lesion, and its margins (bony arrosions, cortical thinning, periosteal reactions, sclerotic margins, and tumor matrix like calcification or ossification). The Lodwick classification is very helpful to obtain a first grading of bone tumors (Table 14.1). Although it is sometimes difficult to differentiate Grade II and III lesions, the precise grading is not that relevant since both describe aggressive growth that requires further evaluation.

Certain radiographic characteristics can give diagnostic clues, like extensive punctuate calcifications being typical, e.g., for enchondroma, whereas small intralesional calcifications are commonly observed in synovial sarcoma.

Furthermore, especially in the case of a fracture, subtle analysis of the adjacent bone for osteolysis and consequent history taking for adequate trauma can point toward underlying metabolic or neoplastic disease.[9]

14.3.4   Computed Tomography

Compared to conventional X-rays, computed tomography (CT) scans can provide additional information on bony detail after MRI and are commonly used to differentiate matrix calcifications from real ossification as well as assessment of cortex integrity (Fig. 14.1). Furthermore, analysis of Hounsfield units allows assessment of

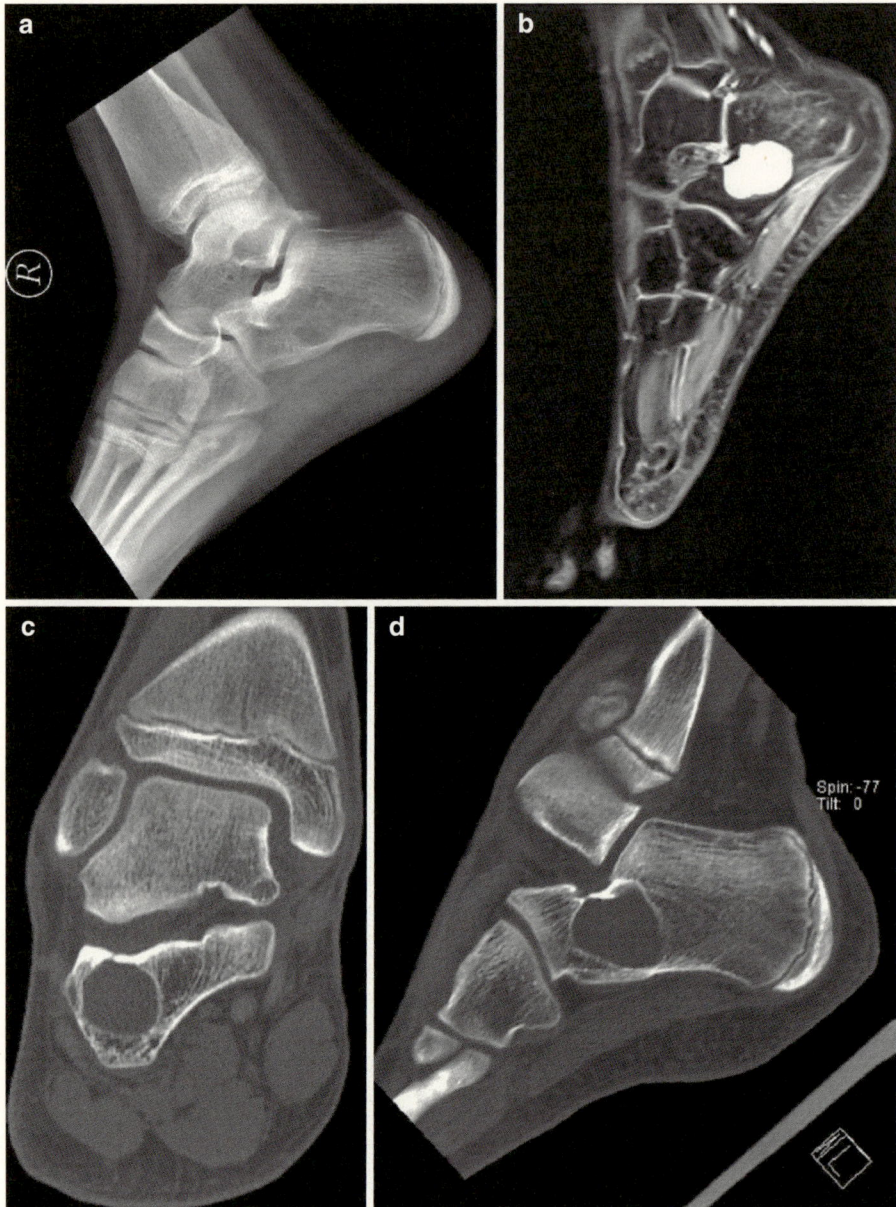

Fig. 14.1 X-ray (**a**), MRI (**b**), and CT (**c, d**) scan of a 16-year-old patient with unicameral bone cyst of the calcaneus. CT scan is the most reliable method to confirm or rule out cortical erosion and penetration into adjacent joints. (**e**) Postoperative radiograph after curettage and filling with autologous bone

Fig. 14.1 (continued)

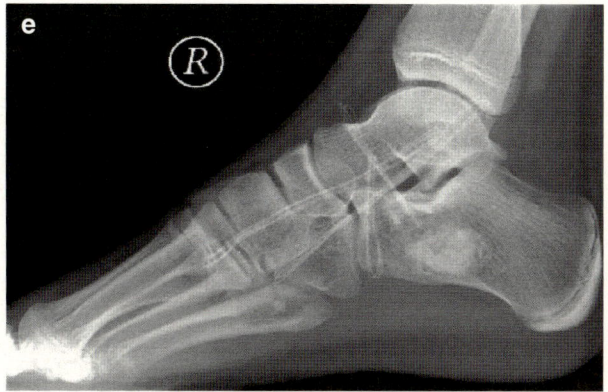

tissue density, especially in comparison with subcutaneous fatty tissue for specific diagnosis of (intraosseous) lipoma. In the case of a metal implant, CT scan is the imaging method of choice to describe tumor expansion and rule out or confirm tumor recurrence.[10]

Finally, CT scan of the thorax is the method of choice in the staging of most malignant tumors of the skeletal system, which commonly metastasize into the lungs.

14.3.5   Magnetic Resonance Imaging

MRI is the standard imaging method for bone and soft tissue tumors.[11] Certain entities – both benign and malignant – can be definitely diagnosed by MRI due to specific resonance characteristics.[8,12,13] Standard protocols have been established, and most commonly native T1, T1 plus intravenous gadolinium, and native T2 sequences in the same orientation are recommended to evaluate the tumor and uptake of contrast medium (Fig. 14.2). Additionally, transverse images of the total tumor expansion are obtained to define the margins of the tumor with regard to major nerves and blood vessels.[13] Depending on the suspected tumor entity, additional sequences can be obtained as necessary (e.g., hem sequences for pigmented villonodular synovitis). Typical MRI features of soft tissue tumors have been summarized in Table 14.2.[6]

There are various diagnostic challenges that require a high level of specialization and experience. For this reason, we recommend regular interdisciplinary conferences with radiologists specialized in musculoskeletal tumors. Soft tissue tumors with bone infiltration can often be distinguished from bone tumors with soft tissue masses by the use of MRI. However, accuracy of MRI to distinguish bone marrow edema from tumor infiltration and postoperative scarring from recurrent tumor is limited.

Vascular infiltration on MRI is defined by encasement of blood vessels by the tumor mass above 180°. Nerves and blood vessels with less contact to the tumor can often be preserved.

Entities that can be specifically diagnosed by MRI alone include hemangioma/lymphangioma, lipoma/low-grade liposarcoma, chondrogenic tumors, benign neurogenic tumors, and various intra-articular tumors.[14] If a specific diagnosis cannot be established by imaging techniques, every tumor has to be regarded "potentially malignant" and a specific diagnosis has to be enforced by biopsy and histopathologic workup.

14.3.6 Biopsy

In any mass with suspected malignancy, indeterminate behavior, or if the diagnosis cannot be specified to one single entity, a biopsy must be obtained (possible differentiation of benign and malignant is not enough!).

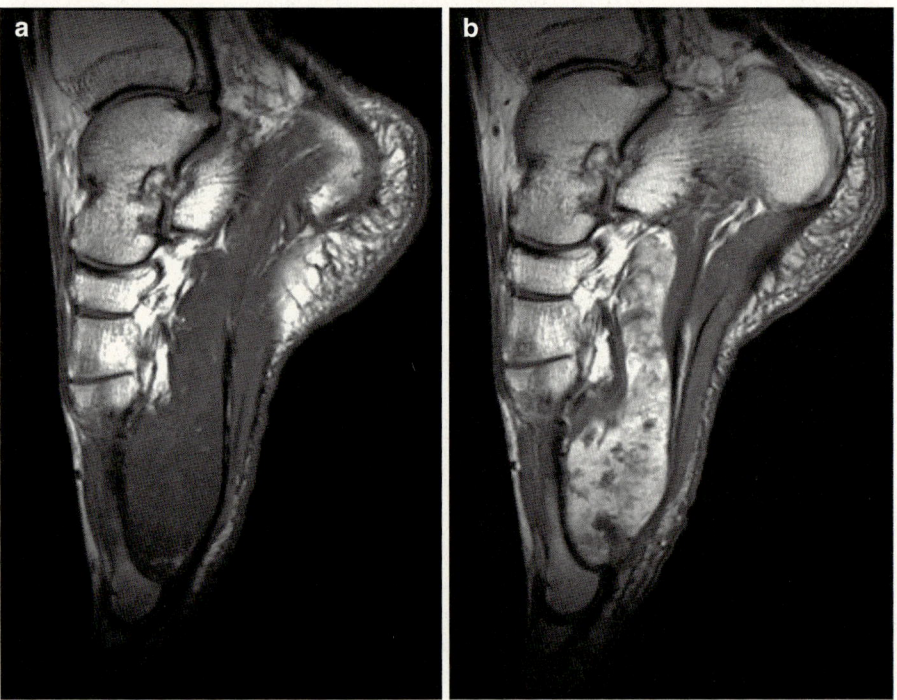

Fig. 14.2 A 48-year-old patient with a chondrosarcoma of the midfoot. Standard MRI with (**a**) native T1-weighted sequence (**b**) T1-weighted sequence with contrast (**c**) T2-weighted sequence, all in the same orientation; (**d**) axial sequence of the complete tumor extension to define the relation to neurovascular structures; (**e**) postoperative X-ray at 2 months after midfoot amputation and fusion of the tilted calcaneus to the distal tibia (Boyd's amputation)

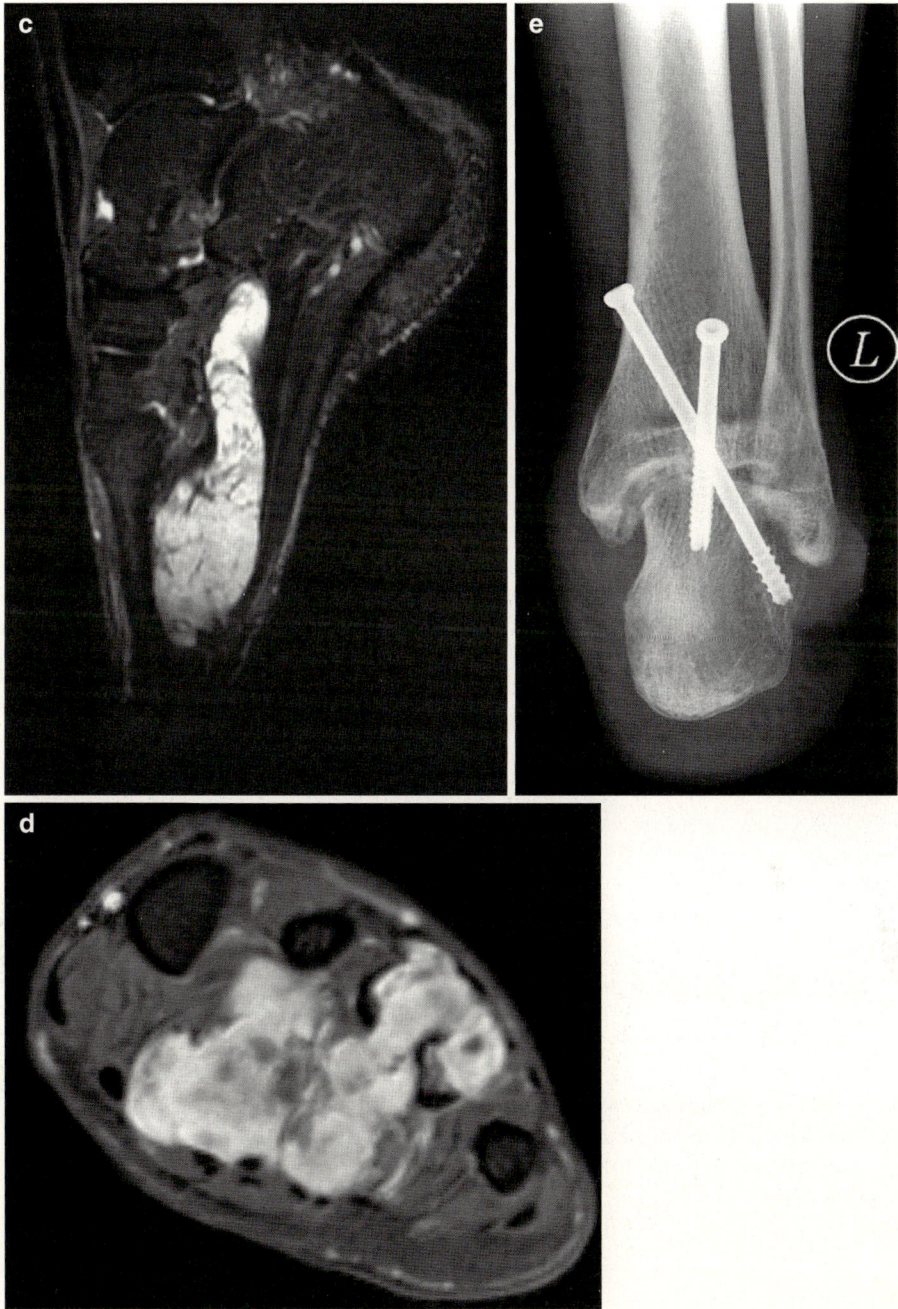

Fig. 14.2 (continued)

Table 14.2 Typical MRI features of soft tissue tumors with corresponding signals

T1+, T2+	T1+, T2+/−	T1−, T2−	T1−, T2+
Hemangioma	Lipoma	Desmoid	Various sarcomas
Lymphangioma	Liposarcoma	Fibromatoses	Neurogenic tumors
Hematoma	Hamartoma	PVNS	Cysts
Small AVM	Elastofibroma	Morton neuroma	Ganglion
Mineralizations	Clear cell sarcoma	Xanthoma	Myxoma
	Melanoma	High-flow AVM	Chondrogenic tumors
		Scar tissue	Myxoid liposarcoma
		Mineralized tumors	Synovial sarcoma
		Amyloid tumors	

T1+ = high signal on T1-weighted MRI images; T1+/− = intermediate signal intensity; T1− = low signal intensity; T2+ = high signal on T2-weighted images; T2+/− = intermediate signal intensity; T2− = low signal intensity; *PVNS* pigmented villonodular synovialitis; *AVM* arteriovenous malformation

Since biopsies can be associated with major complications that might significantly impair prognosis,[15] early referral to a center experienced in musculoskeletal tumors is strongly recommended – even before biopsy! In this context, the Musculoskeletal Tumor Society demonstrated much higher incidence of biopsy-related complications when biopsies were not performed at centers experienced in musculoskeletal tumors.[15,16] Mankin and co-workers demonstrated that out of 17.5% of complications related to biopsy, nearly 10% had negative impact on prognosis; 77.2% of these biopsies with complications had not been performed in oncologic centers.[15,16]

Several important issues have to be regarded when tissue is harvested for histologic workup. Since the tissue that is penetrated during biopsy is potentially contaminated with tumor cells, the biopsy approach has to be excised during final surgery. Thus, the different options and approaches for definitive tumor resection have to be considered already at the time of biopsy! The biopsy approach should be defined by or in accordance with the surgeon who will perform the later definitive tumor resection.

Closed biopsy techniques, such as CT-guided or ultrasound-guided needle biopsies, are especially suitable in deep and larger lesions with homogeneous matrix and in the case of suspected tumor recurrence. Fine needle biopsy has the lowest risk of complication but is limited to cytology, since small size of tissue samples does not allow accurate histologic workup. Core-needle biopsy is appropriate for histology, but has a higher risk of hematoma.[17] Multiple samples should be taken to improve diagnostic accuracy (75–90%).

Open and incision biopsy on the other hand have a higher diagnostic value and allow harvesting of sufficient tissue for histology, immunostaining, and molecular workup. Radical biopsy is appropriate for certain benign lesions and has the advantage that no second surgical intervention is necessary. Areas of vital tumor should be addressed in fast-growing and heterogeneous masses, and margins to healthy tissue as well as cystic membranes are most representative and should also be sent for histopathologic analysis.

Good surgical technique is necessary to avoid complications that can have negative influence on the prognosis for tumor resection and survival. A longitudinal incision facilitates later resection. The skin should not be mobilized to allow complete resection of the biopsy canal at final surgery. A direct approach should be chosen, and additional compartments must not be opened. Neurovascular structures and joints have to be avoided. Bony lesions should be addressed from the dorsum of the foot, whereas a direct approach is appropriate for soft tissue lesions.

Several samples of viable tissue as well as tissue samples for microbiological culture are taken and transported on ice to the pathology department to allow for immunological and molecular analyses. Intraoperative frozen sections are helpful in certain tumors with non-mineralized tissue to make sure that representative tumor tissue has been taken, to check the resection margins for remaining tumor cells, or to verify the diagnosis in case of suspected tumor recurrence. Frozen sections may provide a diagnosis, but often definitive histopathological workup including immunohistochemistry is necessary. If definitive diagnosis is not obtained, discontinue case and perform definitive surgery in a second procedure.

In nonhomogeneous masses, tissue should be taken from different locations within the tumor. Meticulous hemostasis (e.g., with bone wax, acrylic cement, or collagen sponges) is of utmost importance, since hematoma is associated with local uncontrolled tumor cell contamination. In this context, bony biopsies are of special interest because weakening of the bone by tumor and biopsy increase the risk of pathologic fractures which is again associated with tumor cell spreading. Thus, all relevant measures such as splint or cast as well as limited weight-bearing have to be addressed postoperatively. Finally, use of non-resorbable sutures helps to mark the biopsy incision. Drains are used whenever necessary to avoid hematoma, and drains should pass through the skin close to the incision's distal margin in line with the skin incision.

If the diagnosis is not straightforward after definitive histopathology, cases should be discussed in interdisciplinary conferences with pathology consultant, radiologist, and orthopedic surgeon.

14.3.7 Staging

Special considerations have to be used in the staging of foot tumors,[18] because of the special anatomic situation. No real compartments are present at the midfoot, hindfoot, and ankle. Moreover, only thin fascial borders exist along single rays, and thin cortex and periosteum of the tarsals allow early perforation of both bone and soft tissue tumors. In oncologic surgery, the hindfoot and the midfoot are considered single anatomic compartments by the staging system of MSTS.[9,18] Tables 14.3 and 14.4 summarize the classic staging systems for musculoskeletal tumors.[10,11]

Table 14.3 Surgical stages for benign musculoskeletal tumors

Stage	Grade	Site	Metastases	Definition	Behavior
1	G0	T0	M0	Latent or inactive	Remains static or heals spontaneously
2	G0	T1	M0	Active	Progressive growth but limited by natural barriers
3	G0	T2	M0	Aggressive	Progressive growth, not limited by natural barriers

Table 14.4 Surgical stages for malignant musculoskeletal tumors

Stage	Grade	Site	Metastases
IA	Low (G1 and G2)	Intracompartmental (T1)	None (M0)
IB	Low (G1 and G2)	Extracompartmental (T2)	None (M0)
IIA	High (G3 and G4)	Intracompartmental (T1)	None (M0)
IIB	High (G3 and G4)	Extracompartmental (T2)	None (M0)
IIIA	Low (G1 and G2)	Intracompartmental or Extracompartmental (T1–T2)	Regional or distant (M1)
IIIB	High (G3 and G4)	Intracompartmental or Extracompartmental (T1–T2)	Regional or distant (M1)

G is the grade of the tumor as defined by histology. G0 is benign tumor. G1 and G2 are low-grade malignant tumors, and G3 and G4 are high-grade malignant tumors
T is the anatomic extension of the tumor. T0 means a benign tumor contained by a true capsule (intracapsular). T1 is a benign tumor or malignant tumor that is confined inside an anatomical compartment without a true capsule. T2 is a benign or malignant tumor that is originating in an extracompartmental space or expanded extracompartmentally by penetrating the natural barriers
M are the metastases, either regional (skip or lymph nodes) or distant. M0 means absence, M1 means presence of metastases

14.4 Treatment

14.4.1 Surgical Treatment

Adequate resection of any tumor is the *sine qua non* for local tumor control and survival. "Life before limb!" No compromise in resection margins should be tolerated in tumors in which recurrence is associated with decreased survival. Hence, resection has to be adapted to the dignity of the tumor. Reoperations have a statistically worse prognosis, since the extension of the original tumor cannot be determined by the surgeon who is doing the revision. Four general types of tumor resection have been defined: intralesional, marginal, wide, and radical.

Intralesional resection, such as curettage, is appropriate for some benign lesions with none to very low risk of recurrence or good healing potential. Marginal resection is the excision through the reactive zone, and is appropriate for most benign lesions that show a certain potential for recurrence or do not heal spontaneously.

Wide resection is defined as removal of tumor surrounded on all sides with healthy tissue, and this type of resection is adequate for most malignant tumors. Finally, radical resection includes resection of the entire anatomic compartment (metatarsals are the only compartmental boundaries). Since recurrence-free survival after wide and radical resection is similar for most malignant cases, but radical resection is often associated with severe functional impairment, wide resection is the resection of choice in most malignant tumors. However, due to the smaller anatomic situation at the foot with only limited boundaries, radical resection – which is often equivalent with (ray) amputation – is more common at the foot than at other areas.

Again, at the time of definitive surgery for a bone or soft tissue tumor at the foot and ankle, the scar and underlying tissue that has been contaminated during biopsy has to be excised. A tourniquet should be used after exsanguinations by elevation instead of Esmarch to reduce the risk of traumatizing a potentially malignant lesion and possibly promoting metastases. Thereafter, the tumor is excised with appropriate resection margins as described above. If local resection involves sacrificing of plantar nerves, (partial) amputation of the foot may be considered. Resection borders are then unequivocally marked with sutures, and the marked borders are documented on the pathology protocol. The tumor should not be opened during surgery for macroscopic inspection to avoid spreading of tumor cells. After resection, the tumor mass is immediately transported on ice to the pathology department. Similarly to septic surgery, all instruments as well as drapings and gloves should be changed after removal of the tumor mass. Finally, the defect is appropriately reconstructed.

14.4.1.1 Adjuvant Therapy Accompanying Intralesional Procedures

As pointed out before, latent or active benign tumors or tumor-like lesions of the bone, referring to the classification of Enneking,[18] can be treated sufficiently by intralesional curettage in a majority of cases. It is to be noted that the assignment into the three-group classification of latent, active, and aggressive lesions might differ not only from entity to entity but by localization, radiographic appearance, and severeness of symptoms. Optional therapeutical means besides intralesional or marginal resection and the employment of a high-speed burr to clean the cavity in bone tumors might be necessary for successful treatment. Local recurrence after surgical intralesional procedures may be reduced by additional use of local adjuvants, either chemical or thermal. Phenol and alcohol repeatedly have shown to decrease the recurrence rate in the treatment of various bone tumors.[19] Effectivity of phenol on cartilaginous tumor tissue is discussed controversially, though. Lack et al. found no effect of phenol on chondromatous tumor tissue in his studies.[20] Adjuvant thermal procedures include cryotherapy (use of liquid nitrogen) and the use of polymethylmetacrylate (PMMA) by filling the lesion with bone cement. Both methods are widely used and aim at the necrotizing effects of cytotoxical hypo- and hyperthermia.[21] In contrast to liquid nitrogen, the tumoricidal capacity of PMMA is not well investigated. An advantage of bone cement is the stabilizing effect on the curetted cavity and a well-defined and visible demarcation to biological tissue (bone healing, tumor recurrence) on imaging during follow-up.

14.4.1.2 Radiofrequency Ablation

In contrast to traditional surgical tumor therapy with different ways of open tumor resection, radiofrequency thermal ablation allows for a less invasive treatment for a limited number of bone lesions. Image-guided radiofrequency thermal ablation is used in interventional oncology to coagulate and destroy tumor tissue by the direct application of radiofrequency-generated heat,[22] mainly in metastases.

Radiofrequency thermal ablation is well described for the successful treatment of osteoidosteoma and bone metastases for many years, and commonly is guided by CT.[23,24] Osteoidosteoma is characterized by a distinct radiographic appearance, a small tumor volume, superficial localization within the bone, and a latent tumoral behavior and is therefore predestined for minimal-invasive ablation. More active or even aggressive benign bone lesions such as aneurysmatic bone cysts or giant cell tumors and a curative therapeutic concept in singular metastatic bone disease are not suitable for this kind of treatment. Although there have been limited reports of successful radiofrequency therapy of osteoblastoma[24] and chondroblastoma,[25,26] long-term results and larger number of cases are yet to be critically awaited. An obvious disadvantage of this procedure is the lack of adequate sample gathering and subsequent histological verification as well as differentiation of the tumor. Moreover, large tumor formations are less likely to be removed completely by minimal-invasive procedures and higher rates of recurrence thus have to be expected.[27]

14.4.1.3 Amputations

Amputations are more common in malignant tumors of the foot compared to other anatomical sites because functional impairment is less the more distal the amputation is done. Although good results have been reported in limb salvage surgery, compromise in resection margins should not be accepted in foot and ankle tumors, especially, since many different amputation techniques are associated with acceptable functional outcome. Ray amputation of up to three lateral or medial rays leads to good functional results. Other amputation options include transmetatarsal, Lisfranc, Chopart, Boyd, Syme, or transtibial amputation. Figure 14.2 illustrates the case of a 48-year-old patient in whom a Boyd's amputation became necessary due to chondrosarcoma of the midfoot. With good functional result, the patient was able to go downhill skiing 6 months later.

14.4.2   *Nonsurgical Adjuvant Treatment*

Treatment of musculoskeletal tumors requires a multidisciplinary approach. Best results have been reported for specialized surgeons and tumor centers. Each patient should be discussed in interdisciplinary tumor board (with participation of specialized musculoskeletal tumor surgeon, oncologic radiologist, pathologist, radiotherapy specialist, oncology specialist, and plastic surgeon). Neoadjuvant and adjuvant treatment modalities like radiotherapy and chemotherapy have had a major impact on healing rates and long-term survival, especially in primary bone tumors like osteosarcoma and Ewing's sarcoma. In general, neoadjuvant radiotherapy and brachytherapy is indicated in high-grade malignant tumors with limited resection margins or with close contact to neurovascular structures. Preoperative radiation of soft tissue masses that are in direct contact to nerves and blood vessels or that penetrate compartment borders might allow "downgrading" and help to preserve important structures at definitive surgery. Lower doses of radiotherapy are used in the foot because of increased risks of side effects like fibrosis and stress fracture.

14.5   Most Common Entities

14.5.1   *Bone Tumors*

14.5.1.1   Benign

Benign bone tumors are much more common than malignant tumors of the foot and ankle with a rate of approximately 84% vs. 16% in specialized centers.[28] Slowly growing benign bone lesions are often recognized first after the occurrence of a pathologic fracture, after pain due to weakening of the bone with an impending fracture, or by chance. In addition to osteochondroma, which is the most common bone tumor, common foot and ankle lesions are giant cell tumors and intraosseous lipoma of the calcaneus. The most common benign bone tumors have been summarized in Table 14.5.

14.5.1.2   Malignant

Table 14.6 displays typical malignant bone tumors that occur in the foot and ankle. Osteosarcoma[29] and Ewing's sarcoma,[30] which are the most common primary malignant tumors are often misdiagnosed or delayed, since both represent highly variable lesions. Osteosarcomas of the foot occur in a slightly older age group than do osteosarcomas elsewhere. Metastases are the most common malignant lesions in bone. However, metastases of the foot are far less frequent, with foot lesions accounting

Table 14.5 Important benign bone tumors and tumor-like lesions of the foot and ankle

Tumor	Decade/age	Localization	X-ray	CT, MRI[a]	Resection	Recurrence/spreading	Important differential diagnoses
Giant cell tumor	2nd–5th	Distal tibia and fibula, tarsal bones	Intramedullary osteolytic changes, thin sclerotic margin, cortical thinning, pathologic fracture	T1–, T2+	Curettage and grafting; consider bone cement and secondary replacement by bone graft	High risk of recurrence (~10%); rarely pulmonary metastases	Aneurysmal bone cyst, giant cell reparative granuloma, metastasis, osteosarcoma, clear cell chondrosarcoma, multiple myeloma
Giant cell reparative granuloma/solid aneurysmal bone cyst	2nd	Metaphysis of small bones	Osteolytic, no perilesional sclerosis, well-defined margins, cortical thinning	T1–, T2+	Curettage and grafting; radiation therapy in recurrence	Heals with thorough curettage	Osteosarcoma, aneurysmal bone cyst, giant cell tumor
Aneurysmal bone cyst	2nd–3rd	Tubular and tarsal bones, eccentric	Osteolytic, cortical thinning or destruction, no or thin sclerosis	Internal septation, gadolinium enhancement of septa, fluid levels	Curettage and grafting; consider bone cement and secondary replacement by bone graft	High risk of recurrence; often secondary to other tumors; send all tissues to pathology	Chondroblastoma, giant cell tumor, simple bone cyst, osteosarcoma, malignancies
Osteochondroma/osteocartilaginous exostosis	1st–2nd	Tubular bones; not in tarsal bones	Cancellous bone of exostosis blends with cancellous bone of metaphysis, thin outer cortex: pedunculated or broad base; bowing of adjacent bones	Cartilage cap (>2 cm in thickness suspicious for malignancy); T1–, T2+	In cases with mechanical irritation: Marginal excision of the exostosis at the base; complete removal of cartilage component!	Consider multiple hereditary exostoses with higher risk of malignant transformation; risk of recurrence if exostosis is resected in child age	Chondrosarcoma, osteosarcoma, parosteal reactive ossifications
Chondroma/enchondroma	2nd–6th	Tubular bones and tarsals	Pathologic fracture; expansion of affected bone, cortical scalloping, central lysis with well-defined margins and calcifications	CT for cortical perforation; cartilage (T1–, T2+) and calcifications (T1–, T2–)	Rarely required; curettage and bone grafting	Transformation in a chondrosarcoma is controversial	Diagnosis doubtful if calcifications are missing; giant cell reparative granuloma, giant cell tumor, aneurysmal bone cyst, chondrosarcoma

Chondroblastoma	2nd–3rd	Tarsals >> metatarsals, distal tibia	Epiphyseal or small bones; eccentric, well-defined margins, lobulated, thin sclerosis	Parenchimatous, occasionally cystic; T1–, T2+	Curettage and bone grafting or cement, avoid opening joint	Send all tissues for histology; ~10% risk of recurrence (especially if joint is contaminated)	Clear cell chondrosarcoma, giant cell tumor, chondroma, Brodie's abscess
Osteoid osteoma	1st–3rd	Neck of talus, tarsals, phalanges, metatarsals	Eccentric, in or near cortex	CT with thin sections (1 mm) to define characteristic nidus with surrounding sclerosis; characteristic bone scan; highly vascular nidus in CT arteriography	Removal of nidus or percutaneous radiofrequency (histology rarely necessary)	Pain resolves immediately with removal of nidus; no recurrence if nidus is removed	Typical pain at night and early morning, relieve with aspirin or NSARs; osteoblastoma, sclerosing osteoperiostitis
Unicameral bone cyst	1st–2nd	Calcaneus, tubular bones, metaphyseal	Pathologic fracture, central osteolysis, cortical thinning and expansion, sclerosis	Liquid or fatty content, unicameral, sometimes few fibrous septa	Curettage, bone grafting		Aneurysmal bone cyst, fibrous dysplasia

[a]T1+ = high signal on T1-weighted MRI images; T1+/– = intermediate signal intensity; T1– = low signal intensity; T2+ = high signal on T2-weighted images; T2+/– = intermediate signal intensity; T2– = low signal intensity; contrast+ = signal enhancement on gadolinium-enhanced MRI; contrast– = no signal enhancement after gadolinium

Table 14.6 Most common malignant bone tumors of the foot and ankle

Tumor	Decade/age	Localization	X-ray	MRI[a]	Resection	Adjuvant therapy	Spreading	Differential diagnoses
Osteosarcoma	2nd–4th	Tarsals, exceptional in tubular bones and metatarsals; 0.2–2% of all osteosarcomas	Intramedullary, breaching cortex, faded edges, periosteal reactions, both radiolucencies and osseous radiodensity	T1–, T2+, best to show intramedullary tumor extension	Radical	Neoadjuvant and adjuvant chemotherapy	Pulmonary metastases	MFH (malignant fibrous histiocytoma), giant cell tumor, Ewing's sarcoma, lymphoma
Chondrosarcoma	4th–7th	Tarsals and metatarsals	Central osteolysis with signs of slow but permeative growth, "popcorn-like" granular radiodensities due to calcifications and ossifications, scalloping of inner cortex	Cartilage cap >20 mm, lobular pattern of the tumor, T1–, T2+	Wide resection or amputation	Ineffective, radical resection is key	Pulmonary metastases, high rate of local recurrence	Osteochondroma, synovial chondromatosis, chondroblastic osteosarcoma
Ewing's sarcoma (PNET)	1st–3rd	Rare in the foot, localization anywhere possible	Permeative, poorly defined "moth-eaten" and "rotten-wood" osteolysis, often prominent extraosseous mass in flat bones	T1–, T2+, best to study intramedullary tumor extension	Radical resection	Neoadjuvant and adjuvant chemotherapy, radiation	Pulmonary, skeletal and lymphatic (lymph nodes) metastases	Osteosarcoma, lymphoma, mesenchymal chondrosarcoma, osteomyelitis, metastatic neuroblastoma, eosinophilic granuloma

| Metastases | > 5th | Rare in foot and ankle, incidence decreases from proximally to distally | Osteolytic (e.g., kidney, lung, thyroid), osteoblastic (e.g., prostate & bronchial carcinoma) or mixed (breast). Indistinct borders, permeated or eroded cortex with little or no periosteal reaction | T1−, T2+, contrast+ | Intralesional, wide or radical | Radiation, chemotherapy | Hematogeneous, dissemination to multiple skeletal and extraskeletal sites possible | Multiple myeloma, osteolytic sarcomas, lymphoma |

PNET Peripheral neuroendothelial tumor

[a]T1+ = high signal on T1-weighted MRI images, T1+/− = intermediate signal intensity, T1− = low signal intensity; T2+ = high signal on T2-weighted images, T2+/− = intermediate signal intensity, T2− = low signal intensity; contrast+ = signal enhancement on gadolinium-enhanced MRI; contrast− = no signal enhancement after gadolinium

for less than 1% of bony metastases, and lung tumors being the most common[31] (Fig. 14.3).

14.5.2 Soft Tissue Tumors

14.5.2.1 Benign

A soft tissue tumor of the foot and ankle (Table 14.7) has to be considered malignant until proved otherwise, since most malignant soft tissue masses can mimic benign lesions. Clinical characteristics like pain, size of the lesion, and symptom duration are not reliable parameters to distinguish benign and malignant tumors.[32]

The ganglion is the most common mass in the foot and ankle and represents a mucoid cystic degeneration of a joint capsule or a tendon sheath rather than a true neoplasm. Clinically, ganglia are palpable as a firm mass with predisposition to areas of increased mechanical stress. Transillumination is a helpful tool to confirm the presence of a cystic lesion, although further diagnostic measures should be taken if there is any doubt. Diagnosis can be confirmed by needle aspiration, and approximately 50% of ganglia can be adequately treated with the aspiration technique, but MRI is the imaging method of choice. Recurrence of the cyst or failure to aspirate thick fluid may require surgical excision of the ganglion, and all resected tissue should be sent for histopathological workup.

Plantar fibromatosis is the most common real neoplasm of the foot, and bilateral occurrence is common.[33] Clinically, firm cords of small nodules can be palpated in the plantar surface of the foot. Since the neoplasm is in firm contact with the plantar fascia, significant pain can be present with weight-bearing. In symptomatic patients with extensive fibromatosis, resection of the nodules together with the overlying skin and fascia is recommended – even if skin grafting might become necessary – to reduce the risk of recurrence associated with the close contact of fibromatosis and skin.

14.5.2.2 Malignant

Synovial sarcoma is the most common malignant soft tissue tumor of the foot and ankle (Table 14.8). Diagnosis is often delayed, with an average of 21 months between the onset of symptoms and the final diagnosis.[34] The peak incidence of synovial sarcoma is observed in the second to fifth decade. Diagnosis is often challenging since synovial sarcoma can mimic other entities and clinical features are unspecific, with a slowly or rapidly growing, indolent or painful, firm and fixed mass.[35] Risk of pulmonary metastases as well as lymphatic spread is high.

Although generally considered a very rare condition with only 1% of all soft tissue sarcomas, clear cell sarcoma demonstrated a special predilection for the foot with 43% of all clear cell sarcomas involving the foot.[36,37] Similarly, approximately

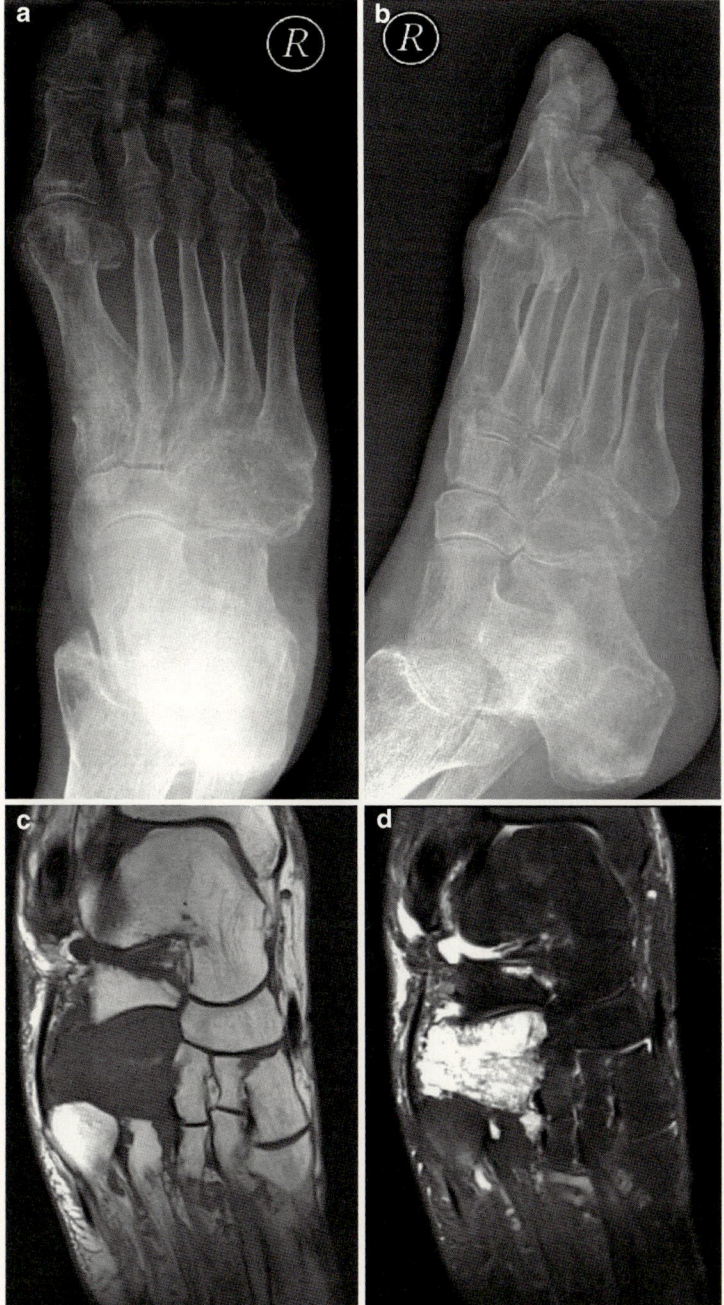

Fig. 14.3 Palliative treatment of a painful and immobilizing metastasis of a lung cancer in the cuboid of an 81-year-old patient with disseminated metastatic disease. Therapy by intralesional resection and filling with bone cement. Postoperative radiotherapy was done to control local tumor recurrence

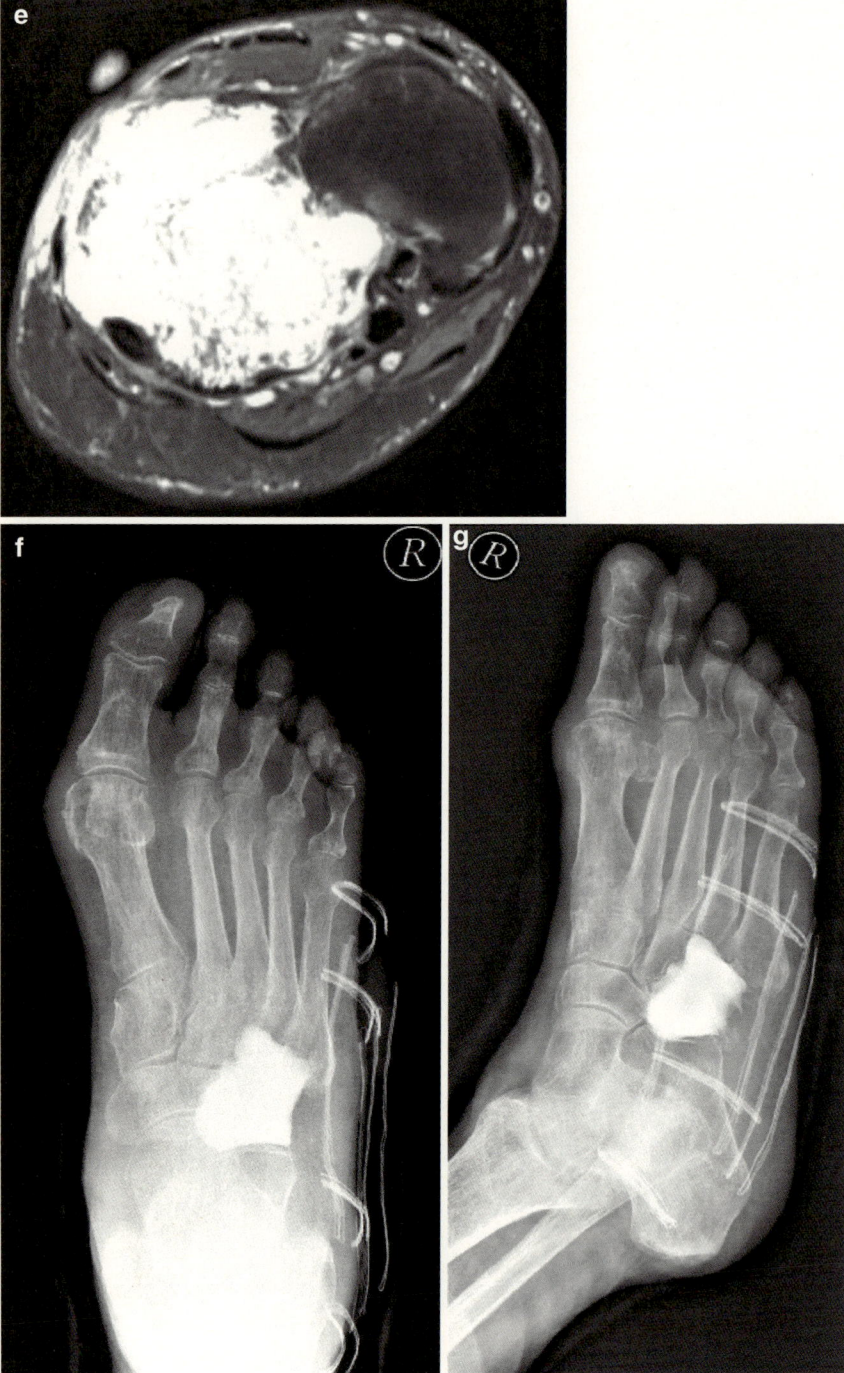

Fig. 14.3 (continued)

Table 14.7 Most common benign soft tissue tumors of the foot and ankle

Tumor	Decade/age	Clinical presentation	X-ray	MRI[a]	Resection	Recurrence/ spreading	Differential diagnoses
Ganglion (= mucous cyst)	All, preferably adult age	Swelling, possible fluctuation, firm on palpation; positive transillumination	Not visible on plain x-rays	Rounded & sharply defined, homogenous and sometimes multilobulated lesion; T1−, T2+, no contrast enhancement	Aspiration technique, marginal resection	Recurrence after aspiration	Synovial cyst, intramuscular myxoma
Lipoma	All, 5th–7th	Painless, soft swelling	Roundish mass, homogeneous translucency	Signal intensity of normal fat, no contrast enhancement, thin fibromuscular traversing septa	Marginal excision	Rare	Well-differentiated liposarcoma, myxoid liposarcoma
Fibromatosis	Any age, more frequent from 2nd–3rd decade	Diffuse or nodular mass, sometimes painful, muscular retraction, limitations in joint function, poorly defined borders	Angiography shows a persistent tumor blush	Highly variable MR imaging pattern, depending on amount of cellular and collagen tissue. Common heterogeneous pattern, with intermediate signal intensity; T1+ and T2+ in hypercellular areas, T1− and T2− in hypocellular areas.	Observation; complete resection of plantar fascia, if necessary with skin	Common if not completely excised	May be accompanied by Dupuytren contractures and Peyronie's disease; fibrosarcoma

(continued)

Table 14.7 (continued)

Tumor	Decade/age	Clinical presentation	X-ray	MRI[a]	Resection	Recurrence/spreading	Differential diagnoses
Pigmented villonodular synovitis (PVNS)	3rd–6th, exceptional in children	Soft to firm on palpation, indolent growth, diffuse or villonodular manifestation; macroscopically yellowish-brown synovium	Bony erosions and subchondral cysts, sharp-edged cortical scalloping	Heterogeneous lobulated masses with contrast enhancement on T1, low signal intensity on both T1 and T2 due to hemosiderin deposits	Complete synovectomy	Common if not completely excised	Synovial hemangioma, traumatic hemarthros, synovial sarcoma
Giant cell tumor of the tendon sheath	3rd–5th	Moderate pain, swelling, tenderness	Typical shell of radiodensity due to reactive ossification at the periphery of the lesion	T1−, T2+	Marginal	Rare	Solid aneurysmal bone cyst, bone metastases, brown tumor of primary hyperparathyroidism
Fibroma (FTS)	3rd–5th	Firm, painless, well-circumscribed and sometimes lobulated, size between 1–2 cm, attached to a tendon or tendon sheath	Usually not visible on plain x-rays	T1−, T2+/−, peripheral contrast enhancement on gadolinium-enhanced MRI	Marginal	Rare	Giant cell tumor of tendon sheaths, nodular fasciitis, tendosynovial chondromatosis

Benign schwannoma (neurilemoma)	3rd–6th	Sharp pain on percussion, radiating distally, slow tumor growth	Small neurilemomas are not visible on plain x-rays, large lesions may appear as radiopaque formations	Homogeneous and isointense to muscle on T1, T2+, moderate enhancement on contrast; large neurilemomas can show inhomogeneous consistency due to hemorrhage, necrosis, and calcification	Longitudinal intracapsular resection[b]	Rare	Neurofibroma, neurofibrosarcoma, hamartoma
Hemangioma	3rd–6th	Deep-seated mass, firm on palpation and painless; changing in size, intermittent pain	Calcifications on plain x-rays possible; angiography shows high vascularity, diffuse capillary blush in the mass, and arteriovenous shunting	Fatty and vascular content; T1+, T2+, strong enhancement after gadolinium	Wide margins as size seems to correlate with malignancy	Common in infiltrating lesions	Sarcoma NOS; synovial sarcoma, mesenchymal chondrosarcoma

[a] T1+ = high signal on T1-weighted MRI images, T1+/− = intermediate signal intensity, T1− = low signal intensity; T2+ = high signal on T2-weighted images, T2+/− = intermediate signal intensity, T2− = low signal intensity; contrast+ = signal enhancement on gadolinium-enhanced MRI; contrast− = no signal enhancement after gadolinium

[b] Longitudinal intracapsular resection with preservation of surrounding nerve fibers (one fiber is always attached to the tumor and has to be excised)

Table 14.8 Most common malignant soft tissue sarcomas of the foot and ankle

Tumor	Decade/age	Clinical presentation	X-ray	MRI[a]	Resection	Adjuvant therapy	Spreading	Differential diagnoses
Synovial sarcoma	2nd–5th	Deep-seated tumor, mostly para-articular, slowly growing within years, pain and tenderness	Calcifications and ossifications may be present (25%);superficial bone erosions, periosteal reaction	Inhomogeneous, T1+/−, T2+, contrast+, triple-signal pattern on T2	Wide or radical	Radiotherapy	Lymphatic, hematogeneous	Ganglion, synovial cyst, PVNS, synovial chondromatosis, clear cell sarcoma, myositis ossificans
Malignant melanoma	2nd–4th	Growth of lesion, deepening pigmentation and ulceration of nevi	Negative	T1+, T2+/−	Wide resection and skin grafting, sentinel lymph node biopsy	Chemotherapy, immunotherapy	Mainly lymphatic	Nevi
Clear cell sarcoma	2nd–3rd	Deep-seated tumor without involvement of the overlying skin; unspecific slow growth	Radiopaque density in case of a large tumor	T1+/−, T2+/−, contrast+	Wide or radical with regional lymph node dissection[b]	Chemotherapy, radiotherapy in case of positive lymph nodes	Mainly lymphatic	Synovial sarcoma, giant cell tumor of the tendon sheaths, metastasis of a melanoma, malignant peripheral nerve sheath tumor; spindle cell melanoma

Epitheloid sarcoma	3rd–4th	Superficial or deeply seated nodule, indolent course, ulcerated skin	Rarely erosion of adjacent bone and/or stippling calcifications	Poorly defined limits, central necrosis	Wide or radical	Radiotherapy	Lymphatic and hematogenous	Chronic inflammatory process, nodular fasciitis, synovial sarcoma
Fibrosarcoma	3rd–8th	Deep soft tissue single roundish mass, firm constancy, usually slow growth	Rarely calcifications and/or erosion of adjacent bone	T1−, T2+, contrast+	Wide or radical	Radio- and chemotherapy with moderate effectiveness	Pulmonary, skeletal, and hepatic metastases common; rarely lymphatic metastases	Sarcoma NOS, malignant peripheral nerve sheaths tumor, leiomyosarcoma, aggressive fibromatosis

[a]T1+ = high signal on T1-weighted MRI images, T1+/− = intermediate signal intensity, T1− = low signal intensity; T2+ = high signal on T2-weighted images, T2+/− = intermediate signal intensity, T2− = low signal intensity; contrast+ = signal enhancement on gadolinium-enhanced MRI; contrast− = no signal enhancement after gadolinium

[b]Sentinel lymph node biopsy for clear cell sarcoma is currently under investigation

31% of all malignant melanomas have been reported to occur at the foot and deserve special consideration in clinical practice.

Squamous cell carcinomas (SCC) of sinus tracts (Marjolin's ulcers) are rare malignant tumors that occur in patients with chronic infections (e.g., osteomyelitis), and represent malignant degeneration of epithelial cells within the sinus tracts.[38] SCC may metastasize rapidly and should be considered particularly if chronic drainage changes to a blood-tinged character. Radical excision or amputation becomes necessary.

14.6 Summary

Although tumors of the foot and ankle are considered uncommon, previous studies have shown an incidence that is consistent with the amount of body mass of the foot and ankle region. In spite of early notice of masses in the foot and ankle due to the confined anatomic areas, diagnosis is often delayed due to late presentation of patients and initial misdiagnosis or neglect. High vigilance to recognize suspicious masses is necessary for the general foot and ankle surgeon. Further diagnostic procedures have to be taken to definitively determine a specific diagnosis. In addition to radiography, MRI represents the method of choice in evaluation of foot tumors. Unfortunately, malignant tumors can also arise with nonaggressive imaging features. Diagnostic errors can be avoided if any lesion that cannot be specifically diagnosed is regarded as potentially malignant until proved otherwise. Biopsies and further treatment should be planned or performed by specialized centers since errors in biopsies often negatively influence outcome and prognosis. Treatment is done after tumor grading and staging with wide resection being the appropriate form of resection in most malignant tumors. No compromise should be accepted in surgical margins, and amputation should be performed if adequate local resection is not possible. Neoadjuvant and adjuvant treatment options like radiotherapy and chemotherapy have significantly improved function and survival after treatment of malignant tumors. Every patient with a musculoskeletal tumor should first be discussed in an interdisciplinary tumor board.[13]

References

1. Dahlin DC, Unni KK, editors. *Bone tumors: general aspects and data on 8,542 cases*. 4th editors. Springfield: Charles C. Thomas; 1986.
2. Kransdorf MJ. Benign soft-tissue tumors in a large referral population: distribution of specific diagnoses by age, sex, and location. *AJR Am J Roentgenol*. 1995;164:395-402.
3. Gerrand CH, Wunder JS, Kandel RA, et al. The influence of anatomic location on functional outcome in lower-extremity soft-tissue sarcoma. *Ann Surg Oncol*. 2005;11:476-82.
4. Chou LB, Ho YY, Malawer MM. Tumors of the foot and ankle: experience with 153 cases. *Foot Ankle Int*. 2009;30:836-41.

5. Ozdemir MH, Yildiz Y, Yilmaz C, Saglik Y. Tumors of the foot and ankle: analysis of 196 cases. *J Foot Ankle Surg.* 1997;36:403-8.
6. Albreski D, Sloan SB. Melanoma of the feet: misdiagnosed and misunderstood. *Clin Dermatol.* 2009;27(6):556-63.
7. Bancroft LW, Peterson JJ, Kransdorf MJ. Imaging of soft tissue lesions of the foot and ankle. *Radiol Clin North Am.* 2008;46(6):1093-103.
8. Llauger J, Palmer J, Monill JM, Franquet T, Bagué S, Rosón N. MR imaging of benign soft-tissue masses of the foot and ankle. *Radiographics.* 1998;18(6):1481-98.
9. Campanacci M, ed. *Bone and soft tissue tumors.* 2nd ed. Padova: Piccin Nuova Libraria and Wien, New York: Springer; 1999.
10. Johnson PT, Fayad LM, Frassica FJ, Fishman EK. Computed tomography of the bones of the foot: neoplastic disease. J Comput Assist Tomogr. 2009;33(3):436-43.
11. De Schepper AM, De Beuckeleer L, Vandevenne J, Somville J. Magnetic resonance imaging of soft tissue tumors. Eur Radiol. 2000;10:213-22.
12. Rhee JH, Lewis RB, Murphey MD. Primary osseous tumors of the foot and ankle. Magn Reson Imaging Clin N Am. 2008;16(1):71-91.
13. Waldt S, Rechl H, Rummeny EJ, Woertler K. Imaging of benign and malignant soft tissue masses of the foot. Eur Radiol. 2003;13(5):1125-36.
14. Woertler K. Soft tissue masses in the foot and ankle: characteristics on MR Imaging. Semin Musculoskelet Radiol. 2005;9(3):227-42.
15. Mankin HJ, Lange TA, Spanier SS. The hazards of biopsy in patients with malignant primary bone and soft-tissue tumors. J Bone Joint Surg Am. 1982;64:1121-7.
16. Mankin HJ, Mankin CJ, Simon MA. The hazards of the biopsy, revisited. Members of the Musculoskeletal Tumor Society. J Bone Joint Surg Am. 1996;78:656-63.
17. Huch K, Röderer G, Ulmar B, Reichel H. CT-guided interventions in orthopedics. Arch Orthop Trauma Surg. 2007;127:677-683.
18. Enneking WF. A system of staging musculoskeletal neoplasms. Clin Orthop Relat Res. 1986;204:9-24.
19. Capanna R, Sudanese A, Baldini N, Campanacci M. Phenol as an adjuvant in the control of local recurrence of benign neoplasms of bone treated by curettage. Ital J Orthop Traumatol. 1985;11(3):381-8.
20. Lack W, Lang S, Brand G. Necrotizing effect of phenol on normal tissues and on tumors. A study on postoperative and cadaver specimens. Acta Orthop Scand. 1994;65(3):351-4.
21. Malawer MM, Dunham W. Cryosurgery and acrylic cementation as surgical adjuncts in the treatment of aggressive (benign) bone tumors. Clin Orthop Relat Res. 1991;262:42-57.
22. Ruiz Santiago F, Del Mar Castellano García M, Guzmán Álvarez L, Martínez Montes JL, Ruiz García M, Tristán Fernández JM. Percutaneous treatment of bone tumors by radiofrequency thermal ablation. Curr Rev Musculoskelet Med. 2009;2(1):43-50.
23. Volkmer D, Sichlau M, Rapp TB. The use of radiofrequency ablation in the treatment of musculoskeletal tumors. J Am Acad Orthop Surg. 2009;17(12):737-43.
24. Simon CJ, Dupuy DE. Percutaneous minimally invasive therapies in the treatment of bone tumors: thermal ablation. Semin Musculoskelet Radiol. 2006;10(2):137-44. Epub 2006 Apr 5.
25. Erickson JK, Rosenthal DI, Zaleske DJ, Gebhardt MC, Cates JM. Primary treatment of chondroblastoma with percutaneous radio-frequency heat ablation: report of three cases. Radiology. 2001;221(2):463-8.
26. Rybak LD, Rosenthal DI, Wittig JC. Chondroblastoma: radiofrequency ablation – alternative to surgical resection in selected cases. Radiology. 2009;251(2):599-604.
27. Ahrar K. The role and limitations of radiofrequency ablation in treatment of bone and soft tissue tumors. Curr Oncol Rep. 2004;6(4):315-20.
28. Murari TM, Callaghan JJ, Berrey BH Jr, Sweet DE. Primary benign and malignant osseous neoplasms of the foot. Foot Ankle. 1989;10:68-80.
29. Fox C, Husain ZS, Shah MB, Lucas DR, Saleh HA. Chondroblastic osteosarcoma of the cuboid: a literature review and report of a rare case. J Foot Ankle Surg. 2009;48(3):388-93.

30. Berliner RA, Guadara J, Adelman H, Conforti J, Uhm K. Extraosseous Ewing's sarcoma in the foot. J Foot Ankle Surg. 1995;34(3):301-4.
31. El Ghazaly SA, DeGroot H III. Metastases to bones of the foot: a case series, review of the literature, and a systematic approach to diagnosis. Foot Ankle Spec. 2008;1(6):338-43.
32. Kirby EJ, Shereff MJ, Lewis MM. Soft-tissue tumors and tumor-like lesions of the foot. An analysis of eighty-three cases. J Bone Joint Surg Am. 1989;71:621-6.
33. Robbin MR, Murphey MD, Temple HT, Kransdorf MJ, Choi JJ. Imaging of musculoskeletal fibromatosis. Radiographics. 2001;21(3):585-600.
34. Brewster MB, Power D, Sumathi VP. Delayed diagnosis of synovial sarcoma of the foot. Orthopedics. 2008;31(2):175.
35. Scully SP, Temple HT, Harrelson JM. Synovial sarcoma of the foot and ankle. Clin Orthop Relat Res. 1999;364:220-6.
36. Malchau SS, Hayden J, Hornicek F, Mankin HJ. Clear cell sarcoma of soft tissues. J Surg Oncol. 2007;95(6):519-22.
37. Sara AS, Evans HL, Benjamin RS. Malignant melanoma of soft parts (clear cell sarcoma). A study of 17 cases, with emphasis on prognostic factors. Cancer. 1990;65(2):367-74.
38. Potter BK, Pitcher JD Jr, Adams SC, Temple HT. Squamous cell carcinoma of the foot. Foot Ankle Int. 2009;30:517-23.

Chapter 15
Postoperative Physical Therapy for Foot and Ankle Surgery

Amol Saxena and Allison N. Granot

Evidence-based studies for foot and ankle rehabilitation mainly focus on preventative and nonsurgical rehabilitation of Achilles and ankle injuries. Postoperative protocols have not been studied for many of the surgical procedures in this text. Only ankle stabilization surgery has been studied comparing 6 weeks of below-knee casting versus earlier range of motion (ROM) with shorter periods of casting. Karlsson et al. studied a randomized group of patients undergoing surgery for chronic (greater than 6 months) ankle instability and found an earlier return to sports and work when patient began controlled ankle ROM at 3 weeks post-surgery and formalized strengthening at 5 weeks, as compared to those who started physical therapy after 6 weeks of below-knee casting.[1] We consider this study a good basis for all types of foot and ankle procedures and therefore use it as justification for our various protocols, i.e., initiation of active ROM at 3 weeks post-surgery and some form of strengthening by 5–6 weeks post-operative, (and often earlier).

When reviewing other studies, postoperative care is often mentioned by authors; however, they state "generically" that physical therapy "is initiated" or "is performed" but do not say exactly what is performed and which modalities or exercises are used. Therefore, the aim of this chapter is to give examples of exercises that we currently utilize for most of the postoperative protocols in our clinics. It is our practice to have patients initiate "home" exercise regimen daily with icing, elevating, and early active ROM exercises even prior to initial evaluation by the therapist, generally at 3 weeks post-operation.

A. Saxena, D.P.M. (✉)
Department of Sports Medicine, PAFMG-Palo Alto Division,
Clark Bldg., 3rd Flr, 795 El Camino Real, Palo Alto, CA 94301, USA
e-mail: heysax@aol.com

A.N. Granot, P.T., M.P.T., O.C.S., C.S.C.S.
Department of Physical Therapy, Palo Alto Medical Foundation,
Palo Alto, CA, USA

A. Saxena (ed.), *Special Procedures in Foot and Ankle Surgery*,
DOI 10.1007/978-1-4471-4103-7_15, © Springer-Verlag London 2013

Fig. 15.1 Stationary bike with cast boot

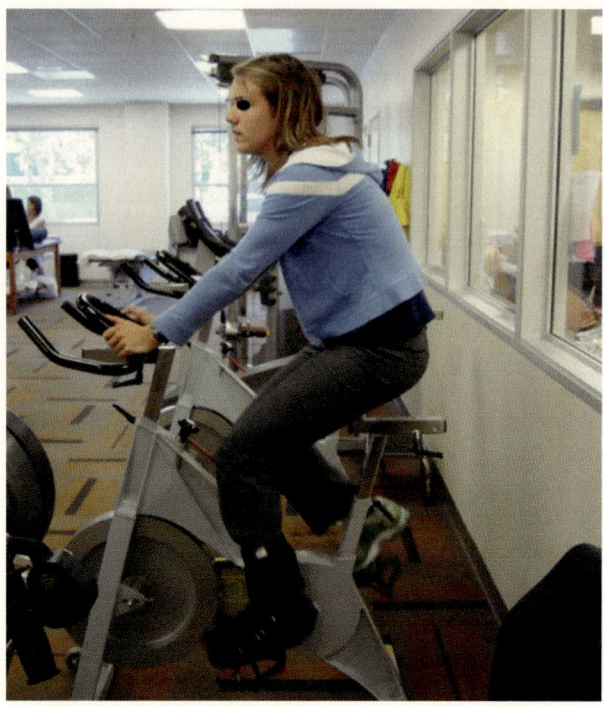

Typical immediate postoperative home instructions include the following:

- Ice for 15 min with an ice pack behind or above the knee (because the surgical dressings insulate and do not allow for vasoconstriction) 4×/day.[2]
- Icing directly with nonchemical ice packs (ice cubes in water) or ice bucket immersion can occur as determined by wound healing and the need for postoperative dressings. Caution with diabetic and neuropathic patients is needed.
- Elevate operative limb, but not above heart (avoids elevation ischemia),[3] and no direct pressure on surgical site such as resting on the heel region after retrocalcaneal surgery.
- When tolerated due to pain and surgically stable, stationary bicycling with the cast or boot on, using the heel region on the pedal, is permitted 15–30 min/day (this can range from less than one to up to 6 weeks post-surgery) (Fig. 15.1).
- When stable and suitable healing has taken place, ankle and foot range-of-motion exercises are initiated using a towel (this can range from less than one to up to 6 weeks post-surgery) (Fig. 15.2).

Formalized physical therapy visits are initiated generally from 2 to 12 weeks post-surgery with an evaluation by a physical therapist.[4-12] In the United States, patients are typically seen 2–3 times/week. A detailed assessment is performed by the physical therapist including history of the injury and surgical procedure, which regions should be protected and not be mobilized (such as with arthrodesis procedures), location of hardware or implants, and generalized situation of the patient.

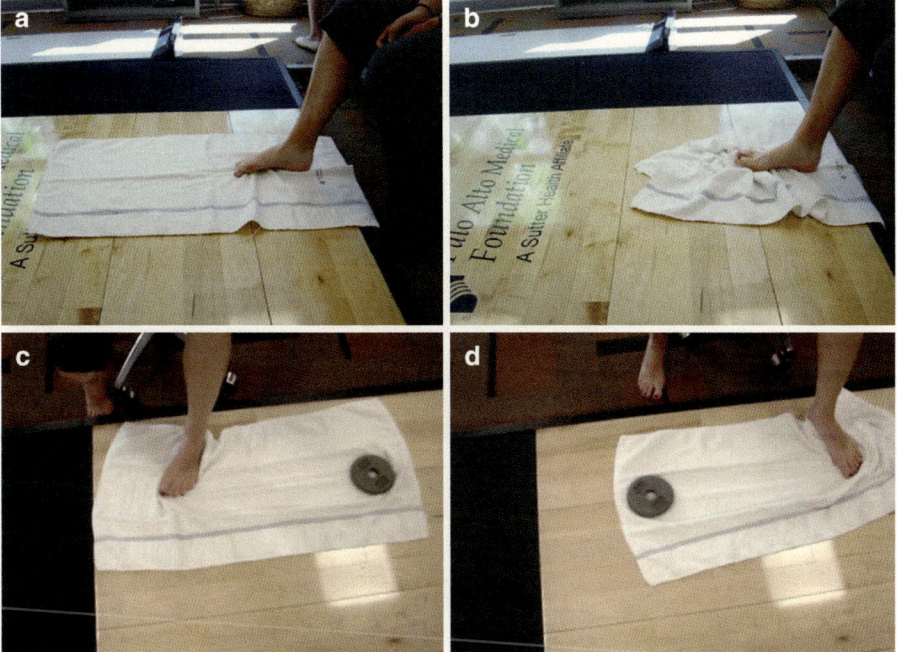

Fig. 15.2 Towel curls for toe (**a**) flexion and (**b**) extension; (**c, d**) Towel "swishes" for ankle inversion/eversion

Table 15.1 Assessment by physical therapist

1. History of injury, date, and type of surgery
2. Length of protection with boot, i.e., when can patient get out of the boot "OOB"
3. Length of protection due to healing such as tendon, fusion site, or bone graft
4. Location of hardware and implants
5. Restriction of motion to be maintained such as with arthrodesis procedures
6. Patients home, work, and activities including sports
7. Degree of pain, swelling, warmth, color of surgical site, presence of external sutures.
8. Disability (needs assistive aids), aggravating and easing factors
9. Patient's current amount of activity, icing, and exercising
10. Patient's goals/sports/occupation
11. Current functional status: ROM, strength, gait, balance, and proprioception
12. Surgeon's expected return to activity "RTA" for procedure
13. Consider objective foot scoring device (i.e., American Orthopedic Foot and Ankle Society, Foot and Ankle Assessment Module, Maryland Foot Score)

Note should be taken as to timing of protection with boots and braces. An appreciation for the stage of the healing must be understood before the therapist determines the effective treatment plan. Different procedures will require strategically timed protection/pain control, while others will call for early motion (Table 15.1).

Fig. 15.3 Game Ready™ ice device and elevation

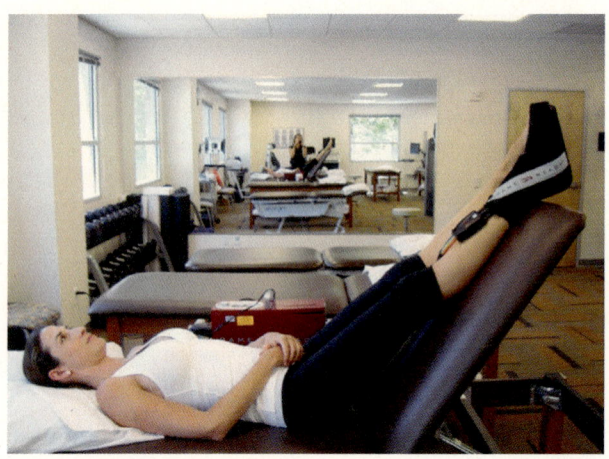

Fig. 15.4 Kinesio™ tape for ankle swelling

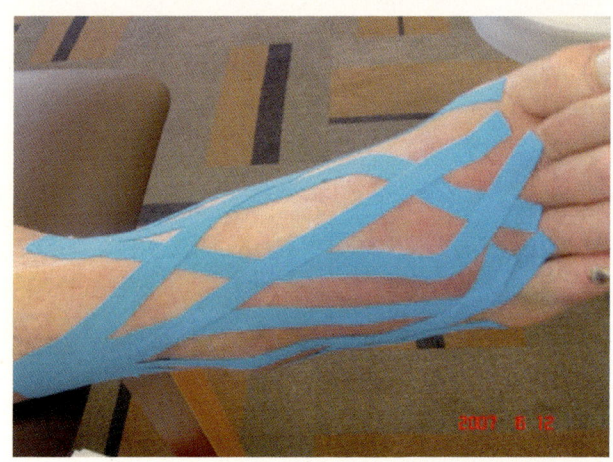

Modalities used postoperatively (such as ultrasound, phono- and iontophoresis, and interferential current) have not been critically studied, and therefore not often used post-surgically in our clinics. Though use of electrical stimulation and ultrasound is common and may be helpful, (for swelling and adhesions, respectively) firmly established protocols have not been performed. Postoperative edema reduction can be enhanced by ice compression devices such as the GameReady™ and Aircast Cryo Cuff™ in a controlled setting (Fig. 15.3).[2] Taping techniques such as Kinesio™ tape for edema control and ankle protection can be helpful (Fig. 15.4). Lymph massage has been proven as helpful and is utilized as needed. This is particularly helpful in patients having multiple surgeries, incisions, and venous stasis.[10]

Ergonomic equipment such as stationary bikes and elliptical trainers is utilized at appropriate times. Strengthening programs have primarily been studied post-ankle sprain and for nonsurgical treatment of Achilles tendonopathy often, withgood success. The eccentric programs for Achilles tendonopathy have not

Fig. 15.5 Runner on
Alter-G™ treadmill

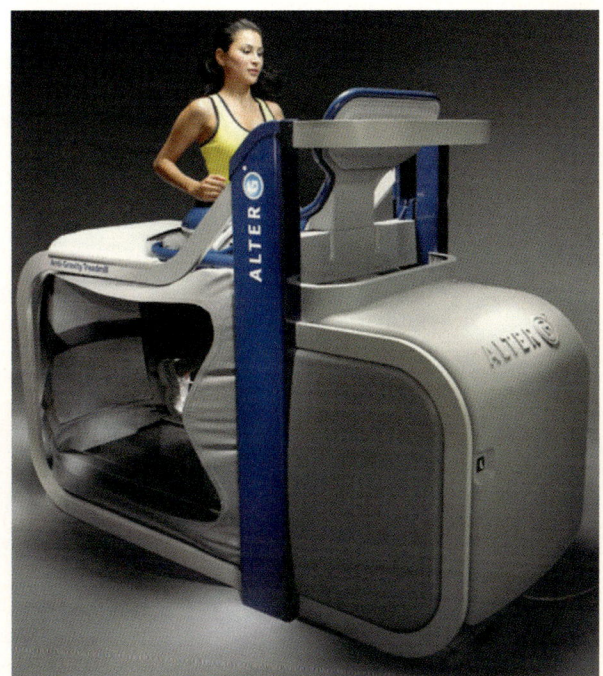

been studied post-surgery. We therefore initiate rehabilitation with concentric strengthening programs post-surgery.[7,8,13,14] Eccentric exercises can be utilized in the later phases of rehabilitation after gait is normalized.[15-18] We also recommend hip stabilization exercises as recent studies point to hip weakness as a factor in ankle injuries.[18-20]

A recent device we have found helpful for lower extremity strengthening and rehabilitation is the "Alter-G™ Treadmill" (Alter-G, Milpitas, CA USA) (Fig. 15.5). This specialized treadmill allows adjustment and reduction of bodyweight such that if a patient is unable to perform lower extremity tasks such as heel raises or walking, the machine can be calibrated to allow them to do so. In our clinic, we typically reduce the body weight 30–50% and initiate single-legged concentric heel raises and restore normal gait (Table 15.2).[8]

15.1   Rehabilitation Programs Used for Ankle Procedures

This program is followed after ankle procedures, i.e., Achilles, posterior tibial tendon reconstruction procedures, peroneal tendon repair, ankle stabilization or fracture repair, and osteochondral defect repair (with bone graft) or chondral lesion (microfracture).

Active ROM is allowed at 3 weeks (generally after cast removal) working on plantarflexion and inversion/eversion with a towel (Fig. 15.6). A below-knee cast

Table 15.2 Concentric heel raise progression (on successive days if pain-free):

3 sets of 10 repetitions single-legged, pain-free
4 sets of 10 repetitions single-legged, pain-free
5 sets of 10 repetitions single-legged, pain-free
3 sets of 15 repetitions single-legged, pain-free
4 sets of 15 repetitions single-legged, pain-free
5 sets of 15 repetitions single-legged, pain-free
3 sets of 20 repetitions single-legged, pain-free
4 sets of 20 repetitions single-legged, pain-free
5 sets of 20 repetitions single-legged, pain-free
3 sets of 25 repetitions single-legged, pain-free
4 sets of 25 repetitions single-legged, pain-free
5 sets of 25 repetitions single-legged, pain-free

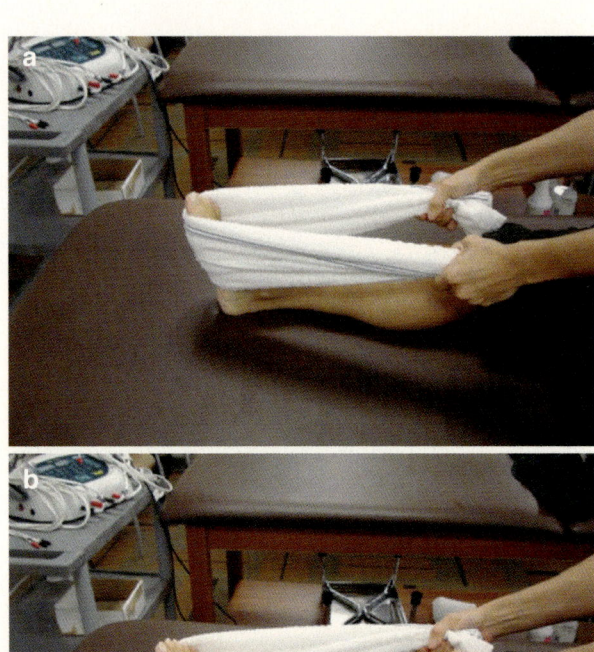

Fig. 15.6 (a, b) Plantarflexion exercises with towel

boot that is maintained for immobilization is removed for exercise. Patients may be non-weight-bearing from 2 to 6 weeks depending on the procedure. Formal physical therapy is initiated between 8 and 10 weeks ("slower healing" procedures start later), though cross-training on a stationary bike is allowed with the boot/cast

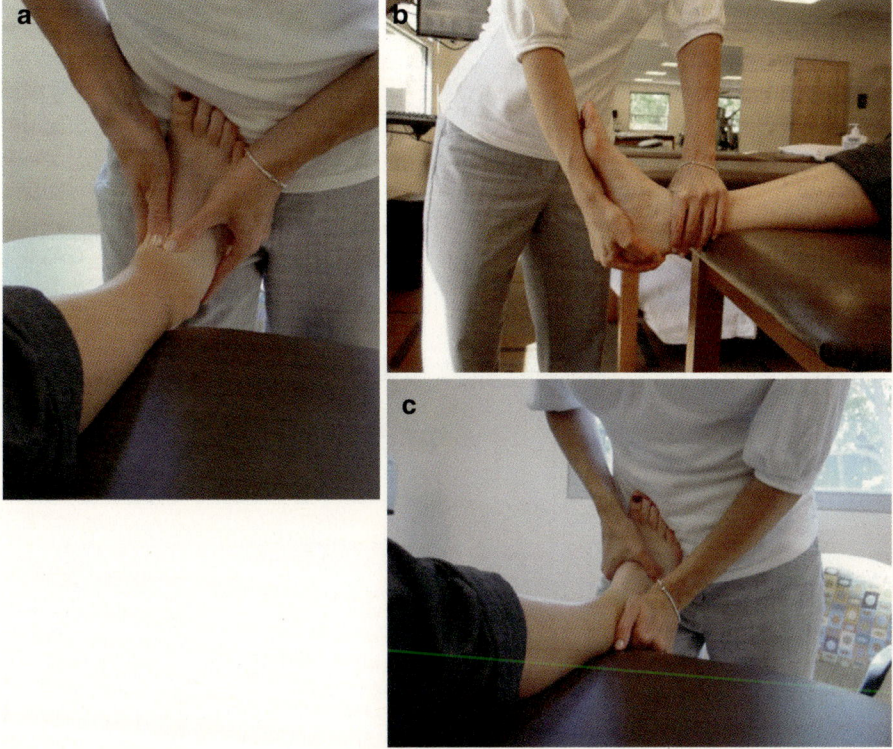

Fig. 15.7 (**a–c**) Distraction with anterior and posterior "glides" (mobilization) of the subtalar joint

(with the heel on the pedal) as soon as 1 week post-surgery.[6,7] Swimming is allowed (without flip-turns) between 4 and 6 weeks post-surgery. Physical therapy includes progressive strengthening with visits on a bi-weekly basis with a physical therapist. It should be noted that stretching, thought to be appropriate post-injury, may have a limited role post-surgery. It must be done under proper supervision.[14,21]

15.1.1 Phase 1

15.1.1.1 Weeks 8–10 Post-surgery

- Initial evaluation;
- Protected mobilization, i.e., dorsiflexion to tolerance with Achilles procedures, no eversion beyond neutral with posterior tibial/medial stabilization, no inversion beyond neutral with peroneal/lateral stabilization procedures. Also, note, no mobilization of fused joints; (Figs. 15.7 and 15.8).

Fig. 15.8 Mobilization (PA glide) of the subtalar joint

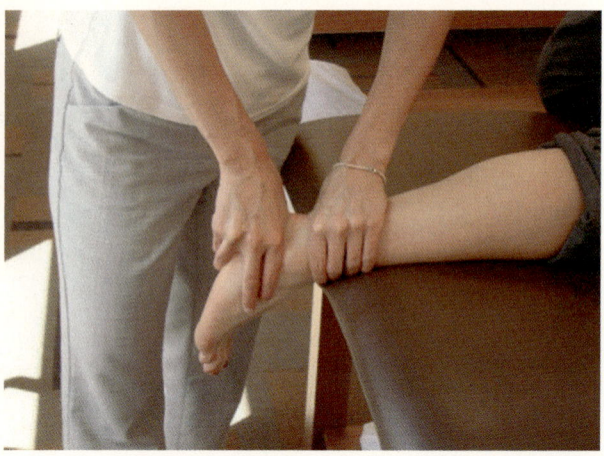

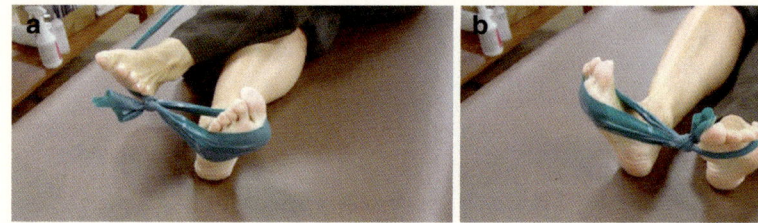

Fig. 15.9 (**a**) Ankle/STJ inversion (*right foot*) and (**b**) Ankle/STJ eversion (*right foot*) with elastic tubing

- Non-weight-bearing ankle strengthening with surgical tubing (inversion, eversion, dorsiflexion and plantarflexion) (Fig. 15.9).
- Cross-friction massage to incision (once fully healed) and posterior ankle (Fig. 15.10).
- Seated and standing calf stretch (Fig. 15.11).
- Introduce single-limb proprioception (Fig. 15.12).
- Bilateral concentric heel raises (can start in a pool, Alter-G™ or on leg press machine if patient is unable to do it on flat ground) (Fig. 15.13).
- Home instruction on strengthening with a towel.
- Cryotherapy for 15 min at session end.

Fig. 15.10 Cross-friction
massage of ankle tendons

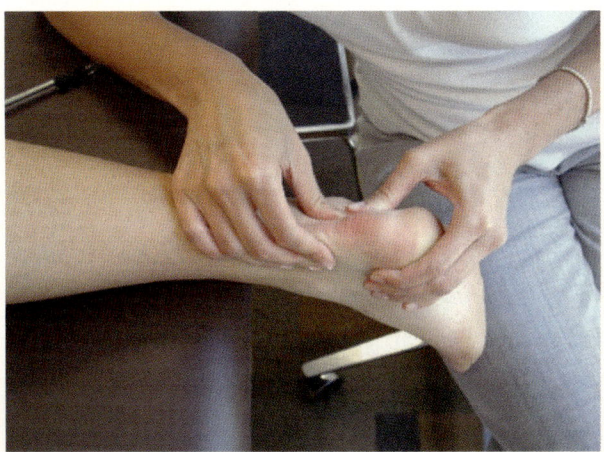

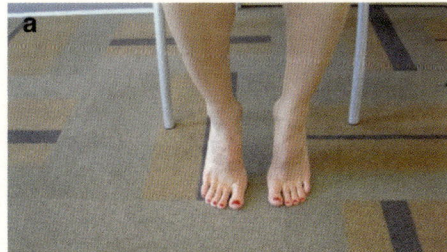

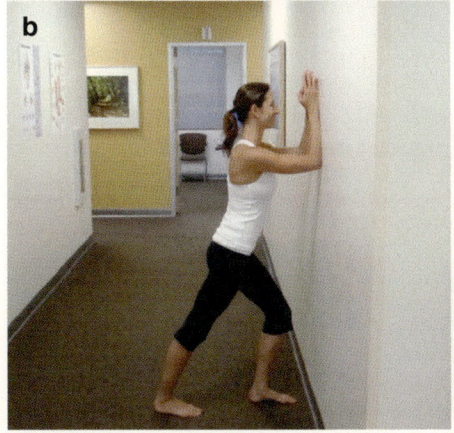

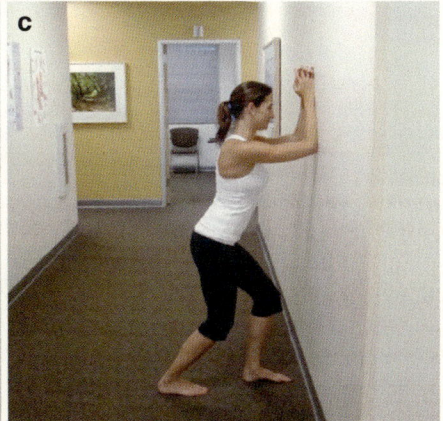

Fig. 15.11 Seated (**a**) and standing with knee straight (**b**) and knee bent (**c**) calf stretch

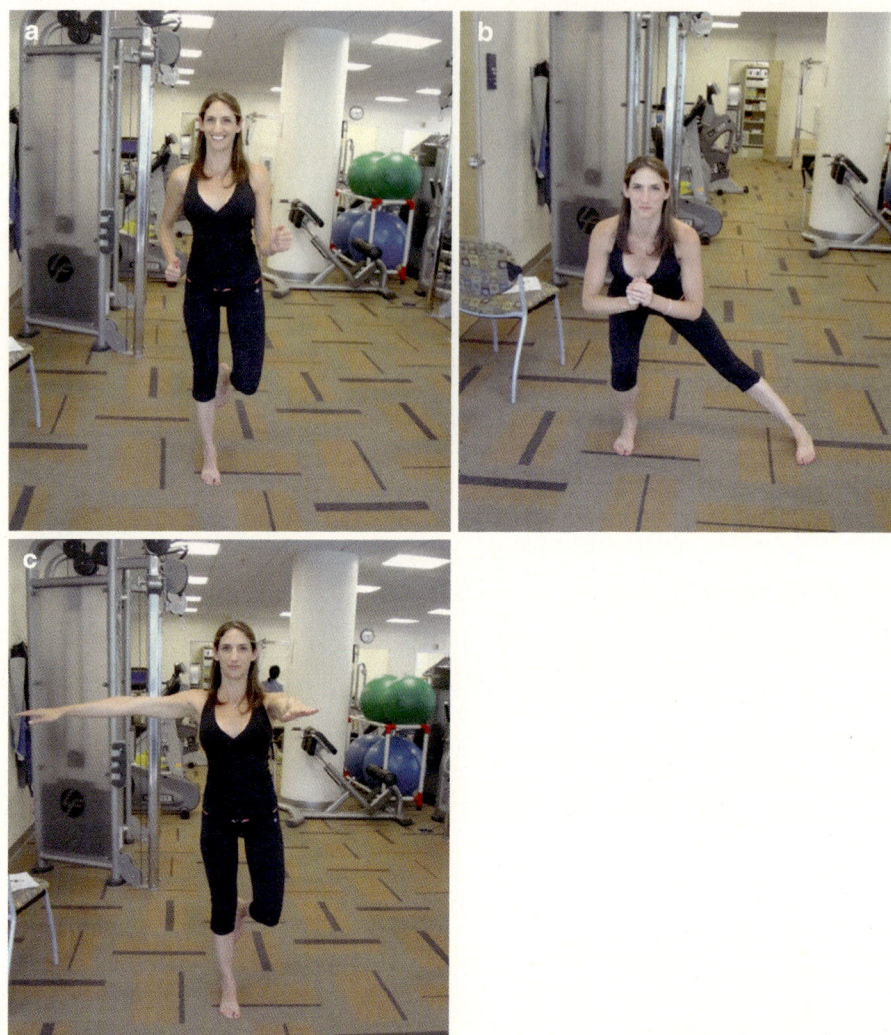

Fig. 15.12 (**a–c**) Single leg, side squat/lateral lunge, back to single leg ankle stability exercise on flat surface, for gluteal strengthening

Fig. 15.13 Bilateral
concentric heel raise

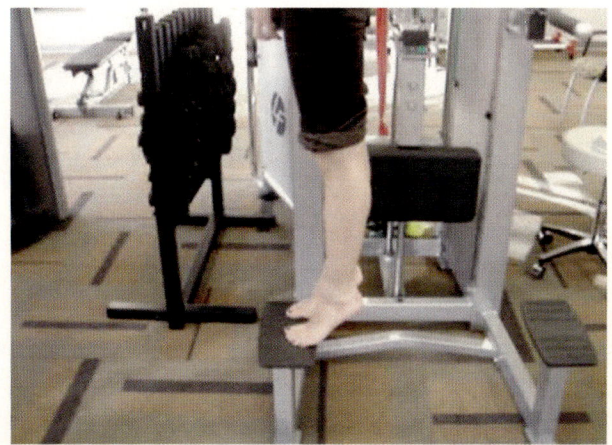

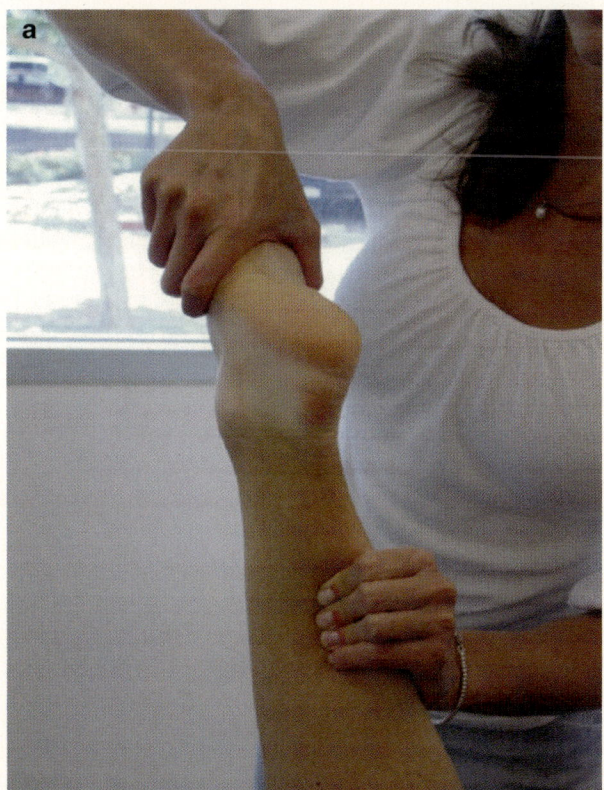

Fig. 15.14 (a, b)
Mobilization of ankle

Fig. 15.14 (continued)

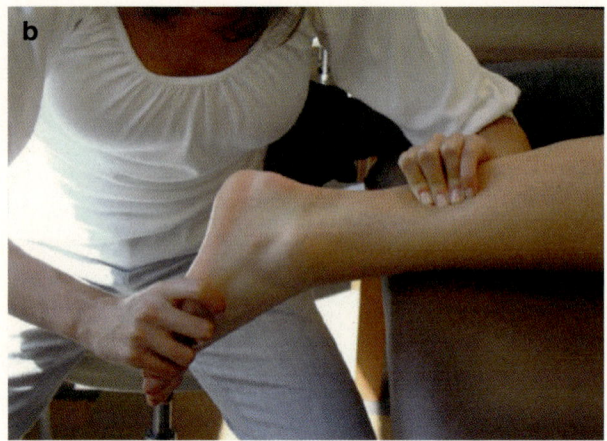

15.1.1.2 Weeks 10–12+ Post-surgery

Same as above, plus:

- Soft-tissue massage to calf muscle and posterior ankle tendons (Figs. 15.14 and 15.15)
- Mobilization of subtalar joint (unless fused) (Fig. 15.8)
- Gluteal strengthening; (Figs. 15.16 and 15.17)
- Unilateral concentric strengthening at 60% bodyweight (BW) in Alter-G™; (Fig. 15.18)
- Stationary bike without boot
- Modalities such as ultrasound and electrical stimulation if needed
- Walking on Alter-G™ @ 40% (BW) for 10 min (minimum). (Can substitute pool workouts)

15.1.2 Phase 2

15.1.2.1 Approximately Week 12 or Later Post-surgery

Same as above plus:

- Standing hip Theraband™ 4 way; (Fig. 15.19)
- Gym ball exercises progressed from above (Fig. 15.20)
- Side steps with tubing (Fig. 15.21)
- Pilates Reformer ™ (leg press, calf raise, hamstring arcs and circles) (Fig. 15.22)
- Ankle proprioceptive neuromuscular facilitation PNF (Fig. 15.23) mobilization of great toe (Fig. 15.24)
- Progression to walking/running at 70% BW in Alter-G™ for 10 min
- Increase home program strengthening

Fig. 15.15 (**a, b**)
Mobilization of calf

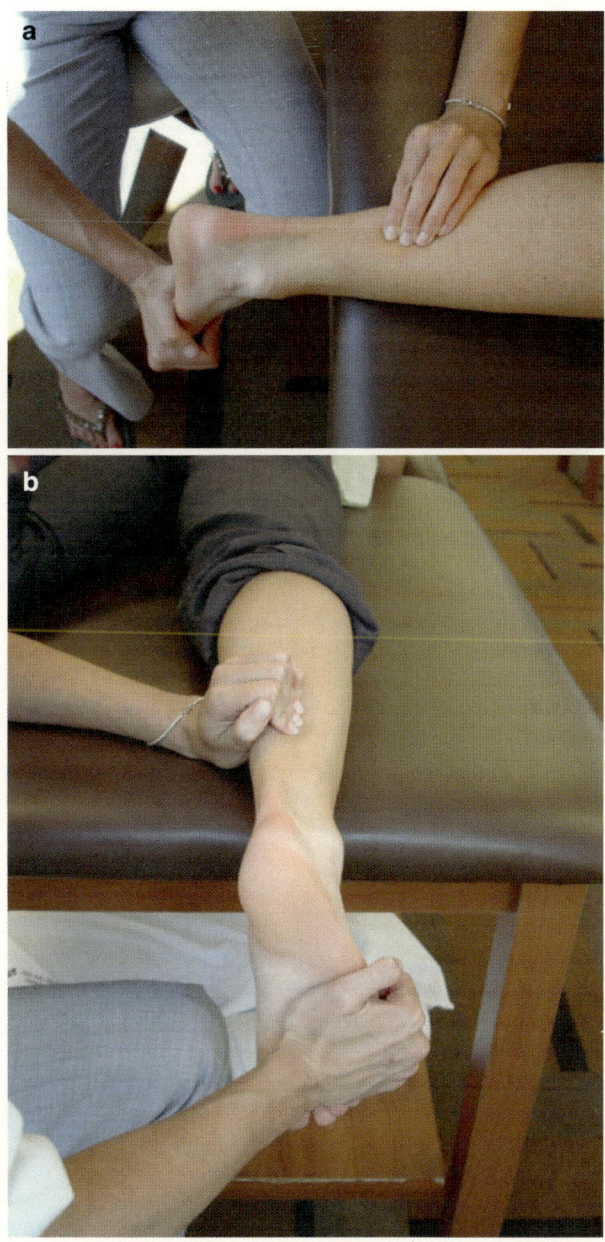

Fig. 15.16 (**a–c**) "1/4" Squats with (**d**) showing 2-legged version for assistance if needed

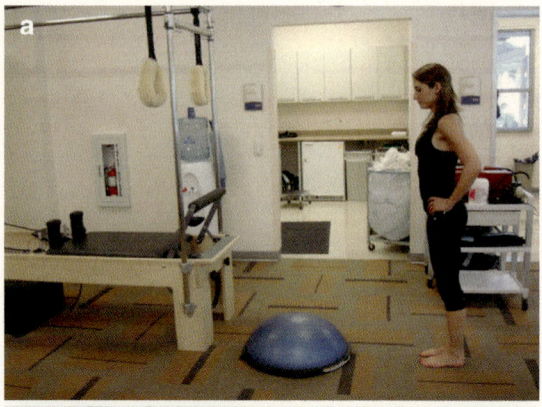

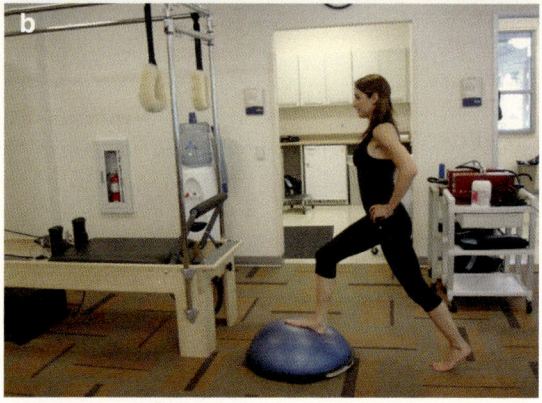

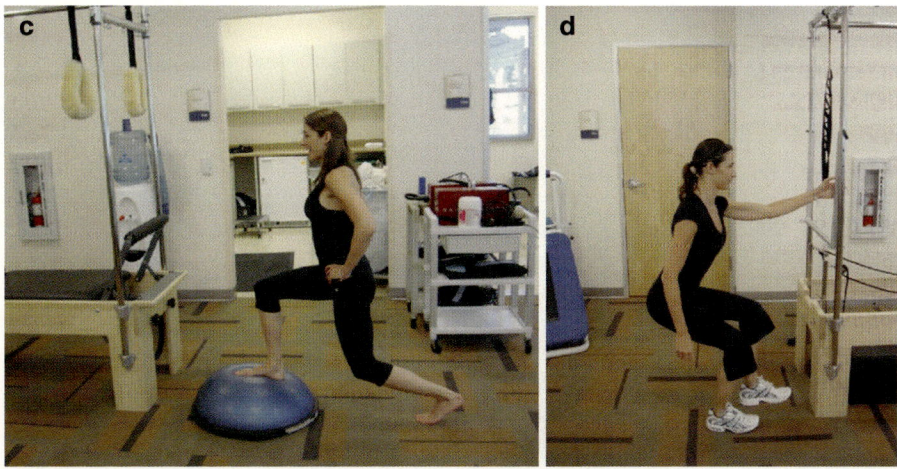

Fig. 15.16 (continued)

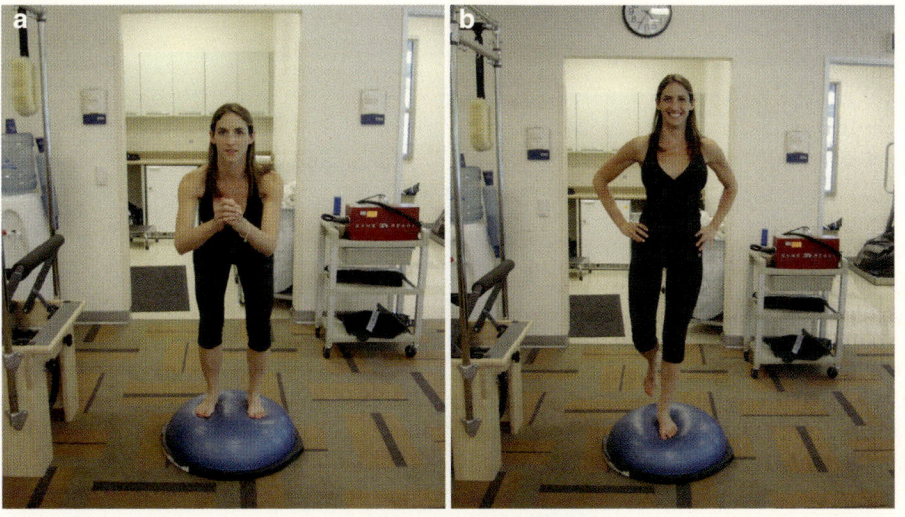

Fig. 15.17 (**a, b**) Double and single legged BOSU™ ball exercise

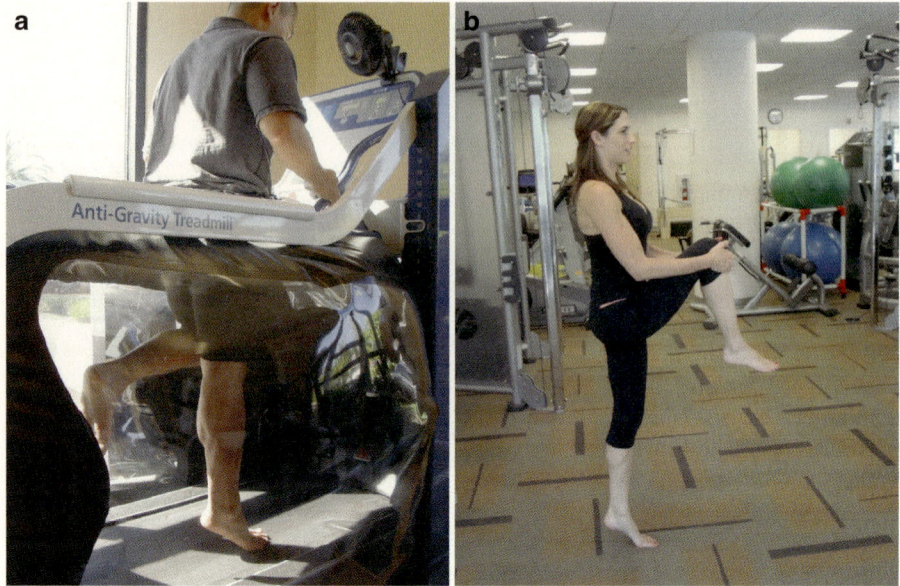

Fig. 15.18 (**a**) Unilateral leg strengthening on flat surface (shown utilizing Alter-G™ to reduce body weight or can do in shallow swimming pool if needed) (**b**) More advanced single-legged strengthening and balance

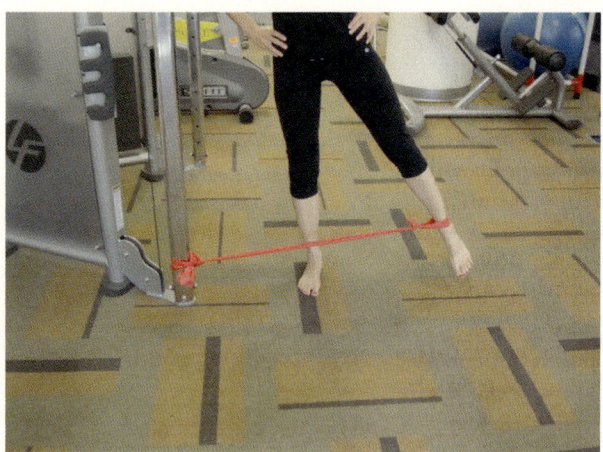

Fig. 15.19 Hip abduction with elastic band

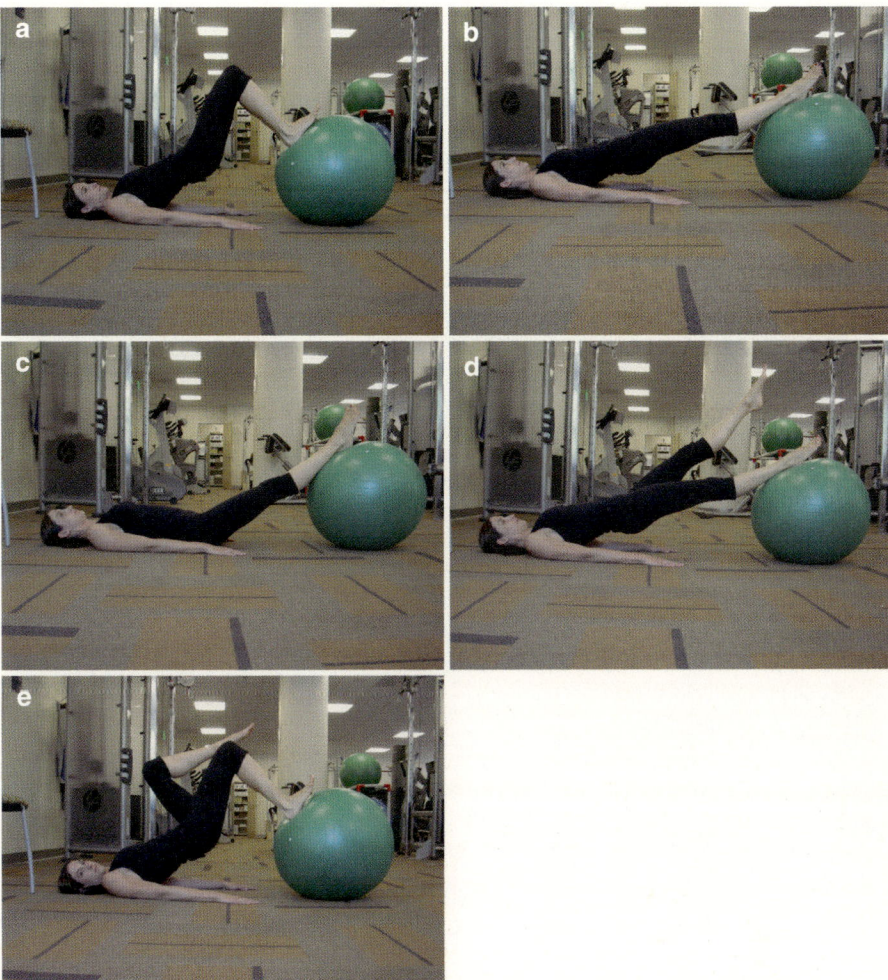

Fig. 15.20 (**a–e**) "Gym ball" hamstring strengthening

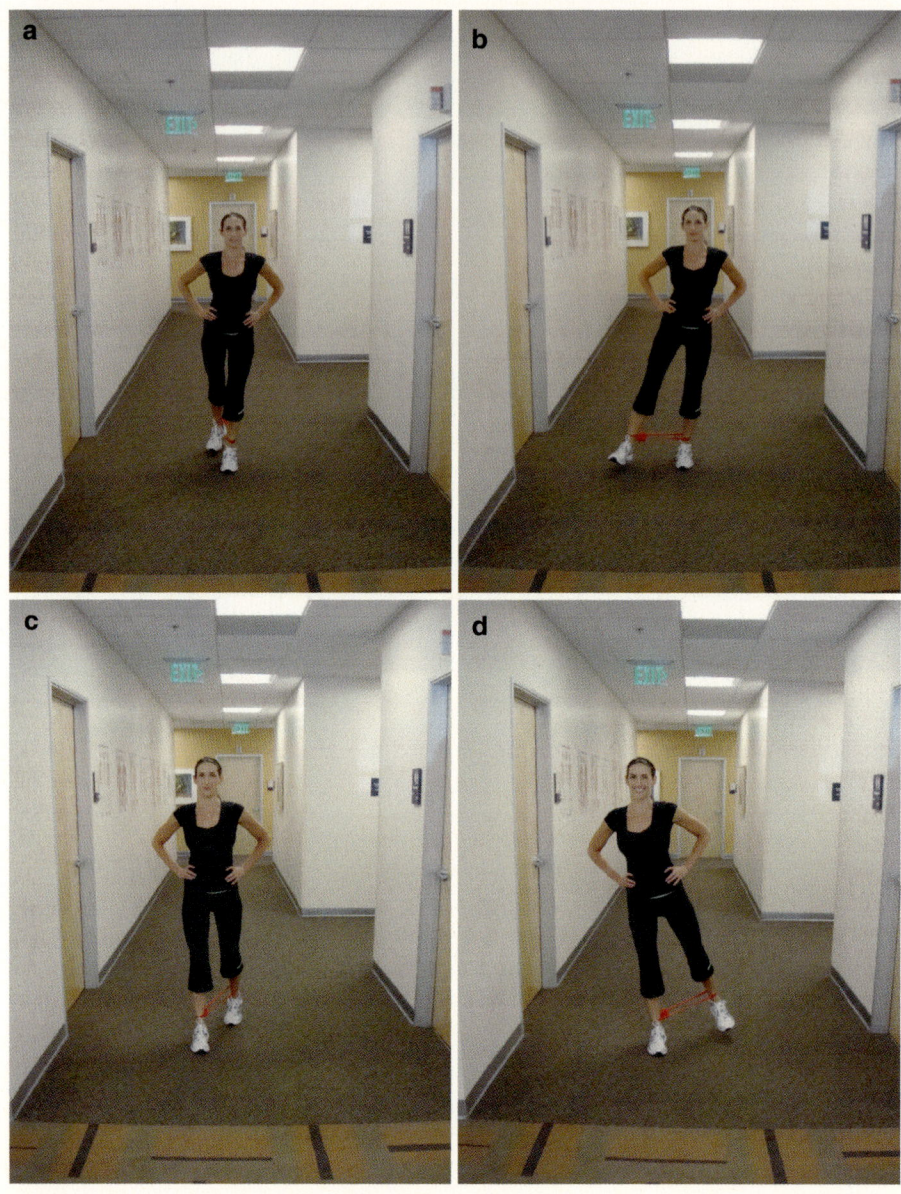

Fig. 15.21 (**a–d**) Figure-of-eight walk with elastic band

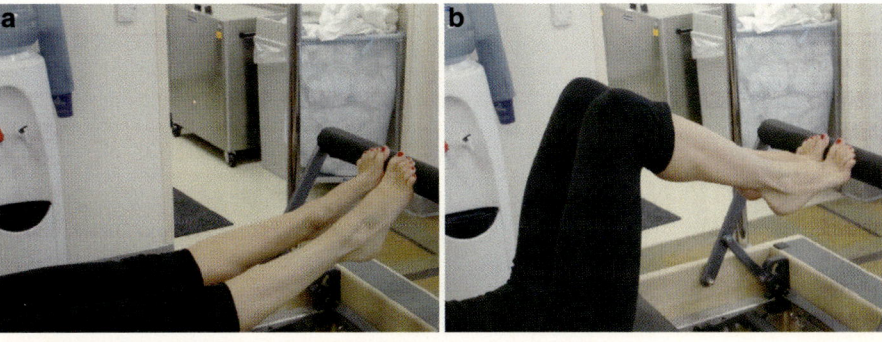

Fig. 15.22 (**a, b**) Pilates Reformer™ exercises

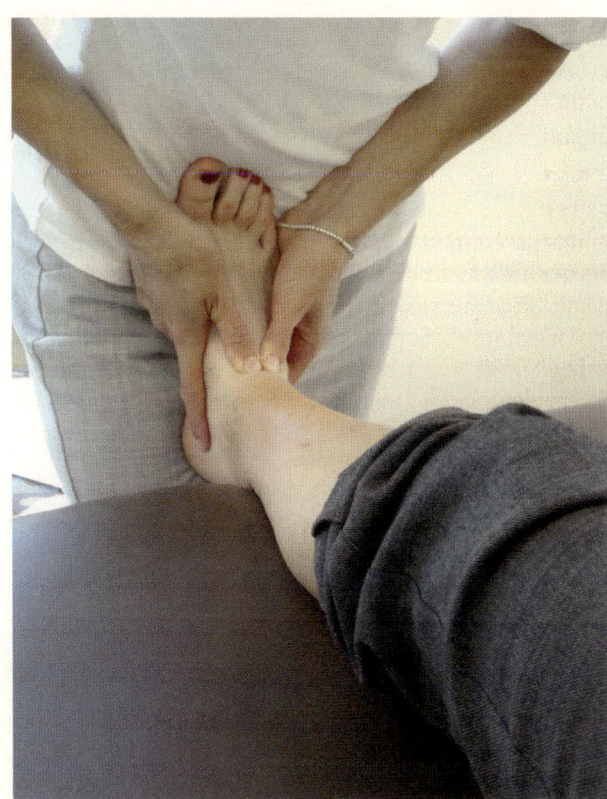

Fig. 15.23 Talar AP
mobilization

Fig. 15.24 Mobilization of first MPTJ

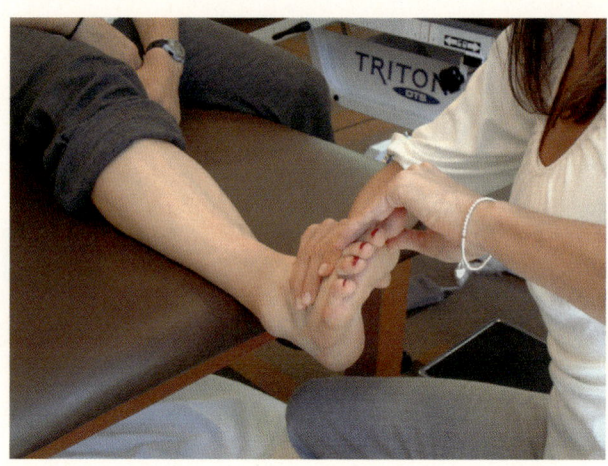

15.1.3 Phase 3

15.1.3.1 Approximately Week 14 or Later Post-surgery

Same as above with:

- Progression of single-limb strengthening from 70% to 90% BW in Alter-G™ or in pool (starting w 3× 10 reps, progress to 5× 25).
- Walking/running up to 2 mi at 70% BW.
- Depending on patient's individual progress: dynamic balance and BOSU™ squats (Figs. 15.25 and 15.26); step-downs; calf eccentrics if pain-free, first with the knee straight and can progress to knee bent (Fig. 15.27); lunges; single leg heel raises and leg press and ankle PNF as shown above.
- Taping may be helpful either laterally (Fig. 15.28), medially (Fig. 15.29), or posteriorly (Fig. 15.30) as necessary with elastic tape (Darco Body Armour Tape™, Darco International, West Virginia, USA).

15.1.3.2 Week 15 or Later Post-surgery

Same as above with progression to walking/running 75–85% BW in G-trainer or in pool for 30 min. Increase strengthening concentrically full bodyweight with surgical limb including active hip stabilization (Fig. 15.31).

15.1.3.3 Week 16 or Later

Same as above plus begin walk/jog program progress 75–85% BW in G-trainer for 10–20 min or in pool 30–40 min. Patients are typically discharged at this time with their home program of strengthening, proprioception, stretching, and

Fig. 15.25 Ankle stability on pillow. Rotating an object increases the "demand." Ball sports athletes can throw a ball against a wall or rebounding apparatus and try to catch it, which further improves balance

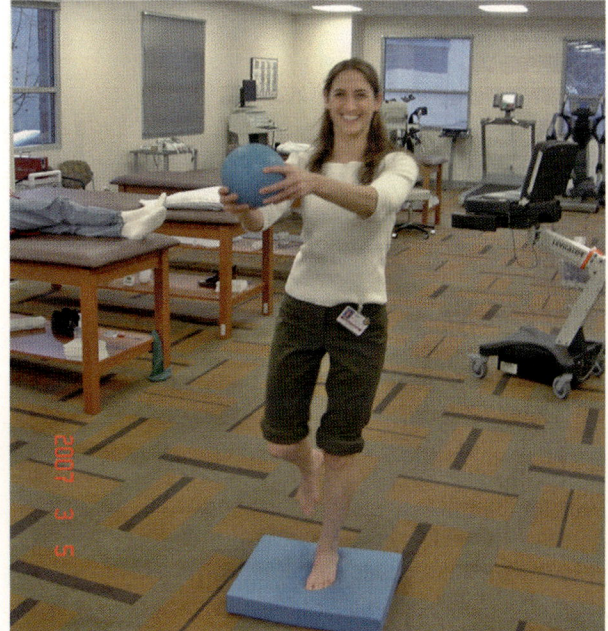

cryotherapy to be maintained until they are able to return to their full activity level. Please see the respective chapters in this text for more specifics as to typical return to activity (RTA) time frames as many reconstructive procedures require up to a year to return to full activity. Athletes often have an accelerated RTA, as have been found in some studies.[5,6,8] A continuation of specific strengthening and proprioception for the entire lower quarter is continued for over a year postoperatively.

15.2 Rehabilitation of Midfoot Surgeries and Fusions (Lisfranc's Injuries, Navicular Injuries, and Lapidus Procedure)

Postoperative course is nearly identical to the surgeries discussed above. Patients may be non-weight-bearing from 4 to 6 weeks. Formalized appointments start generally around 8–10 weeks post-surgery (Phase 1), when alignment and/or bony consolidation is confirmed. Similar postoperative rehabilitation progression as above with the exception that no mobilization is performed on the midfoot, and barefoot proprioception is delayed especially on the BOSU™ ball. Seated heel raises (Fig. 15.32) and first metatarsal–phalangeal joint (MPJ) mobilization techniques described in the next section are utilized for the Lapidus procedure. The physical

Fig. 15.26 (**a**, **b**) Ankle
stability on balance board

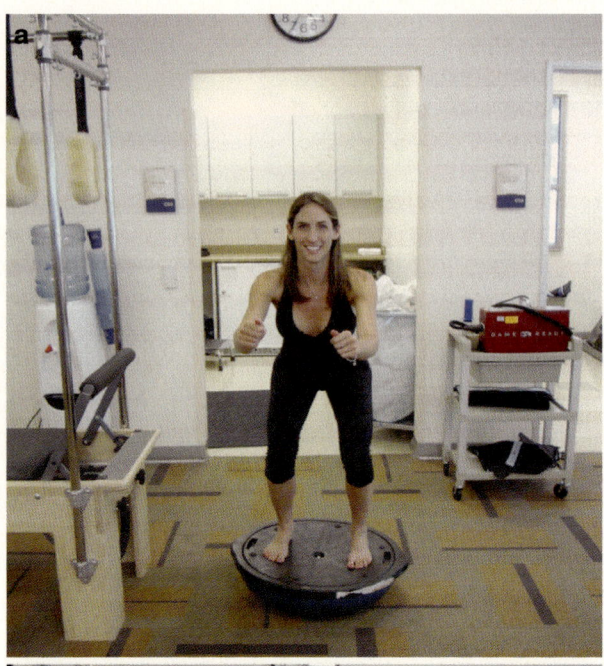

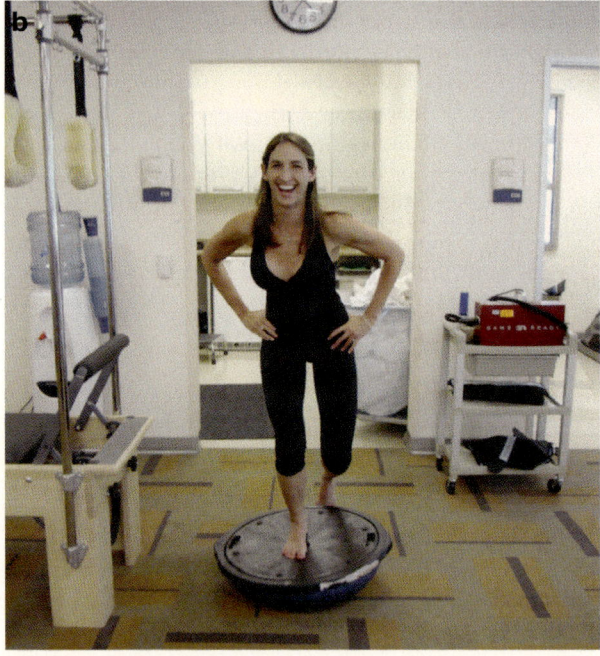

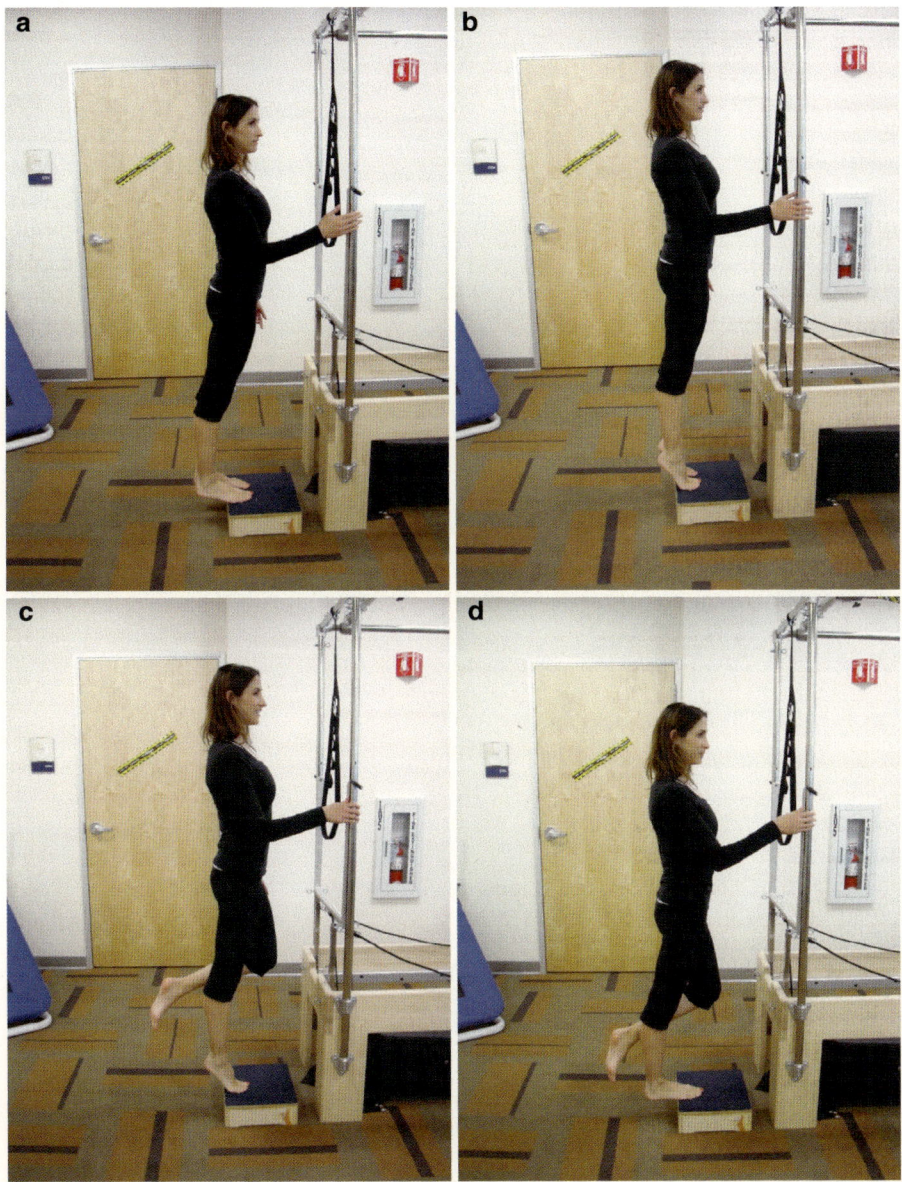

Fig. 15.27 Eccentric strengthening with knee straight. Heel raise with two legs, and lowering with one leg below the platform (achieve negative heel). (**a** through **d**) Side and (**e** through **g**) front views. Start with three sets of 10 repetitions

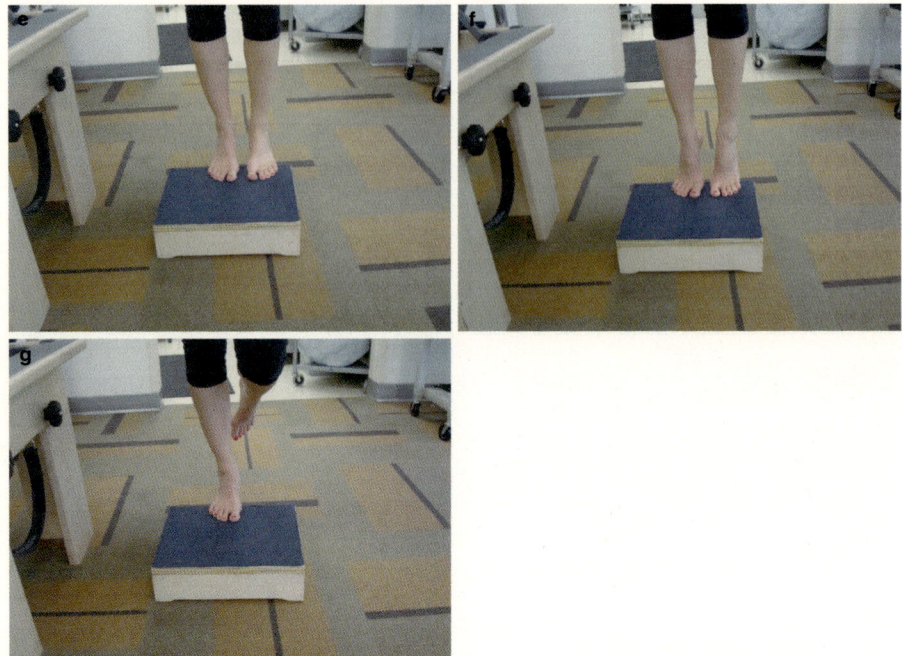

Fig. 15.27 (continued)

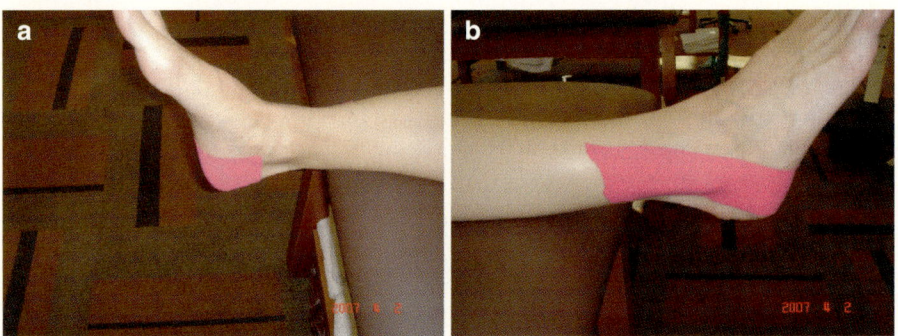

Fig. 15.28 (**a**, **b**) Taping from medial to lateral with Kinesio™ tape for lateral ankle stability. (**c**, **d**) Applying a second layer of tape perpendicular to the 1st, again medial to lateral

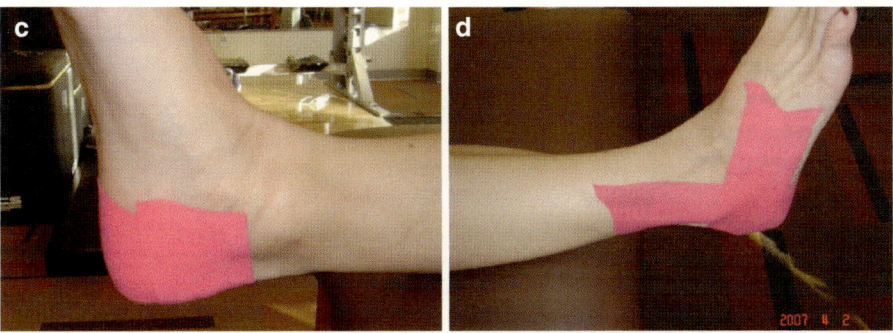

Fig. 15.28 (continued)

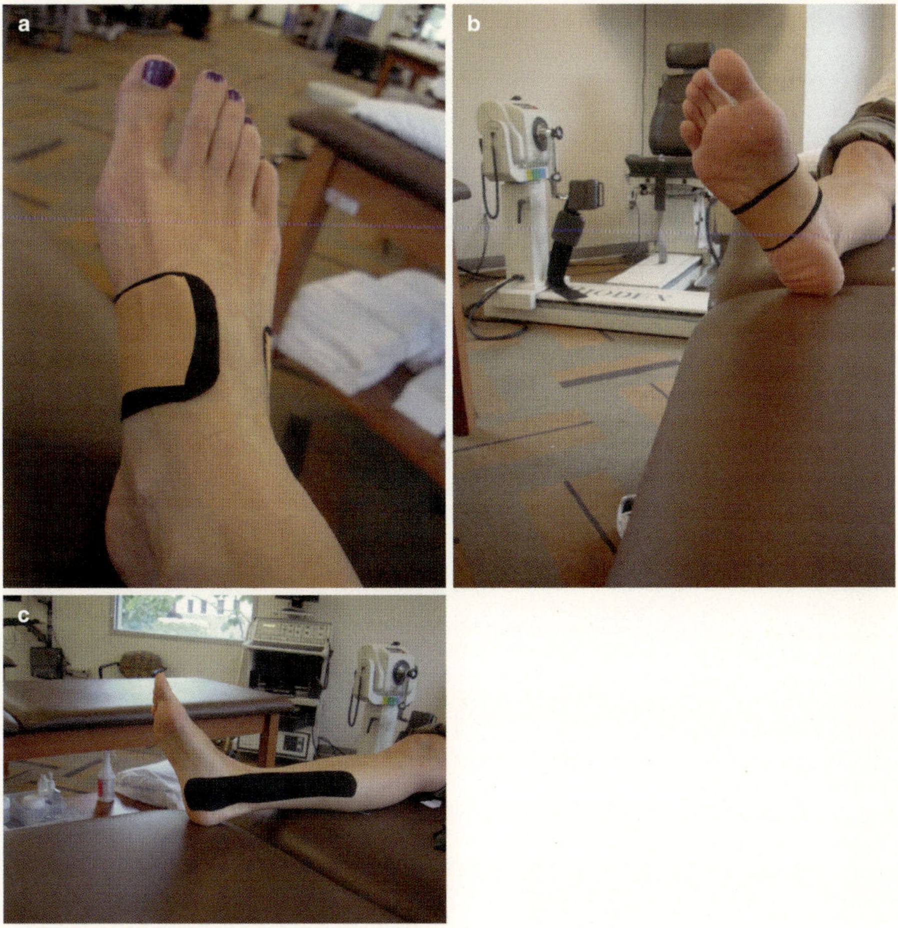

Fig. 15.29 Kinesio (TM) tape for medial arch support (**a**, **b**) and for posterior tibial support (c)

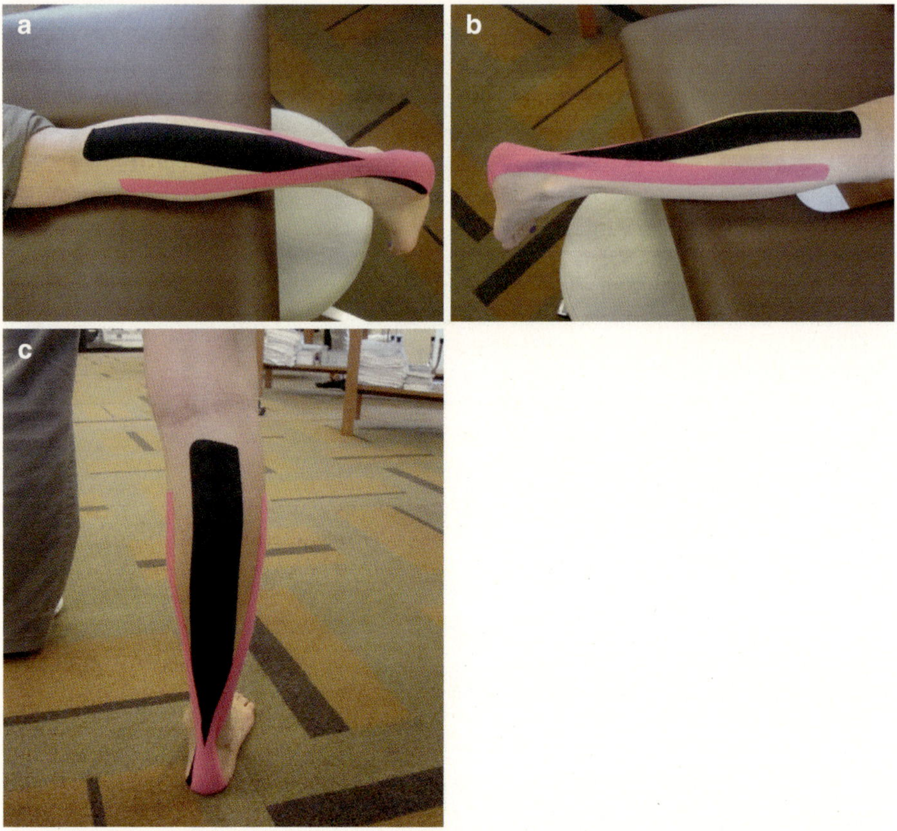

Fig. 15.30 (**a–c**) Kinesio™ tape for Achilles support

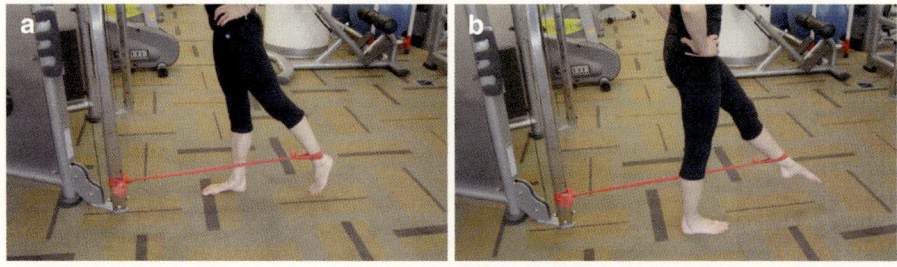

Fig. 15.31 Hip extension (**a**) and flexion (**b**) with elastic tubing for Core/dynamic strengthening

Fig. 15.32 Seated dorsiflexion for MPTJs

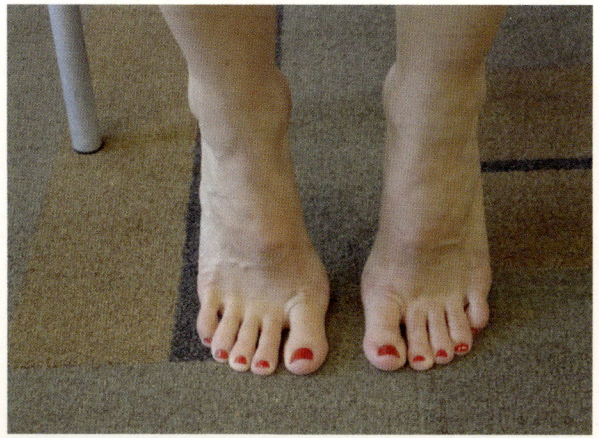

therapyprogression is similar as above, though patients with Lisfranc's injuries, particularly those requiring significant reconstruction, may take more than 6 weeks of sessions. Therefore, patients may not enter Phase 2 until 16 or more weeks post-surgery. Phase 3 may take 26 or more weeks.

15.3   Rehabilitation of Forefoot Surgeries

The program for forefroot surgeries (i.e.,hammertoe, neuroma, bunionectomy/hallux rigidus surgery with or without osteotomy, lesser metatarsal osteotomy, and sesamoidectomy) is similar to the postoperative rehabilitation described above, though cast or boot immobilization may be shorter or not needed. Patients are able to use a stationary bike with a cast, cast boot, or even athletic shoe often within the first postoperative week with their heel on the pedal. Between 2 and 3 weeks post-surgery, patients begin towel exercises including curling, and seated dorsiflexion exercises. Patients with some forefoot procedures may be weight-bearing within 2–5 days, such as with hammertoe or primary neuroma surgeries; other forefoot surgeries may non-weight-bearing for 3 weeks. Formalized physical therapy sessions begin between 4 and 6 weeks post-op, (Phase 1), except for the Lapidus procedure discussed above in "Midfoot." Postoperative mobilization and physical therapy gains also focus on improving metatarsophalangeal motion. This may be assisted by applying mobilization (Figs. 15.33 and 15.34). The progression of the physical therapy sessions is similar as described above, though may be more rapid, and sometimes courses for 3–4 weeks duration for some more minor forefoot procedures starting at 6 or more weeks post-surgery. Phases 2 and 3 occur around 10 and 12 weeks or later post-surgery. Arch taping/support may be helpful for some procedures postoperatively (Fig. 15.35).

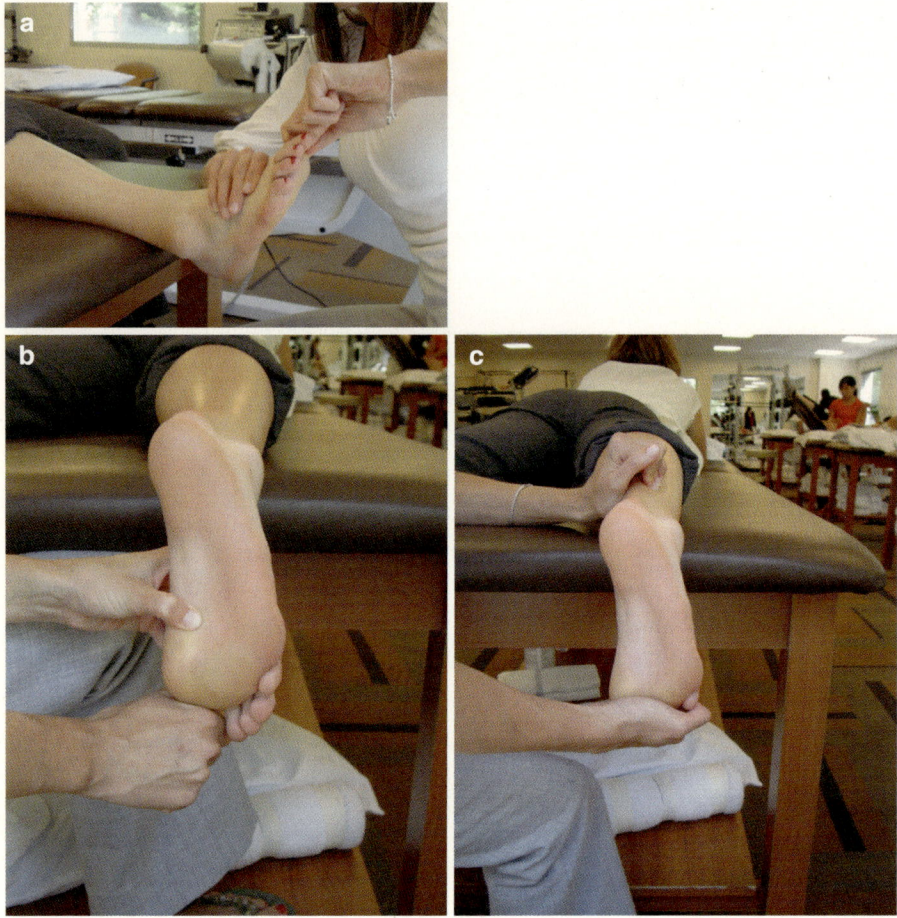

Fig. 15.33 Mobilization of the first MPTJ (**a**, **b**) and FHL/soleous (**c**)

15.4 Return to Running Sports

Lower extremity rehabilitation postoperatively includes not only surgical site strengthening but core stabilization as well. We are including diagrams of exercises to be considered post foot and ankle surgery. Combination of some of these and individualization of the treatment plan should be determined by the surgeon and therapist as needed. The criteria for returning to sports have not been firmly established for all types of foot and ankle surgeries.[6,15] We utilize the following parameters based on research on rehabilitation of the Achilles tendon to clear patients to return to running sports[6-8]:

- Calf girth within 5 mm of nonoperative limb measured 10 cm distal to an adult's tibial tuberosity.

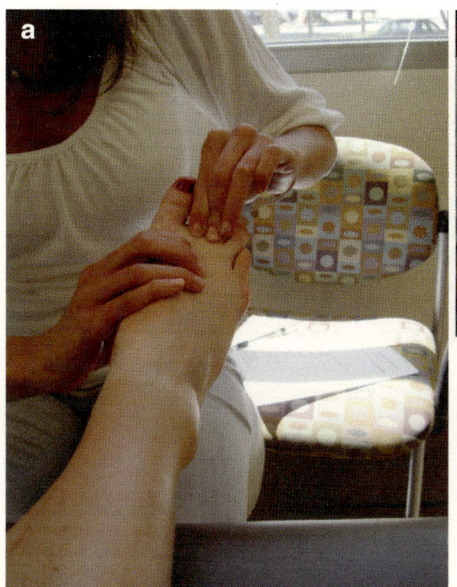
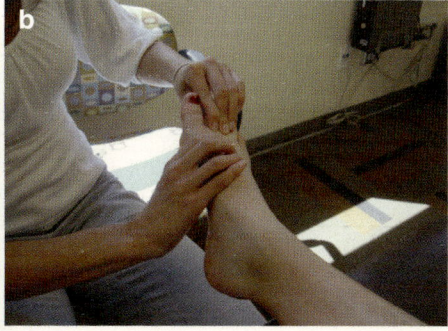

Fig. 15.34 (**a**, **b**) Mobilization of lesser MPTJ

Fig. 15.35 Arch taping

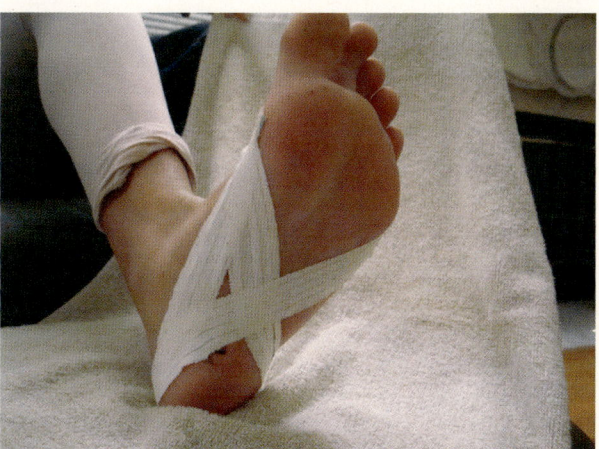

- Affected joint ROM within 5° of nonoperative limb.
- Ability to perform 5 × 25 concentric heel raises pain-free with operative limb.
- Include vertical leap testing and broad jump testing (3 hop test). The patient should be able to show you they can and are willing to bound on that leg prior to release.[18]
- 10 step-downs from an 8-in. step without discomfort.[18]

Table 15.3 Sample return to "LAND" running

Day 1 (min)	Day 2	Day 3 (min)	Day 4	Day 5	Day 6	Day 7 (min)
15	Rest	15	Rest	20 min	Rest	20
20	Rest	25	Rest	25 min	Rest	30
20	Rest	30	Rest	40 min	Rest	40
20	Rest	40	Rest	50 min	Rest	50
20	Rest	50	30 min	Rest	60 min	20

Table 15.4 Sample return to running using the Alter-G™ treadmill

	Outside running		Alter-G time (min)	Alter-G body weight (%)	
Week 1			30–>40	70–>85	
Week 2			30–>60	75–>90	
Week 3	20 min qod 3 days		40–60	75–90	1 day off
Week 4	30–40 min qod 3 days		60–75	75–90	1 day off
Week 5	40–50 min qod 3–4 days		60–90	75–90	1 day off
Week 6	50–60 min 4 days	Strides on grass	60–90	75–90	1 day off
Week 7	60+ min 4 days	Strides on grass	60–90	75–90	Tempo/speed on alter-g 1 day off
Week 8	60+ min 4 days	Strides on grass	60–90	75–90	Tempo/speed on alter-g 1 day off
Week 9	Gradual Full training				

qod = every-other day

A typical return to running program would be as follows: Have the patient alternate walking and jogging for 2 min each, completing four cycles (16 min of total activity). Have them take a rest day and then reassess 2 days later. If they felt challenged, have them repeat this every-other day for a week. If this was not challenging, then have the patient alternate 3-min jogging with 1-min walking, again for four cycles. Again have the patient reassess and repeat this every-other day for a week. If the patient experiences any increase in pain accompanied by swelling, they should refrain from running until the symptoms subside. Running can then be re-initiated.

As the running program progresses, the patient and therapist should monitor symptoms of compensatory symptoms such as lateral foot pain after first MPJ procedures or excessive contra-lateral limb soreness from favoring the surgical side or "vaulting." Once the patient can run every-other day, they can begin other sports drills. Increased ball handling skills can be performed. If running is the primary sport, the patient can begin with the running schedule outlined in Table 15.3. If the therapist has access to an Alter-G™ treadmill, they can utilize Table 15.4 as a guideline.

15.5   Summary

Postoperative physical therapy is often currently done in a non-structured approach across the world. In our clinic, we are currently establishing protocols based on surgical rationale, published RTA of common procedures, and previous evidence-based findings on other studies with ankle rehabilitation. A good dialogue between therapist, surgeon, and patient, including a fundamental understanding of the procedure and goals, is needed. We hope to verify our protocols in the future, and therefore, for now, use the above guidelines as suggestions and to provoke more study.

Acknowledgments   The authors would like to thank Matt Richardson, DPT and Marc Guillet, MSPT for their assistance with this chapter.

References

1. Alfredson H, Pietila T, Jonsson P, Lorentzon R. Heavy-load eccentric training for the treatment of chronic Achilles tendinosis. *Am J Sports Med.* 1998;26:360-6.
2. Cook JL, Purdam CR. Rehabilitation of Achilles and patellar tendinopathies. *Best Pract Res Clin Rheumatol.* 2007;21:295-316.
3. Saxena A, O'brien T. Post-operative physical therapy for podiatric surgery. *J Am Podiatr Med Assoc.* 1992;82(8):417-23.
4. Saxena A. Retrospective review of 91 surgeries for chronic achilles pathology. *J Am Podiatr Med Assoc.* 2003;93(4):283-91.
5. Saxena A. Results of achilles tendon surgery in elite and sub-elite track athletes. *Foot Ankle Int.* 2003;24(9):712-20.
6. Hansen ST. Acute compartment syndromes. "Elevation ischemia". In: *Functional reconstruction of the foot and ankle*. Philadelphia: Lippincott; 2000. p.37, chap 2.
7. Knight K. Orthopedic surgery and cryotherapy. In: *Cryotherapy in sports injury management*. Champaign: Human Kinetics; 1995. p. 99-105.
8. Saxena A, Guillet M, Maffulli N. Rehabilitation of the operated Achilles Tendon: parameters for predicting return to activity. *J Foot Ankle Surg.* 2011;50(1):37-40.
9. Saxena A, Granot A. Use of a novel treadmill in the rehabilitation of the operated Achilles tendon: a pilot study. *J Foot Ankle Surg.* 2011;50(5): (epub).
10. Adler SS, Beckers D, Buck M. Proprioceptive neuromuscular facilitation in practice: an illustrated guide. 3rd ed. Berlin: Springer; 1993.
11. Voss DE, Ionta KI, Myers BJ. Proprioceptive neuromuscular facilitation. 3rd editors. Philadelphia: Harper and Row; 1985.
12. Proprioceptive Neuromuscular Facilitation 1: the functional approach to proprioceptive neuromuscular facilitation. Institute of Physical Art. Course Notes Jan 1992.
13. Karlsson J, Lundin O, Lind K, Styf J. Early mobilization versus immobilization after ankle ligament stabilization. Scand J Med Sci Sports. 1999;9(5):299-303.
14. Donatelli R, Hall W, Prell B, Ferkel R. Lateral ligament repair. In: Maxey L, Magnusson J, editors. Rehabilitation for the postsurgical orthopedic patient. 2nd ed. St. Louis: Mosby; 2007. p.401-32.
15. Donatelli R, Hall W, Prell B, Ferkel R. Open reduction and internal fixation of the ankle. In: Maxey L, Magnusson J, editors. Rehabilitation for the postsurgical orthopedic patient. 2nd ed. St. Louis: Mosby; 2007:433-446.
16. Cozen D, Ferkel R, Maxey L. Ankle arthroscopy. In: Maxey L, Magnusson J, editors. Rehabilitation for the postsurgical orthopedic patient. 2nd ed. St. Louis: Mosby; 2007. p.447-60.

17. Zachazewski J, Gruber J, Giza E, Mandelbaum B. Achilles tendon repair. In: Maxey L, Magnusson J, editors. Rehabilitation for the postsurgical orthopedic patient. 2nd ed. St. Louis: Mosby; 2007.
18. Prelaz C. Transitioning the jumping athlete back to the court. In: Maxey L, Magnusson J, editors. Rehabilitation for the postsurgical orthopedic patient. 2nd ed. St. Louis: Mosby; 2007. p. 513-24.
19. Nicholas JA, Marino M. The relationship of injuries of the leg, foot, and ankle to proximal thigh strength in athletes. Foot Ankle. 1987;7:218-28.
20. Friel K, McLean N, Myers C, Caceres M. Ipsilateral hip abductor weakness after inversion ankle sprain. J Athl Train. 2006;41:74-8.
21. Small K, McNaughton L, Matthews M. A systematic review into the efficacy of static stretching as part of a warm-up for the prevention of exercise-related injury. Res Sports Med. 2008;16(3):213-31.

Index

Printed by Printforce, the Netherlands